Textbook of
Endocrine Physiology

Textbook of Endocrine Physiology

Fifth Edition

Edited by

JAMES E. GRIFFIN, M.D.
Professor of Internal Medicine
University of Texas Southwestern Medical Center at Dallas

SERGIO R. OJEDA, D.V.M.
Head, Division of Neuroscience
Oregon Regional Primate Research Center

OXFORD
UNIVERSITY PRESS
2004

OXFORD
UNIVERSITY PRESS

Oxford   New York
Auckland   Bangkok   Buenos Aires   Cape Town   Chennai
Dar es Salaam   Delhi   Hong Kong   Istanbul   Karachi   Kolkata
Kuala Lumpur   Madrid   Melbourne   Mexico City   Mumbai   Nairobi
São Paulo   Shanghai   Taipei   Tokyo   Toronto

Copyright © 1988, 1992, 1996, 2000, 2004 by Oxford University Press, Inc.

Published by Oxford University Press, Inc.
198 Madison Avenue, New York, New York, 10016
http://www.oup.com

Oxford is a registered trademark of Oxford University Press

Library of Congress Cataloging-in-Publication Data
Textbook of endocrine physiology /
edited by James E. Griffin, Sergio R. Ojeda.—5th ed.
p. ; cm.   Includes bibliographical references and index.
ISBN 0-19-516565-9 (cloth) — ISBN 0-19-516566-7 (pbk.)
1. Endocrine glands—Physiology. 2. Endocrinology.
I. Griffin, James E. (James Emmett), 1944- II. Ojeda, Sergio R.
[DNLM: 1. Endocrine Glands—physiology.
2. Hormones—physiology.
WK 102 T355 2004]
QP187.T43 2003   612.4—dc22   2003060957

1 2 3 4 5 6 7 8 9

Printed in the United States of America
on acid-free paper

Preface

During the past 16 years this textbook of endocrinology has been widely used by graduate and medical students as they learn physiology, anatomy, biochemistry, and cell biology. The aim of the book is to provide a solid, clear, and succinct account of basic endocrine function, emphasizing the impact that advances in the biological sciences have on our understanding of physiological processes. It addresses clinical disorders only as a means of illustrating the divergence from normal physiology and normal regulation of endocrine function but the book offers basic insights into endocrinology that should lead to a better understanding of the complex array of endocrine disorders that medical students will encounter in later years. It should also provide a framework for those, planning to pursue a career in research who are seeking to identify subjects of investigation directly relevant to human health.

The contributors are well-recognized authorities in the fields of neuroendocrinology, reproductive endocrinology, endocrinology of growth and pregnancy, intermediary metabolism, diabetes and lipid physiology, calcium homeostasis, adrenal steroidogenesis, immunoendocrinology, and mechanisms of both peptide and steroid hormone action. They have taken a consistent approach in writing their chapters.

The first five chapters deal with general aspects of endocrine physiology: the organization of the endocrine system, genetic control of hormone synthesis, mechanisms of hormone action, immune–endocrine interactions, and assessment of endocrine function. The next two chapters concern the neuroendocrinology of the hypothalamus and its relationship to the pituitary gland. Subsequent chapters are devoted to reproductive physiology (sexual differentiation, female reproductive function, male reproductive function, and endocrinology of pregnancy), somatic growth and development, thyroid gland physiology, and the adrenal glands. The last two chapters deal with the multihormonal control of calcium homeostasis and of glucose, lipid, and protein metabolism. Clinical examples of altered endocrine physiology are provided throughout the book, without clinical jargon. As in previous editions, we have tried to keep the level of discussion in each chapter appropriate for students who are just beginning their medical and graduate education. Despite this necessary simplicity, the authors present the latest advances in the areas of genetic control of hormone synthesis, hormone action, energy metabolism, obesity and control of appetite; discuss novel interactions between the immune and endocrine systems and their implication for tumor growth; and describe the discovery of new peptides involved in the regulation of feeding behavior and pituitary function. They also discuss in a simple, but accurate manner the recent advances in understanding fluid and electrolyte balance and in hormones of the heart and brain, as well as the importance of newly discovered molecules involved in the regulation of gonadal, adrenal, and thyroid development and function.

For this fifth edition, there are some new authors and three chapters have been completely rewritten. Robert Munford is the new author of Chapter 4 (Cytokines and Immune-Endocrine Interactions), Keith Parker and William Rainey wrote a new version of Chapter 14 (The Adrenal Glands), and Howard Heller is the new author of Chapter 15 (Calcium Homeostasis). Richard Auchus joined James Griffin as a coauthor of Chapter 5, Khurram Rehman joined Bruce Carr in writing Chapter 11, while Robert Dobbins and Michael Cowley now coauthor Chapter 16 with Daniel Foster. Overall, this edition has 41 new or significantly revised figures. We would like to express our special appreciation to all the contributors, new and old.

Dallas, TX   J.E.G.
Beaverton, OR   S.R.O.

Contents

Contributors

RICHARD J. AUCHUS, M.D., PH.D.
Assistant Professor of Internal Medicine
University of Texas Southwestern Medical Center

BRUCE R. CARR, M.D.
Professor of Obstetrics and Gynecology
University of Texas Southwestern Medical Center

PINCHAS COHEN, M. D.
Professor of Pediatrics
University of California Los Angeles

MICHAEL A. COWLEY, PH.D.
Assistant Scientist
Oregon National Primate Research Center-Oregon Health & Sciences University

ROBERT L. DOBBINS, M.D., PH.D.
Assistant Professor of Internal Medicine
University of Texas Southwestern Medical Center

DANIEL W. FOSTER, M.D.
Professor and Chair of Internal Medicine
University of Texas Southwestern Medical Center

JAMES E. GRIFFIN, M.D.
Professor of Internal Medicine
University of Texas Southwestern Medical Center

HOWARD J. HELLER, M.D.
Associate Professor of Internal Medicine
University of Texas Southwestern Medical Center

CAROLE R. MENDELSON, PH,D.
Professor of Biochemistry
University of Texas Southwestern Medical Center

ROBERT S. MUNFORD, M.D.
Professor of Internal Medicine
University of Texas Southwestern Medical Center

SERGIO R. OJEDA, D.V.M.
Head, Division of Neuroscience
Oregon National Primate Research Center-Oregon Health & Sciences University

KEITH L. PARKER, M.D., PH.D.
Professor of Internal Medicine
University of Texas Southwestern Medical Center

WILLIAM E. RAINEY, PH.D.
Professor of Obstetrics and Gynecology
University of Texas Southwestern Medical Center

KHURRAM S. REHMAN, M.D.
Fellow in Reproductive Endocrinology
University of Texas Southwestern Medical Center

RON G. ROSENFELD, M.D.
Senior VP for Medical Affairs
The Lucile Packard Foundation

WILLIS K. SAMSON, PH.D.
Professor of Pharmacology and Physiological Sciences
St. Louis University School of Medicine

PERRIN C. WHITE, M.D.
Professor of Pediatrics
University of Texas Southwestern Medical Center

Textbook of
Endocrine Physiology

1

Organization of the Endocrine System

SERGIO R. OJEDA
JAMES E. GRIFFIN

The evolutionary appearance of multicellular organisms dictated the necessity of establishing coordinating systems to regulate and integrate the function of the different cells. Two basic regulatory mechanisms developed to perform this delicate function: the nervous system and the endocrine system. Whereas the former employs electrochemical signals to send commands to peripheral organs and to receive information from them, the latter performs its regulatory function by producing chemical agents that, in general, are transported by the bloodstream to the target organs.

The two systems are, nevertheless, closely linked. The best-known connection is that of the hypothalamus and the pituitary gland. Hypothalamic neurosecretory cells produce substances that are delivered to the portal blood vessels (see Chapter 6) and transported to the anterior pituitary (adenohypophysis), where they regulate the secretion of adenohypophyseal hormones. Other hypothalamic neurons send their axons to the posterior pituitary, where they end in close proximity to the vascular bed of the gland and release their neurosecretory products directly into the bloodstream. The nervous and endocrine systems are further related by the innervation of endocrine glands. Most, if not all, endocrine glands, including the gonads, the thyroid, and the adrenals, receive nerves that appear to control both their blood flow and their secretory activity. In turn, the endocrine system regulates the function of the nervous system. For example, the gonadal and adrenocortical steroids act directly on the central nervous system either to inhibit or stimulate the secretory activity of those neurons that produce releasing hormones involved in the control of the pituitary–gonadal and pituitary–adrenal axes, respectively (i.e., luteinizing hormone-releasing hormone [LHRH] and corticotropin-releasing hormone [CRH]; see Chapter 6).

Although conventional definitions of the nervous and endocrine systems clearly delineate their differences, an absolute distinction between the two systems cannot be made. For instance, the nervous system produces substances that do not act across synapses, but rather are released into the bloodstream and travel to distant target cells. Among these substances of neural origin are the hypothalamic-releasing factors that control the secretion of anterior pituitary hormones; epinephrine of adrenomedullary origin, which upon release into the bloodstream can affect the function of various organs, such as the liver and muscle; and oxytocin and vasopressin, which are secreted by hypothalamic neurons and act on the mammary gland and uterus (oxytocin) to stimulate the activity of contractile tissue and on the kidney (vasopressin) to regulate extracellular fluid volume. Conversely, several peptides originally discovered in the gastrointestinal tract, where they exert hormonal actions, are produced in neurons of both the central and peripheral nervous systems, where they appear to act as neurotransmitters or neuromodulators. Examples of these hormones are gastrin, secretin, ghrelin, and vasoactive intestinal peptide.

Because of their interrelationships, endocrine glands and the components of the nervous system that regulate endocrine function are referred to as the *neuroendocrine system*. The discipline devoted to the study of this system is called *neuroendocrinology* (see Chapter 6). It is now clear that the neuroendocrine system does not operate alone; instead, it is subjected to regulatory input from an unexpected source, the immune system (see Chapter 4). The relationship between the neuroendocrine system and the immune system is reciprocal: hormones influence the immune system, and cytokines (the secretory products of the immune system) affect neuroendocrine functions. Most remarkably, immunologically reactive cells have been found to secrete certain hormones such as adrenocorticotropin (ACTH), β-endorphin, prolactin, and LHRH, which until recently were thought to be produced only in the brain and/or the pituitary gland.

Perhaps the best-characterized neuroendocrine–immune system relationship is that of the immune–hypothalamic–pituitary–adrenal axis. Cytokines, particularly interleukin-1 (produced by antigenically challenged macrophages), act on the hypothalamus to stimulate the secretion of CRH, which, in turn, stimulates the pituitary gland to secrete ACTH. This hormone acts on the adrenal cortex to elicit glucocorticoid secretion. Glucocorticoids then promote the formation of neutrophils in the bone marrow, decrease the formation of monocytes/macrophages and lymphocytes, and inhibit both cytokine and antibody production.

The immune system also affects the secretion of other pituitary hormones via the hypothalamus. Thus, in addition to the stimulatory effect of interleukin-1 on CRH release, cytokines have been shown to depress thyrotropin-releasing hormone (TRH) and LHRH production. In turn, several pituitary hormones and neuroendocrine peptides, including somatostatin, thyroid-stimulating hormone (TSH), and growth hormone (GH), are able to affect specific immunological functions (such as immunoglobulin synthesis, which is enhanced by TSH, and lymphocyte production, which is increased by GH).

The ovary provides another example of the interrelationships between the endocrine and the immune systems. Cytokines directly regulate certain ovarian functions and, as in the case of the neuroendocrine system, ovarian hormones have the ability to affect the immune system. For instance, interleukin-1 synthesis increases in the ovary during the hours preceding ovulation, resulting in a greater production of progesterone and prostaglandins, which in turn have a stimulatory effect on ovulation. Conversely, low doses of progesterone enhance the expression of the interleukin-1 gene in macrophages.

In their definition of a hormone, Baylis and Starling specified that for a substance to be considered a hormone, it should meet the requirement of being produced by an organ in small amounts, released into the bloodstream, and transported to a distant organ to exert its specific actions. This definition indeed applies to most of the *classical hormones* produced by the endocrine glands. It is now apparent, however, that hormones can act on contiguous cells, performing a paracrine function, and that they can modify the secretory activity of the same cells that produce them, performing an autocrine function. In acting locally, hormones do not need to be transported in the bloodstream, but they still can exert their action in a manner commensurate with their hormonal nature, that is, through binding to specific receptors.

Still, other *nonclassical hormones*, such as growth factors of the epidermal growth factor (EGF) family of trophic polypeptides, can affect cellular function in a nondiffusible, *juxtacrine* manner. This mode of communication is established when a membrane-anchored growth factor precursor on one cell is cleaved to yield the mature form of the growth factor, which then interacts with its membrane-bound receptor located on an adjacent cell.

ENDOCRINE GLANDS AND HORMONES

The endocrine system is composed of several glands located in different areas of the body that produce hormones with different functions. The major morphological feature of endocrine glands is that they are ductless, that is, they release their secretory products directly into the bloodstream and not into a duct system. Because they are richly vascularized, each secreting cell can deliver its products efficiently into the circulation.

The classical endocrine glands and their known secretory products are listed in Table 1-1. In recent years, the traditional view of the endocrine system's glandular nature has been broadened to include production of recognized hormones in

Table 1-1 Classical Endocrine Glands and Their Hormones

Gland		Hormone
Pituitary	Anterior lobe	Luteinizing hormone (LH), follicle-stimulating hormone (FSH), prolactin (PRL), growth hormone (GH), adrenocorticotropin (ACTH), β-lipotropin, β-endorphin, thyroid-stimulating hormone (TSH)
	Intermediate lobe	Melanocyte-stimulating hormone (MSH), β-endorphin
	Posterior lobe	Vasopressin (AVP) or antidiuretic hormone (ADH), oxytocin
Thyroid		Thyroxine (T_4), 3,5,3'-triiodothyronine (T_3), calcitonin
Parathyroid		Parathyroid hormone (PTH)
Adrenal	Cortex	Cortisol, aldosterone, dehydroepiandrosterone, androstenedione
	Medulla	Epinephrine, norepinephrine
Gonads	Testis	Testosterone, estradiol, androstenedione, inhibin, activin, müllerian-inhibiting substance
	Ovary	Estradiol, progesterone, testosterone, androstenedione, inhibin, activin, FSH-releasing peptide, relaxin, follistatin
Placenta		Human chorionic gonadotropin (hCG), human placental lactogen (hPL), progesterone, estrogen
Pancreas		Insulin, glucagon, somatostatin, pancreatic polypeptide, gastrin, vasoactive intestinal peptide (VIP)
Pineal		Melatonin, biogenic amines, several peptides

Table 1-2   Nonclassical "Endocrine Organs" and Their Hormones

Organ	Hormone
Brain (especially hypothalamus)	Corticotropin-releasing hormone (CRH), thyrotropin-releasing hormone TRH), luteinizing hormone-releasing hormone (LHRH), growth hormone-releasing hormone (GHRH), somatostatin, growth factors[a] (fibroblast growth factors, transforming growth factor-α (TGF-α), transforming growth factor-β (TGF-β), insulin-like growth factor I (IGF-I)
Heart	Atrial natriuretic peptides
Kidney	Erythropoietin, renin, 1,25-dihydroxyvitamin D
Liver, other organs, fibroblasts	IGF-I
Adipose tissue	Leptin
Gastrointestinal tract	Cholecystokinin (CCK), gastrin, ghrelin, secretin, vasoactive intestinal peptide (VIP), enteroglucagon, gastrin-releasing peptide
Platelets	Platelet-derived growth factor (PDGF), TGF-β
Macrophages, lymphocytes	Cytokines, TGF-β, pro-opiomelanocortin (POMC)-derived peptides
Various sites	Epidermal growth factor (EGF), TGF-α, neuregulins, neurotrophins

[a]Not considered to be hormones, but they can act as such.

organs whose primary function is not endocrine. Perhaps the earliest example of this was the recognition that hormones are produced by cells scattered along the mucosa of the stomach and small intestine. The brain, heart, kidney, liver, and certain blood elements also produce peptides or form active steroid metabolites from circulating precursors that deserve the designation of *hormones* (Table 1-2). Not all of these hormones will be considered in this textbook.

CHEMICAL NATURE OF HORMONES

Chemically, the hormones fall into three general categories. The first comprises hormones derived from single amino acids. They are the amines, such as norepinephrine, epinephrine, and dopamine, which derive from the amino acid tyrosine, and the thyroid hormones, 3,5,3'-triiodothyronine (T_3) and 3,5,3',5'-tetraiodothyronine (thyroxine, T_4), which derive from the combination of two iodinated tyrosine amino acid residues.

The second category is composed of peptides and proteins. These can be as small as TRH (three amino acids) and as large and complex as GH and follicle-stimulating hormone (FSH), which have about 200 amino acid residues and molecular weights in the range of 25,000–30,000.

The third category comprises the steroid hormones, which are derivatives of cholesterol and can be grouped into two types: (*1*) those with an intact steroid nucleus such as the gonadal and adrenal steroids and (*2*) those with a broken steroid nucleus (the B ring) such as vitamin D and its metabolites. Figure 1-1 provides examples of these three categories of hormones.

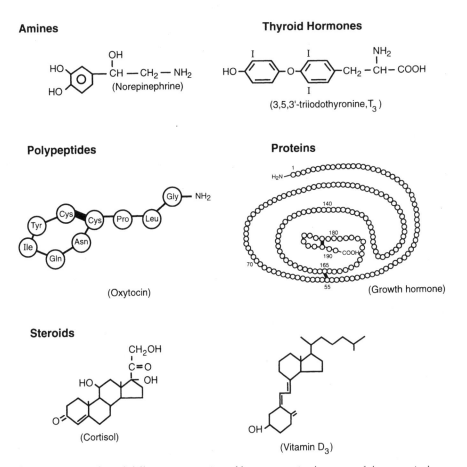

Fig. 1-1 Examples of different categories of hormones. In the case of the protein hormone, each circle represents an amino acid, as shown for the polypeptide hormone.

FUNCTION OF HORMONES

Regardless of their chemical nature, hormones are present in the bloodstream in very low concentrations (10^{-7} to 10^{-12} M). Thus, it is not surprising that a prerequisite for any hormone to exert its actions is that it must first bind to specific high-affinity cellular receptors. These receptors may be located on the cell membrane, as in the case of protein hormones and amines, or in the nucleus, as with thyroid and steroid hormones (see Chapter 3). Another characteristic feature of hormones is that a single hormone can exert various effects in different tissues; conversely, several hormones can regulate a single function. Estradiol exemplifies the versatility of some hormones. It is produced by the ovary and can act on the ovarian follicles themselves to promote granulosa cell differentiation, on the uterus to stimulate its growth and maintain the cyclic change of the uterine mucosa, on the mammary gland to simulate ductal growth, on bone to promote linear growth and closure of the epiphyseal plates, on the hypothalamic–pituitary system to regulate the secretion of gonadotropins and prolactin, and on general metabolic processes to affect adipose tissue distribution, volume of extracellular fluid, and so on. In each case, estradiol acts through the same common mechanism, namely, binding to high-affinity, specific nuclear receptors followed by attachment of the receptor–steroid complex to DNA regions of genes that are expressed in a tissue-specific manner.

An example of a single function regulated by more than one hormone is the release of fatty acids (lipolysis) from adipose tissue stores. A variety of hormones including catecholamines, glucagon, secretin, prolactin, and β-lipotropin stimulate lipolysis within minutes by activating, via cyclic adenosine monophosphate (AMP), a rate-limiting triglyceride hydrolase known as *hormone-sensitive lipase*. Growth hormone and glucocorticoids also stimulate lipolysis, but only after a time lag of 2 hours because they induce the synthesis of hormone-sensitive lipase instead of activating the hydrolase. Other hormones such as insulin, insulin-like growth factors (IGFs) or somatomedins, oxytocin, and gastric-inhibitory polypeptide inhibit lipolysis.

An example of a complex function regulated by different hormones is the development of the mammary gland, which is under the primary influence of prolactin, estradiol, and progesterone and the permissive influence of glucocorticoids, thyroid hormones, and insulin. The effect of these latter hormones is considered permissive because, by themselves, they have little effect, but when they are present the actions of prolactin, estrogen, and progesterone become fully manifested.

Hormones exert their functions in four broad physiological areas: reproduction, growth and development, maintenance of the internal environment, and the regulation of energy balance.

Reproduction

Hormones produced by the gonads (androgens, estrogen, progestogens) and the anterior pituitary gland (luteinizing hormone [LH], FSH, GH, and prolactin) interact to regulate the growth and structural integrity of the reproductive organs, the production of gametes, the patterns of sexual behavior, the phenotypic difference between the sexes, and the continuation of the species (through their effects on ovulation, spermatogenesis, pregnancy, and lactation).

Several examples of these interactions can be provided. For instance, estradiol induces hypertrophy and hyperplasia of both the muscular and endothelial layers of the uterine wall; in turn, the secretion of estradiol from the ovary is under the control of the pituitary gonadotropins. Testosterone, which in males is under the control of LH, exerts tropic effects on sex accessory glands such as the prostate and seminal vesicles. Both estradiol in females and testosterone in males play fundamental roles in determining the female and male external appearance at puberty. Testosterone promotes the growth of the testes, scrotum, and penis and stimulates muscle development, particularly that of the pectoral region and shoulders. Estradiol promotes the development of the female external genitalia and the redistribution of adipose tissue, which localizes more noticeably in the thighs, hips, and breasts (see Chapter 9). Although in humans gonadal steroids do not induce a stereotyped pattern of sexual behavior, as in animals, there is no doubt that they are important in maintaining the libido.

Both ovulation and spermatogenesis are processes tightly controlled by the pituitary gonadotropins LH and FSH, which act either directly on the gonads to promote follicular development (ovary) and formation of sperm (testis) or indirectly through their stimulatory effects on estrogen and testosterone secretion. During pregnancy various hormones of placental origin including estradiol, progesterone, chorionic gonadotropin, placental lactogen, and several others (see Chapter 11) contribute to maintaining the normal progression of pregnancy. After delivery, another group of hormones, most noticeably prolactin (see above), maintains the structure and function of the lactating breast.

Growth and Development

Various hormones play primary and permissive roles in the timing and progression of growth, both for overall body size and for individual tissues. In many cases the local production of growth factors is a result of hormone action. In other instances the production of a growth factor may be hormone independent, but the growth factor interacts with hormones to promote or reduce growth.

The classical hormones involved in the process of growth are GH, thyroid hormones, insulin, glucocorticoids, androgens, and estrogens. Although the stimulatory effect of GH on bodily growth is mediated by a family of peptides known collectively as *insulin-like growth factors* (IGFs; see Chapter 12), it is unclear to what extent these growth factors are involved in mediating the stimulatory effect of androgens and estrogens on linear growth and acquisition of muscle mass. An example of a hormone that plays both permissive and primary roles in growth is T_4. In its absence, GH fails to stimulate skeletal growth, a phenomenon that appears to be related to a reduced ability of the tissue to respond to IGFs. In the central nervous system, however, T_4 plays a primary role in inducing growth and cellular differentiation. Some of its actions in the brain appear to be mediated by the production of a issue-specific growth factor, nerve growth factor (NGF). Specific hormones (GH, T_4, sex steroids) can also regulate the synthesis of peptide growth factors such as the IGFs, NGF, and EGF. A more detailed discussion of the hormones and peptide growth factors involved in regulating growth is presented in Chapter 12.

Maintenance of Internal Environment

The maintenance of the internal environment involves the control of extracellular fluid volume and blood pressure, the electrolyte composition of bodily fluids, the regulation of plasma and tissue levels of calcium and phosphate ions, and the maintenance of bone, muscle, and body stores of fat.

A multitude of hormones participates in the regulation of these processes. For example, vasopressin or antidiuretic hormone, which is synthesized in the hypothalamus and released from the posterior pituitary, acts on the kidney to induce water reabsorption; aldosterone produced in the adrenal cortex stimulates sodium reabsorption and potassium excretion in the kidney. Thus, both hormones contribute to regulating blood pressure, extracellular fluid volume, and the electrolyte composition of bodily fluids.

Plasma levels of calcium and phosphate ions are controlled by parathyroid hormone (PTH) from the parathyroid glands (see Chapter 15). The PTH increases the serum calcium concentration mainly through its stimulatory actions on calcium transport in bone and kidney, but also by enhancing intestinal calcium absorption through its stimulatory influence on the renal formation of 1,25-dihydroxyvitamin D. Also, PTH acts on the kidney to increase phosphate excretion.

The functions of bone, muscle, and adipose tissue are regulated by hormones as diverse as PTH, estrogens, androgens, and GH (bone) and catecholamines, insulin, glucagon, and glucocorticoids (muscle and adipose tissue). Pertinent details are given in Chapters 14, 15, and 16.

Regulation of Energy Balance

For an organism to survive, it must be able to convert the calories contained in food into energy, to store part of that energy for subsequent use, and to mobilize it when necessary. Maintenance of energy homeostasis is of paramount importance for the proper regulation of body weight, which requires a balance between food consumption and energy expenditure. The hypothalamus plays a central role in this process by integrating a variety of afferent sensory, visual, biochemical, and hormonal signals reflecting the nutritional status of the organism. Processing of these signals results in the activation of efferent signals that regulate both feeding behavior and energy expenditure. The latter is regulated via mechanisms controlling the metabolic rate, such as those influenced by the sympathetic and parasympathetic nervous systems, and by insulin, glucagon, and thyroid hormones.

In recent years, several of the afferent signals controlling energy balance have been identified. For instance, leptin, a hormone produced by white adipose tissue, has been shown to act on the brain to decrease food intake and increase energy expenditure. Leptin acts through specific receptors, which are particularly abundant in hypothalamic nuclei, such as the ventromedial nucleus and the arcuate nucleus, known to be involved in the control of feeding behavior. Thus, leptin serves as a "lipostat" or "adipostat" that—acting via its strategically located receptors—informs the brain of the status of energy storage in adipose tissue and modifies the efferent wing of energy homeostasis. One target of leptin action are the neurons of the arcuate nucleus of the hypothalamus that produce neuropeptide Y (NPY), an appetite-stimulating neuropeptide. An increase in plasma leptin levels leads to decreased production of NPY and a corresponding decrease in food intake.

In addition to leptin, at least three centrally originated peptides have been shown to suppress feeding behavior: melanocortinergic neurons of the arcuate nucleus acting via a melanocyte-stimulating hormone receptor known as *MC4-R*; a corticotropin-releasing-factor–related peptide known as *urocortin*, produced in the lateral hypothalamus; and an orphan receptor known as *bombesin receptor type-3*. It is possible that at least part of the suppressive effects of leptin on feeding behavior is mediated by one or more of these systems. Accordingly, they should be considered as part of the efferent mechanisms controlling energy balance.

Counteracting the suppressive effect of these peptides on feeding behavior are other peptides produced by either hypothalamic neurons or peripheral cells that stimulate feeding. Two of these peptides, termed *orexin A* and *orexin B*, and their receptors are are produced in neurons of the lateral hypothalamus. In addition, a peptide termed *ghrelin*, produced in the stomach and small intestine, is secreted in response to fasting and stimulates feeding. It is thus clear that the the mechanisms underlying the regulation of energy balance are being unraveled at an ever-increasing rate.

SYNTHESIS AND RELEASE OF HORMONES

Peptide and protein hormones are synthesized in the rough endoplasmic reticulum. As with all proteins, the amino acid sequence of protein hormones is determined by specific messenger RNAs that are synthesized in the nucleus and have a nucleotide sequence dictated by a specific gene. We shall see in Chapter 2 that translation of the specific messenger RNA sequence results in the ribosomal synthesis of a protein larger than the mature hormone. This precursor form may be either a prohormone or a preprohormone. Prohormones are extended at their amino termini by a hydrophobic amino acid sequence called *leader* or *signal peptide*. Preprohormones are also extended by a signal peptide, but in addition contain internal cleavage sites that upon enzymatic action yield different bioactive peptides. In some instances, preprohormones contain peptide sequences that may not have a known biological activity. These sequences are called *cryptic peptides*. In other instances these peptides may act as *spacers* between two bioactive peptides.

Because of its hydrophobic nature, the leader peptide sequence of both preprohormones and prohormones permits the newly synthesized protein to move across the membrane of the endoplasmic reticulum to be transported to the Golgi apparatus. The leader peptide is removed from the hormone before the synthesis of the polypeptide chain is ended, and this permits the protein to assume its secondary structure during its transport to the Golgi apparatus. Once it arrives at this organelle, the hormone may be further processed by proteolytic enzymes, which cleave the prohormone generating one or more mature hormones and/or by other enzymes that add nonprotein residues such as carbohydrates. Whatever the case, the hormone is always stored in granules that fuse with the cell membrane during the release process and allow their contents to be extruded into the extracellular perivascular space. This process is called *exocytosis* and involves the participation of microtubules and the mobilization of calcium across the cell membrane. During release, not only the hormone but also the cleaving enzymes and peptides associated with the prohormone are discharged from the granule.

Amine and steroid hormones are synthesized in a manner much different from that of proteins. They originate from precursor molecules (tyrosine and cholesterol, respectively) that are either totally (tyrosine) or partially (cholesterol) transported to the cell of synthesis via the bloodstream. Once inside the cell, these precursor molecules are subjected to the sequential action of several enzymes, resulting in the formation of various intermediate products that themselves may be hormones. Like proteins, amines are packed into granules and are released by a similar process of exocytosis. In contrast to protein hormones, thyroid hormones and steroids, once produced, can freely cross the cell membrane without having to be packed in granules and actively exocytosed.

Although we have discussed mechanisms involved in the formation of hormones at their site of origin, well-documented examples exist of hormones that are produced at sites other than those in which their precursor is formed, using these same mechanisms (i.e., proteolytic cleavage of peptide hormone precursors and enzymatic modification of steroid hormones). In some instances, a hormone with little activity is converted into an active or a more active form by the action of enzymes in the circulation or other tissues. For example, angiotensin II is formed in the circulation through the sequential action of the enzyme renin, produced in the kidney to convert angiotensinogen to angiotensin I, and a converting enzyme produced in the lungs that cleaves two amino acids from angiotensin I to form angiotensin II. The androgen androstenedione (produced by both the gonads and adrenal glands) can be metabolized to the estrogen estrone in adipose tissue, and testosterone is converted into the more potent androgen dihydrotestosterone in androgen target tissues such as the prostate.

Although protein, amine, and steroid hormones differ in their mechanisms of synthesis and release, a feature they all share is the variability of their blood levels. As we shall see next, fluctuating plasma hormone levels are the consequence of the episodic nature of hormone secretion.

PATTERNS OF HORMONE SECRETION

The concentration of hormones in the circulation is generally regulated by control loops or feedback mechanisms to allow a response to physiological needs (see below). In addition, the basal secretion of most hormones is not a continuous process but rather has a pulsatile nature. When hormone release is induced by a secretagogue, the pattern of response is episodic. Conversely, inhibition of hormone secretion by other hormones always results in suppression of the episodic increases in hormone levels. The pulsatile pattern of hormone secretion is characterized by episodes of release that can be as frequent as every 5–10 minutes; each episode is followed by a quiescent period during which plasma levels of the hormone fall toward basal values. Another discharge then occurs and the cycle repeats itself, often varying in both amplitude and frequency of the pulses. In the case of hormones subjected to negative feedback control (see below), removal of the inhibitory feedback signal results in a marked enhancement of the amplitude and frequency of the episodes of secretion.

Secretory episodes may occur with different periodicities. For example, the most prominent episodes of release may occur with a frequency of about 1 hour. This mode of release is called *circhoral*. If the episodes of release occur at intervals longer than 1 hour but less than 24 hours the rhythm is called *ultradian*; if the periodicity is about 1 day the rhythm is called *circadian*; and if it recurs every day it is called *quotidian*. Release patterns of the latter type are usually referred to as *diurnal* because the increase in secretory activity becomes expressed at defined periods of the day. For example, ACTH has a characteristic diurnal pattern of release, with plasma levels rising sharply during the early morning hours.

The release pattern of a hormone may have a much less frequent periodicity. For example, the monthly preovulatory discharge of gonadotropins recurs approximately every 30 days, a pattern of release that has been called *circatrigintan*. Other hormones such as T_4 exhibit changes in plasma levels that occur over months. If the changes take place on a yearly basis the rhythm is called *circannual* or *seasonal*, as it occurs in relation to the seasonal phases of the year.

Although it is clear that these low periodicity rhythms of hormone release are dictated by either environmental or hormonal cues, the mechanisms underlying the pulsatile release of hormones are unknown. It does appear, however, that secretory cells, including neurosecretory neurons, have the ability to secrete their products in a discontinuous, episodic manner. Superimposed on this basic mode of release, the amount of hormone produced and the frequency of the secretory episodes are modulated by specific negative and positive feedback mechanisms (see below).

The physiological importance of pulsatile hormone release has been best demonstrated in humans and nonhuman primates treated with LHRH, the hypothalamic peptide that stimulates the secretion of gonadotropins from the anterior pituitary (see Chapter 6). Only when LHRH is given in a pulsatile fashion at a frequency of about one pulse per hour is gonadotropin secretion and gonadal function maintained normally; a slower frequency fails to maintain gonadotropin secretion at a level sufficient to support normal gonadal production of steroids and gametes; a faster frequency or continuous administration of LHRH inhibits the secretion of gonadotropins and prevents normal gonadal function. This latter phenomenon, which results from a reduced sensitivity of the pituitary to frequent or continuous LHRH stimulation, has been applied to the treatment of precocious puberty and to fertility control using long-acting LHRH analogs (see Chapters 9 and 10).

TRANSPORT AND METABOLISM OF HORMONES

Once a hormone is released into the bloodstream it may circulate freely, if it is water soluble, or it may be bound to a carrier protein. In general, amines, peptides, and proteins circulate in free form, whereas steroids and thyroid hormones are bound to transport proteins. A well-known exception to this rule is provided by the IGFs, which, despite being polypeptides, circulate tightly attached to specific binding proteins. Some plasma proteins such as albumin and prealbumin have the capacity to transport nonselectively a variety of low molecular weight hormones. In contrast, specific transport proteins that are globulins have saturable, high-affinity binding sites for the hormones they carry. These proteins include thyroid hormone-binding globulin (TBG), testosterone-binding globulin (TeBG), and cortisol-binding globulin (CBG).

Binding of hormones to carrier proteins has a profound impact on the hormone clearance rate from the circulation. The greater the binding capacity of the specific protein carrier, the slower the clearance rate of the hormone. Thus, hormones that circulate mostly in bound form, such as T_4, disappear much more slowly from the plasma than do hormones that circulate either in free form or only weakly bound. In general, changes in the plasma levels of binding proteins are rapidly followed by adjustments in the secretion rate of the corresponding hormone, so that the fraction of hormone readily available for tissue delivery remains constant and endocrine function remains normal. One well-known example of this is the increase in CBG

Table 1-3 Half-Life of Protein, Amine, and
Steroid Hormones in Plasma

Hormone	Half-life
Amines	2–3 minutes
Thyroid hormones	
T_4	6.7 days
T_3	0.75 day
Polypeptides	4–40 minutes
Proteins	15–170 minutes
Steroids	4–120 minutes

concentration that occurs during pregnancy as a consequence of estradiol stimulation. While the total plasma cortisol level rises as a result of the increased CBG levels, the cortisol available to the tissues remains normal. This is because, as the concentration of CBG increases, there is a temporary decrease in the cortisol available to target tissues, as more is bound to CBG. This results in a temporary increase in ACTH by activation of feedback mechanisms (see below) and increased cortisol secretion to increase the total plasma concentration of cortisol and return tissue delivery of cortisol to normal. Thus, in the steady state with intact control mechanisms, alterations in hormone-binding proteins do not affect endocrine status.

The metabolic clearance rate (MCR) of a hormone defines quantitatively its removal from plasma. Under steady-state conditions, the MCR represents the volume of plasma cleared of the hormone per unit of time; usually the units employed are milliliters per minute. If a radioactive hormone is infused into the bloodstream until a constant level is reached and the infusion is then stopped, the disappearance rate of the labeled hormone from the plasma can be determined and the plasma half-life of the hormone calculated. The plasma half-life of a hormone is inversely related to its MCR. Table 1-3 lists the half-lives of several hormones.

Only a small portion of the circulating hormones is removed from the circulation by most target tissues. The liver and the kidneys perform the bulk of hormone clearance. This process includes degradation by a variety of enzymatic mechanisms such as hydrolysis, oxidation, hydroxylation, methylation, decarboxylation, sulfation, and glucuronidation. In general, only a small fraction (<1%) of any hormone is excreted intact in the urine or feces.

The interaction of hormones with their target tissues is apparently followed by intracellular degradation of the hormone. In the case of protein hormones and amines, degradation occurs after their binding to membrane receptors, internalization of the hormone–receptor complex, and dissociation of this complex into its two components (see Chapter 3). In the case of steroid or thyroid hormones, degradation may occur after binding of the hormone–receptor complex to nuclear chromatin.

FEEDBACK MECHANISMS

The secretion of most, if not all, hormones is regulated by closed-loop systems known as *feedback mechanisms*. Indeed, the endocrine system as a whole is organized in a hierarchy of closed-loop systems that not only operate between cells but also constitute an essential feature of intracellular regulation. Feedback mechanisms are of two types: negative and positive. Negative feedback is the prevailing control mechanism regulating endocrine function; in its simplest form it is a closed loop in which hormone A stimulates the production of hormone B, which in turn acts on the cells producing hormone A to decrease its rate of secretion. An example of this type of feedback can be found in the stimulation of adrenal cortisol secretion by the adenohypophyseal hormone ACTH (hormone A) and the resulting inhibition of ACTH release by the increased plasma cortisol (hormone B) levels (Fig. 1-2). In the less common positive feedback mechanisms, hormone B further stimulates the production of hormone A instead of diminishing it (Fig. 1-2). A typical example of a positive feedback loop is that which exists between LH and estradiol. During the menstrual cycle a gradual increase in plasma LH levels stimulates the production of estradiol by the ovary; after reaching a certain level, estradiol induces an abrupt increase in LH secretion, known as the *preovulatory surge* of LH, because it induces ovulation. Upon reaching maximal levels, plasma LH declines despite the presence of still elevated estrogen concentrations. This latter phenomenon exemplifies the self-limiting nature of positive feedback systems. The secretion of hormone A declines rapidly after its initial activation because the secretory cell has a limited capacity to produce the hormone and because there are always additional negative feedback loops that limit the magnitude of the response.

Endocrine control systems also have feedforward loops directing the flow of hormonal information. These feedforward loops can be negative or positive. They are intrinsically unstable because they do not function as closed-loop systems. Because feedforward loops always form part of a large, more complex feedback circuit, their performance is closely regulated by subserving closed-loop mechanisms. This concept is diagrammed in Figure 1-3, which shows a feedforward loop that accelerates the conversion of product 2 into product 3. The latter results in product 4, which then inhibits the formation of product 2.

A well-recognized example of a feedforward loop is the release of insulin by the β-cells of the islets of Langerhans in response to an increase in plasma glucose concentration. Upon stimulation of its secretion by the elevated glucose levels, insulin acts on the liver to enhance the uptake of glucose. When plasma glucose levels fall to basal levels, insulin mobilization decreases and glucose uptake is reduced.

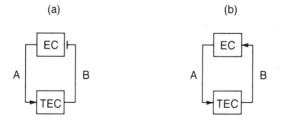

Fig. 1-2 Schematic representation of a negative (a) and a positive (b) feedback loop. The arrows represent stimulation. The blunt-ended lines represent inhibition. EC, endocrine cells; TEC, target endocrine cell; A, hormone A; B, hormone B.

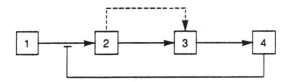

Fig. 1-3 Schematic representation of a feedforward loop (broken line) that activates the progression of the reaction in a hypothetical metabolic pathway. The loop, however, operates within a system tightly controlled by negative feedback systems (blunt-ended line). (Adapted from Rasmussen H: In: *Textbook of Endocrinology,* 5th ed., RH Williams, ed., Saunders, Philadelphia, p. 2, 1974, with permission.)

As one would suspect, different levels of complexity exist in the organization of endocrine control systems. The simplest is that of a single negative feedback loop. Much more complex is the situation in which one hormone controls the production of another hormone from a different cell type, which, in turn, controls a third secretory cell that produces a hormone(s) that both feeds back upon the first and/or second component of the system and regulates the function of still another cell type. An example of such a system is the hypothalamic control of gonadotropin secretion from the anterior pituitary (Fig. 1-4). While the hypothalamus stimulates the secretion of gonadotropins through the delivery of LHRH to the pituitary gland, the gonadotropins control the secretion of ovarian steroids, which in turn feed back on the hypothalamus and anterior pituitary to regulate the secretion of LHRH and gonadotropins, respectively.

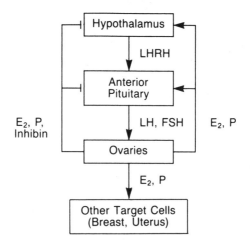

Fig. 1-4 The hypothalamic–pituitary–gonadal axis as an example of a complex endocrine control system. Arrows indicate stimulation and blunt-ended lines represent inhibition. E_2, estradiol; FSH, follicle-stimulating hormone; LH, luteinizing hormone; LHRH, luteinizing hormone-releasing hormone; P, progesterone.

MECHANISMS OF ENDOCRINE DISEASE

Endocrine disorders can result from hormone deficiency, hormone excess, or hormone resistance. With some notable exceptions (e.g., calcitonin), hormone deficiency always causes disease. Hormone deficiency is usually the result of a destructive process occurring in the gland in which the hormone is produced. Thus, infection by viruses or bacteria, infarction due to an impaired blood supply, physical compression by tumor growth, or attack by cellular or humoral immune mechanisms all may lead to impaired hormone production in most endocrine glands. Alternatively, hormone deficiency states can result from genetic defects in hormone formation such as gene deletion or mutation, failure to cleave a peptide hormone precursor to the active hormone, or a specific enzymatic defect in the formation of thyroid or steroid hormones. Inactivating mutations in cell surface receptors for hormones that stimulate endocrine glands can also cause hormone deficiency (e.g., LHRH in the anterior pituitary, LH in the testes, and TSH in the thyroid).

Hormone excess usually results in disease. The hormone may be overproduced by the gland that normally secretes it or by a tissue that is not normally an endocrine organ. Malignancies are often involved in each of these types of hormone excess. Some tumors of endocrine glands (e.g., pituitary, adrenal) are functional and secrete the appropriate hormone for the gland but in an unregulated manner. In some instances, activating mutations in cell surface receptors for stimulating hormones have been found (LH, TSH). In the malignant transformation occurring in nonendocrine tissues (e.g., lung cancer), dedifferentiation may lead to the production of certain peptide hormones. Other mechanisms of hormone excess include the effects of antireceptor antibodies stimulating a receptor instead of blocking its activation, as in the common form of hyperthyroidism, and the ingestion of exogenous hormones, as in the glucocorticoid excess resulting from its therapeutic use.

Hormone resistance as a mechanism of disease has now been described for almost all hormones. In these disorders the hormone is present in normal or increased amounts, but the expected actions of the hormone do not occur. In some cases, because of a mutation, a structurally abnormal peptide hormone is present, causing the resistance (e.g., insulin, PTH). In other instances, there are antibodies to the hormone or hormone receptor (e.g., insulin and its receptor). Finally, hormone resistance may occur as the result of primary receptor defects (e.g., androgen and vitamin D receptors) or defects in the postreceptor mechanisms of hormone action (e.g., insulin, PTH).

SUGGESTED READING

Ahima RS and Flier JS: Leptin. Annu Rev Physiol 62:413–437, 2000.
Cahill GF: Origin, evolution, and role of hormones. In: *Endocrinology*, 2nd ed., LJ Degroot, ed., Saunders, Philadelphia, pp. 3–5, 1989.
Igaz P, Falus A, Glaz E, and Racz K: Cytokines in diseases of the endocrine system. Cell Biol Int 24:663–668, 2000.
Merriam GR and Wachter KW: Analysis of the temporal coincidence of hormonal pulses. In: *Pulsatility in Neuroendocrine Systems* (*Methods in Neuroscience*, Vol. 20), J Levine, ed., Academic Press, San Diego, pp. 326–335, 1994.

Pardridge WM: Transport of protein-bound hormones into tissues in vivo. Endocr Rev 2:102–123, 1981.

Rasmussen H: Organization and control of endocrine systems. In: *Textbook of Endocrinology*, 5th ed., RH Williams, ed., Saunders, Philadelphia, pp. 2–30, 1974.

Schwartz MW, Woods SC, Porte D Jr, Seeley RJ, and Baskin DG: Central nervous system control of food intake. Nature 404:661–671, 2000.

Turek FW and Van Cauter E: Rhythms in reproduction. In: *The Physiology of Reproduction*, 2nd ed., E Knobil and JD Neill, eds., Raven Press, New York, pp. 487–540, 1994.

2

Genes and Hormones

PERRIN C. WHITE

Much of the knowledge presented in the following chapters has been gained using molecular genetic techniques to analyze the structure, synthesis, regulation, and effects of hormones. This chapter provides an overview of some of the relevant techniques and associated concepts.

GENE EXPRESSION

Deoxyribonucleic acid (DNA) and *ribonucleic acid* (RNA) consist of *nucleotides*. A nucleotide consists of a *base*, a sugar moiety (either deoxyribose or ribose), and a phosphate group. The sugars and phosphates alternate in the backbone of a nucleic acid strand. In general, there are four possible bases. In DNA, these are *adenine* (A), *cytosine* (C), *guanine* (G), and *thymine* (T). Adenine and guanine are *purines*, whereas cytosine and thymine are *pyrimidines*. The corresponding nucleotides are *adenosine, cytidine, guanosine,* and *thymidine.* In RNA, *uracil (uridine)* is substituted for thymine (thymidine).

DNA is double stranded. Each strand has a direction because the deoxyribose molecules forming the backbone are asymmetrical, with the phosphate bonds linking each two sugar molecules going from the 3′ position of one to the 5′ position of the next. Thus the 5′ position of a sugar molecule is free at one end (the 5′ end) of the strand, and the 3′ position is free at the other. The two strands of a DNA molecule run in opposite directions, so that the 5′ end of one strand is opposed to the 3′ end of the complementary strand.

The DNA strands interact with each other through *complementary (Watson-Crick) base pairing*, in which A and T or C and G are paired through hydrogen bonds. Thus the sequence of one DNA strand unambiguously determines the sequence of the complementary strand during DNA replication.

The length of a DNA segment is typically given in bases or nucleotides (nt) or, if double-stranded, in *base pairs* (bp). A longer segment is measured in thousands of bases (kilobases, kb) or millions of bases (megabases, mb).

A *gene* may be defined as a segment of DNA within a chromosome that can be *transcribed* to yield RNA that serves a particular function. Many transcripts are *messenger RNAs* (mRNA) that are *translated* into proteins. Others function directly as RNA, including ribosomal RNA and transfer RNA, which are required for protein synthesis, and small nuclear RNAs required for splicing introns out of primary mRNA transcripts (see below).

Genes encoding proteins consist of several components (Fig. 2-1). *Exons* are regions that are retained in mRNA. These are usually interspersed with *introns*, sequences spliced out of the primary transcript before it leaves the nucleus. Exons consist of coding sequences that are translated into protein and untranslated regions at both ends of the gene. Transcriptional regulatory regions (or *cis* regulatory elements) may be near, anywhere within, or at some distance from a gene, but most often are located within a few hundred nucleotides of the start of transcription.

A *hormone*, broadly defined, is a soluble substance that is secreted in a regulated manner by one cell in a multicelled organism and has defined effects on a second cell. Many but not all of these effects directly or indirectly modify levels or patterns of gene expression in the target cell. Thus studies of gene expression comprise an important part of modern endocrinology.

Transcription

Messenger RNA is single stranded. Its sequence corresponds to the *coding* or *sense* strand of DNA. During transcription, it is synthesized in the 5′ to 3′ direction by a

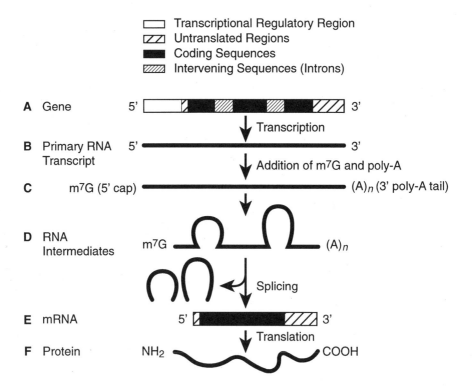

Fig. 2-1 Steps in expression of a protein product of a gene. Different parts of a generic gene are diagrammed in *A*. The same shadings are used in *E*, but they are omitted in *B–D*, which schematically illustrate RNA processing.

transcriptional apparatus that "reads" the complementary or *antisense* strand of DNA and synthesizes an mRNA molecule complementary to it. This process is mediated by the interactions of many proteins with defined sequences, or *elements*, of DNA.

DNA (Cis) Elements

Promoters. Transcription is invariably controlled at least in part by sequences located in the 5' flanking region of the gene before (5' or upstream of) the start of transcription. These sequences fall into two categories. Those whose function is dependent on their location and orientation are collectively referred to as the *promoter* of the gene (although this term is also sometimes used for all transcriptional regulatory sequences in the 5' flanking region of the gene). One element of the promoter is the binding site for RNA polymerase II. In many genes this region includes a short nucleotide sequence known as a *TATA box* (TATAAA or a related sequence) approximately 30 bases upstream from the site at which transcription begins. Some genes do not contain this element but instead have one or more *GC boxes* (GGGCGGGG); often these are *housekeeping* genes that are transcribed at a relatively constant level in different cell types.

Enhancers and Silencers. The *cis* elements that increase transcription independently of their position and orientation are termed *enhancers*, whereas those that decrease transcription are called *silencers*. Such elements can be located within a gene itself, usually in an intron, or at some distance (up to thousands of nucleotides) from a gene. When tested using reporter constructs (see below), such elements are found to be functional even when inserted backward or 3' of the reporter gene, or even when the reporter gene is expressed from a different (heterologous) promoter.

Locus Control Regions. *In situ*, locus control regions are required to establish a tissue-specific open chromatin domain (see below) in the vicinity of a particular locus and thus permit appropriate tissue-specific expression; the first one identified is in the b-globin cluster. The open chromatin configuration is detected experimentally as tissue-specific hypersensitivity of DNA to digestion with deoxyribonuclease (DNase) I. In transgenic mice, locus control regions direct high-level, tissue-specific expression that is independent of the site of chromosomal integration but dependent on copy number. Locus control regions can exert effects over tens of kilobases and may consist of complex DNA elements themselves spaced over several kilobases. In addition to their effects on chromatin, elements within certain locus control regions can act as transcriptional enhancers in reporter constructs, and so the distinction between these categories is not absolute.

DNA Methylation. In addition to defined DNA *cis* elements, modification of DNA by cytosine methylation at CpG dinucleotides is associated with gene inactivation. Each such dinucleotide is paired with another on the opposite DNA strand, and usually both cytosines are methylated. This serves as a signal for a DNA methylase to methylate the cytosines on daughter strands whenever DNA is replicated. This minimizes expression of permanently inactivated genes when differentiated cells divide. Conversely, hypomethylation of DNA in CpG-rich regions in the 5' ends of genes is associated with active transcription. In some genes, the copies derived from each parent (i.e., the parental *alleles*) are differently and permanently methylated, or *imprinted*, leading to differences in gene expression. Several diseases such as Prader-Willi syndrome are caused by heterozygous deletion of a particular gene inherited from one parent because the remaining gene copy has been permanently inactivated by imprinting.

Protein Factors

Chromatin. Within chromosomes, eukaryotic DNA is organized into *nucleosomes*, each consisting of eight positively charged histone molecules (two each of histones H2A, H2B, H3, and H4) with 160–200 bp of DNA wound around it. Higher-order winding organizes nucleosomes into chromatin. This organization renders DNA relatively inaccessible to transcription factors, so that transcription is enhanced by remodeling of nucleosomes to permit assembly of transcription complexes. This remodeling or activation is mediated in part by acetylation of histones. Histone molecules interact with DNA and with each other in part via positively charged amino terminal domains, and acetylation of lysine residues in these domains reduces their positive charge. Conversely, deacetylation of histones represses transcription.

General Transcription Factors. The promoter of a gene is bound by general transcription factors (TFs) to form a transcription initiation complex that ultimately has a molecular weight of greater than 2 million (Fig. 2-2). Although preformed complexes may exist, stepwise assembly is usually postulated. TFIID binds to the TATA box. TFIID is a complex of proteins consisting of TATA-binding protein (TBP) and at least a half dozen TBP-associated factors. This complex separates the DNA strands, allowing TFIIA and TFIIB to bind adjacent to the TATA box. This is followed by binding of TFIIF-α and RNA polymerase II. Transcription begins following binding of TFIIE, TFIIH, and TFIIJ and subsequent release of RNA polymerase II from the initiation complex.

RNA polymerases I and III transcribe genes for ribosomal RNA and small RNAs (such as transfer RNAs), respectively. They are not regulated in the same way as RNA polymerase II and bind distinct sets of transcription factors.

Transcriptional Regulatory Factors. Many different factors bind to enhancer elements including nuclear hormone receptors and factors phosphorylated by kinases that are activated by hormone-dependent signaling pathways. These are described in greater detail in Chapter 3. In general, each consists of a DNA-binding domain and at least one activation domain that interacts with elements of the transcriptional apparatus. Almost all DNA-binding domains include an α-helical protein segment that fits into the major groove between two turns of the DNA helix. Many of these domains (including those of nuclear hormone receptors) are stabilized by chelated zinc atoms and are termed *zinc fingers*. *Leucine zipper* domains have leucine residues at every seventh position in the α-helix, which results in them all being on the same side of the helix. An example of such a protein is SREBP-1 (sterol regulatory element binding protein-1), which mediates transcriptional regulation by sterols. *Homeodomains* are 60 amino acid motifs that are most often found in transcription factors

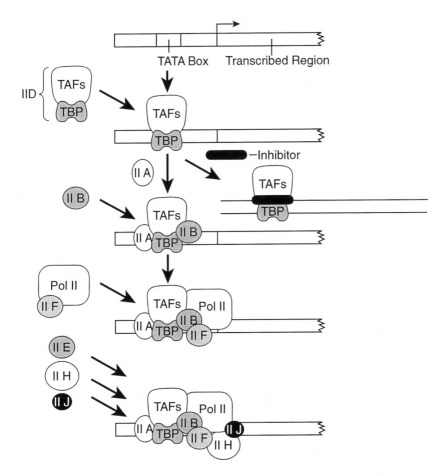

Fig. 2-2 Diagram of the sequential assembly of a transcription initiation complex. TAFs, TBP-associated factors, II A–J, transcription factors II A–J; Pol II, RNA polymerase II; TBP, TATA-binding protein. (Adapted from Lodish et al., p. 454, 1995.)

regulating embryonic development. Examples of such factors in mammals include Pit1 (defective in some cases of panhypopituitarism) and HESX1 (defective in some cases of septooptic dysplasia).

Many transcription factors bind DNA at adjacent sites as homo- or heterodimers. Factors that bind DNA elements separated by hundreds of base pairs may nevertheless be in physical contact because DNA is not completely rigid and can form loops. Enhancer factors may interact with general transcription factors to promote the assembly of the preinitiation complex. In addition, they interact with large complexes of proteins that act as *coactivators* or *corepressors*. Coactivators may interact with general transcription factors to stabilize the preinitiation complex, and several also have histone acetyltransferase activity. Others have ATPase activity and apparently remodel higher-order structures (involving many nucleosomes) in chromatin. Conversely, corepressors destabilize the preinitiation complex, may have histone deacetylase activity, and may remodel higher-order chromatin structures. Several corepressors have ubiquitin ligase activity that may target other transcriptional factors for degradation by the proteosome. The individual proteins in coactivator and corepressor complexes have overlapping and somewhat redundant activities so that functional specificity may result from particular combinations of factors. Clearly, coactivators and corepressors act to integrate signals from different pathways (such as intracellular second messengers and ligands for nuclear hormone receptors) into coherent effects on expression of particular genes.

RNA Processing

The primary RNA transcript of a gene is modified in several ways in the nucleus before being exported as mRNA to the cytoplasm, where it is translated into protein (Fig. 2-1).

Cap Structure. The first posttranscriptional event during the course of RNA maturation is the addition of a cap, a methylated structure at the 5′ end of the RNA molecule. The cap structure is formed by addition of a guanosine to the 5′ end of the mRNA through an unusual 5′,5′ triphosphate bond followed by methylation of this guanosine in the N-7 position and subsequent methylation of the adjacent nucleotide(s). This structure is required for export of mRNA from the nucleus, and it also facilitates the binding of eukaryotic RNA to ribosomes and thus enhances the initiation of translation.

Poly(A) Tail. Eukaryotic transcription does not terminate at well-defined sequences. However, most transcripts are clipped 12–16 bases downstream from a consensus poly(A) addition site, AAUAAA or AUUAAA. Then a nucleotide sequence consisting entirely of repeated adenosines is added to the 3′ end of the RNA. It may play a role in RNA stability. Poly(A) tails generally range between 50 and 250 bases and are found in virtually all mRNAs except those coding for histones.

Splicing of Introns. A key aspect of the maturation of RNA is the removal of introns by *splicing*. This process is mediated by *spliceosomes*, which are large complexes of small RNA molecules and proteins called snRNPs (*small nuclear ribonucleoproteins*, pronounced "snerps"). The RNA molecules in snRNPs recognize specific sequences at intron–exon boundaries, thereby signaling precisely where the RNA sequence cleavage will occur. Consensus sequences are found at both the 5′ (splice donor) and 3′ (splice acceptor) ends of introns. The last nucleotide of the exon is usually a G, and the first two nucleotides of the intron are almost invariably GT. The last two nucleotides of the intron are almost invariably AG; this is usually proceeded by several pyrimidine (C or T) nucleotides.

Intron excision consists of two transesterification reactions. In the first, a phosphate ester bond at the splice donor is transferred to the 2' hydroxyl group of a specific adenosine located approximately 50 nucleotides 5′ of the splice acceptor, leaving the intron in a looped or *lariat* configuration and a free 3' hydroxyl at the end of the splice donor. Then a phosphate ester bond at the splice acceptor is transferred to the splice donor.

The reason for the presence of intervening sequences in eukaryotic genes has not been established. However, in some genes they serve to separate specific structural and/or functional domains of the resultant protein. This may facilitate evolution by allowing segments coding for such domains to be transferred from one gene to another by genetic recombination. When genes encoding the same protein are compared among different species, the nucleotide sequences within introns are found to be much less similar than the coding sequences, suggesting that the exact sequence of an intron is relatively unimportant except for sequences involved in splicing.

Translation

Within the nucleotide sequence of the mature mRNA transcript lies an *open reading frame*, which is *translated* into protein by the ribosomal protein synthesis apparatus that reads the mRNA nucleotide sequence in *triplets* or *codons* (Fig. 2-3). Translation begins at an initiator methionine codon (AUG) in an adequate sequence *context* for initiation, the most important feature of which is a purine (an A or G) three nucleotides 5' of the AUG. The ribosome reads the subsequent sequence without internal punctuation until it reaches a stop codon (UAA, UGA, or UAG), at which point the ribosome dissociates from the mRNA. Because there are four ribonucleotides, the *genetic code* consists of 64 codons. Besides the initiator and stop

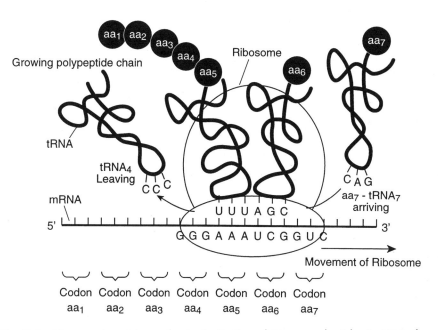

Fig. 2-3 Ribosomal protein synthesis. A, C, G, and U are nucleotides in RNA; they are illustrated in mRNA only in the region in contact with the ribosome, and only in transfer RNA (tRNA) in the region of the anticodon that interacts with mRNA through complementary base pairing. aa_{1-7} represent successive amino acids in the nascent polypeptide. (Adapted from Lodish et al., p. 120, 1995.)

codons, there are 60 other codons to encode 19 other amino acids; thus, an average of 3 codons (range, 1–6; usually 2–4) can encode each amino acid. The code is thus *degenerate*.

Codons are actually read by small *transfer RNA* (tRNA) molecules that are specific for each amino acid. A tRNA molecule is charged with the appropriate amino acid at its 3′ end by a specific *aminoacyl tRNA synthase*. The tRNA molecule has an *anticodon* that is complementary to the codon. Degeneracy in the code lies mostly in the third nucleotide of the codon (e.g., alanine may be encoded by GCA, GCC, GCG, or GCT); the interaction between the first nucleotide of the tRNA's anticodon and the third nucleotide of the mRNA's codon is relatively weak or *wobbly*, permitting a single tRNA to accommodate degeneracy in the third position of the codon.

Posttranslational Processing

Many proteins of interest to endocrinologists are either secreted from cells (such as peptide hormones) or are integral membrane proteins (such as many hormone receptors). Such proteins are synthesized on ribosomes bound to the *endoplasmic reticulum* and undergo post-translational processing.

All such proteins contain an N-terminal segment termed a *signal peptide* that contains approximately 20 amino acids, most of which are hydrophobic. Synthesis of such proteins begins on free ribosomes, but after the first 70 or so amino acid residues have been synthesized, the N terminus is bound by a ribonucleoprotein complex, the *signal recognition particle*. This is then bound by the signal recognition particle receptor, which is inserted in the membrane of the endoplasmic reticulum and recruits specific proteins to form a transmembrane channel to begin transporting the protein across the membrane of the endoplasmic reticulum as it is being synthesized (Fig. 2-4).

Secreted proteins are usually synthesized as *prepeptides*, meaning that the signal peptide is cleaved by a signal peptidase shortly after it is inserted into the endoplasmic reticulum membrane. The nascent protein is then transported through the transmembrane channel. In many integral membrane proteins, the signal peptide is not cleaved; in some cases the N terminus ends up in the lumen of the endoplasmic reticulum, whereas the orientation is reversed in others so that the N terminus remains on the cytoplasmic side of the membrane.

The nascent protein is transported across the endoplasmic reticulum membrane in an unfolded state and must then assume the correct conformation. This often requires interactions with chaperone proteins, the formation of disulfide bonds between cysteine sulfhydryl groups, and glycosylation, all of which occur within the endoplasmic reticulum. Sugars may be attached to either the amide groups of asparagines (*N-glycosylation*) or the hydroxyl groups of serine and threonine (*O-glycosylation*); glycosylation may be required for proper folding or stability of proteins and/or for proper targeting to subcellular organelles such as lysosomes.

Secretory and cell surface proteins are transported in specific vesicles to the *Golgi apparatus,* where they may undergo additional processing such as modification of glycosylation. They are sorted within the Golgi apparatus into vesicles containing proteins destined for the cell surface, those for proteins that are continuously secreted (such as albumin), and those for proteins that are secreted in a regulated

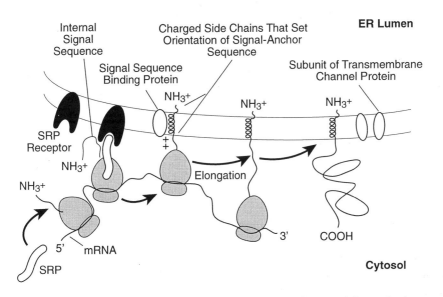

Fig. 2-4 Insertion of a nascent polypeptide into the membrane of the endoplasmic reticulum (ER). This is one of several possible modes of protein processing by the ER. The gray shapes represent ribosomes. SRP, signal recognition particle. NH_3^+ and COOH denote the amino and carboxy termini of a polypeptide. (Adapted from Lodish et al., p. 681, 1995.)

manner such as insulin. Sorting is an energy-requiring process involving specific GTP-binding proteins.

Certain peptide hormones such as insulin are synthesized as *preprohormones*; they require additional proteolytic steps that usually take place within secretory vesicles. Some preprohormones contain multiple peptide hormones within their primary sequence, such as proopiomelanocortin (POMC), the precursor for adrenocorticotropin (ACTH) α-, β- and γ-melanotropin (MSH), γ-lipotropin (γ-LPH), and γ-endorphin (see Chapter 6).

Some proteins, particularly enzymes like cytochromes P450, are synthesized as *apoproteins* requiring addition of functional groups like heme before they are active. This typically occurs at the site (e.g., mitochondria) at which the enzyme is to function. Many additional types of posttranslational processing exist, including phosphorylation at serine, threonine, or tyrosine residues, binding of lipids, and chemical modification of amino acids (e.g., hydroxylysine residues in collagen).

CLONING AND RELATED TECHNIQUES

Although many different molecular genetic techniques have been used to analyze the structure and function of hormones, they can be classified into a small number of broad categories.

Hybridization

Southern blot hybridization (Fig. 2-5) identifies DNA segments corresponding to a specific *probe* segment in a more complex mixture of DNA such as total human DNA. DNA is treated with a *restriction endonuclease*, an enzyme that can digest DNA at a defined sequence 4–8 bp in length. The DNA is fractionated on the basis of size by electrophoresis in an agarose gel; the smaller the fragment, the faster it migrates. The DNA is then denatured (rendered single-stranded) by treating the gel with alkali and is transferred to a nylon membrane by blotting; this preserves the spatial information in the gel (i.e., how far each fragment has migrated). Next, the membrane is hybridized with the probe, a labeled segment of cloned DNA that is rendered single-stranded by boiling. During hybridization, the two strands of the probe may reanneal, but some probe molecules will instead anneal to complementary fragments of DNA immobilized on the membrane. After the membrane is washed, these bound probe molecules can be detected as distinct bands. If the probe has been radioactively labeled, the membrane is autoradiographed. As an alternative to radioactivity, it is possible to label the probe chemically with groups such as biotin or digoxigenin. These groups are detected by binding with a specific anti-

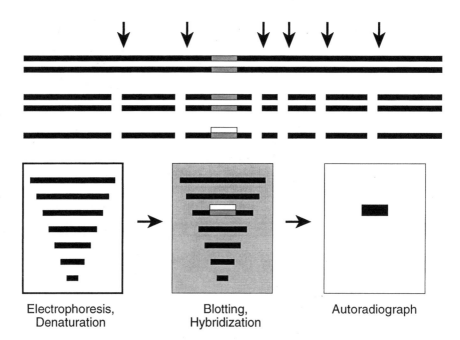

Electrophoresis, Denaturation

Blotting, Hybridization

Autoradiograph

Fig. 2-5 Schematic of Southern blot hybridization. The double line at the *top* of the figure represents DNA; the shaded segment denotes the DNA segment to be detected. Arrows denote digestion by a restriction endonuclease; the products of digestion are the second set of double lines. The DNA fragments are then denatured (rendered single-stranded, denoted by single lines) and hybridized with a labeled probe, represented by the short white line. The three rectangles at the *bottom* of the figure denote (from *left* to *right*) DNA fragments within an agarose gel, DNA fragments after transfer to a membrane and hybridization, and an autoradiogram of the hybridized membrane.

body that is linked to an enzyme such as alkaline phosphatase. This can mediate a chemoluminescent reaction that is detected by exposure to film.

Northern blots are conceptually similar, except that RNA is subjected to electrophoresis instead of DNA (see below).

Fluorescent *in Situ* Hybridization

A gene or other DNA segment is fluorescently labeled and hybridized to metaphase spreads of chromosomes. The chromosome(s) to which the labeled probe hybridizes and the approximate location on the chromosome can be determined with a suitable microscope. This technique, *fluorescent in situ hybridization* (FISH), has supplanted earlier, more laborious, and less sensitive approaches using radioactive probes. It is a highly sensitive way of detecting genetic deletions and rearrangements at the scale of whole genes or chromosomal segments.

Cloning

As applied to DNA (rather than to cells or whole organisms), *cloning* refers to the isolation of a desired segment of DNA so that it can be indefinitely replicated within an easily grown *host* organism such as *Escherichia coli* and large quantities thereby obtained. This involves *ligation* of the desired insert in a *vector* that contains sequences required for DNA replication in the host, and some marker gene that permits identification and selection of cells carrying the vector (Fig. 2-6). Vectors usually have a series of recognition sites for restriction endonucleases so that a DNA insert can be ligated to the vector after the vector is digested with the enzyme. In

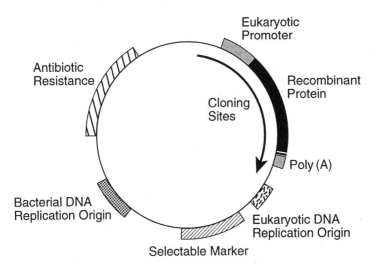

Fig. 2-6 Schematic of a plasmid vector used for expression of a complementary DNA (cDNA) encoding a recombinant protein. A plasmid is a double-stranded circular DNA molecule; this is not shown. Segments with specific functions are denoted by various shadings.

some cases, digestion with a restriction endonuclease yields DNA molecules with short (2–4 nucleotides) single-stranded segments at the ends; in such cases DNA molecules can be ligated only if they have compatible, complementary ends.

Many vectors are plasmids, circular DNA molecules that replicate separately from the bacterial chromosome. Plasmid vectors usually carry at least one gene for antibiotic resistance, allowing bacterial cells carrying the plasmid to be selected by growth in a medium containing the appropriate antibiotic. Other vectors are bacteriophage, viruses that infect bacteria. Bacteria infected with bacteriophage can be readily identified on culture plates as plaques of bacterial lysis or poor growth.

Whereas intact bacteriophage can infect bacteria in culture, plasmids cannot enter bacteria unless the bacteria have been chemically treated to make them *competent* to take up DNA. Bacteria that have absorbed the plasmid are selected by plating on the appropriate antibiotic.

Some vectors have additional desirable properties, such as the ability to grow in mammalian cells or to direct the synthesis of a protein encoded by the insert in bacterial, yeast, insect, or mammalian cells.

Polymerase Chain Reaction (PCR)

As long as the sequences at the ends of a DNA segment are known, it may not be necessary to clone the segment into a vector in order to obtain large quantities of it. Instead, the segment can be replicated *in vitro* (Fig. 2-7). It is rendered single-stranded (i.e., *denatured*) by heating, and then a short (usually 17–21 bp) synthetic oligonucleotide *primer* is annealed near the 5′ end of each original strand, creating a short double-stranded segment. The primer (and thus the double-stranded region) is extended using a DNA polymerase that incorporates deoxynucleotide triphosphate (dNTP) precursors (i.e., dATP, dCTP, dGTP, dTTP) complementary to the original strand. Thus, there will be two completely double-stranded DNA molecules at the end of this process for every original molecule in the reaction. These two molecules are again denatured by heating, primers again annealed, and each molecule copied

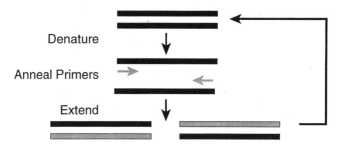

Fig. 2-7 Polymerase chain reaction (PCR). A double-stranded DNA molecule (black double line) is denatured, and complementary primers (gray arrows) are annealed to each strand. These are extended by a DNA polymerase to yield two completely double-stranded molecules (black plus gray lines at the bottom of the figure) corresponding to each starting molecule. Each of these molecules is then subjected to the same procedure.

by the polymerase, yielding a total of four molecules. Because the number of molecules doubles with every cycle, any desired quantity of DNA can be obtained by running a reaction of appropriate size for a sufficient number of cycles.

In practice, PCRs are run in a *thermocycler*, which can raise and lower temperatures in a heating block to optimal levels for DNA denaturation, primer annealing, and strand extension. A special DNA polymerase is used that can withstand high temperatures without itself being denatured.

DNA Sequence Analysis

Almost all sequence analysis uses the Sanger (*dideoxy* or *chain termination*) method (Fig. 2-8). As with the polymerase chain reaction (PCR), sequencing reactions involve extension of a primer annealed to a single-stranded *template* DNA molecule. As originally conceived, four reactions (*A, C, G,* and *T*) are run, each containing a dideoxy analog of one of the four dNTPs in addition to all four dNTPs. When one of the dideoxy molecules is incorporated instead of the corresponding dNTP, the newly synthesized DNA strand can no longer be extended. The concentration of the dideoxy analog is adjusted so that a dideoxy molecule is likely to be incorporated at any of the first few hundred positions where the corresponding dNTP would normally be used. Thus, when completed, the reaction contains an assortment of newly synthesized chains of different lengths, each length corresponding to the location of the appropriate base. The chains of various length are resolved by gel electrophoresis, with the four A, C, G, and T reactions in adjacent lanes. If a radioactive dNTP was included in the reactions, the fragments can be detected by autoradiography. They

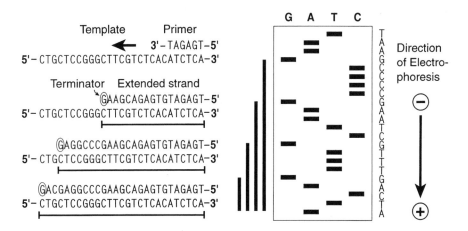

Fig. 2-8 DNA sequencing. *Left,* illustration of a sequencing reaction. A short, single-stranded *primer* (actually, primers are usually 15–20 nucleotides long) is annealed to a complementary, longer single-stranded *template* molecule. The primer is then extended with a DNA polymerase until a dideoxy *terminator* nucleotide (the circled *G* in the figure) is randomly incorporated into the elongating DNA strand, at which point elongation stops. This produces a collection of terminated strands of various lengths that can be resolved by electrophoresis (illustrated on the *right*). A set of four reactions is usually run, one for each of the four dideoxy nucleotide terminators.

appear as a ladder with a band in one of the four lanes at each *rung*. By reading from the bottom of the gel (fastest-migrating and smallest fragments), the sequence of the template can be deduced, starting from a point near the primer.

Most large laboratories and core facilities now carry out DNA sequencing using automated equipment. In the most widely used protocol, each template is analyzed in a single reaction that includes a mix of all four dideoxy analogs, each labeled with a fluorescent dye of a different color. Sequencing reactions are resolved by gel or capillary electrophoresis, and fragments are detected by photomultipliers as they pass the bottom of the gel; the color at which each fragment fluoresces indicates which dideoxynucleotide is incorporated at the end. The sequence information is captured directly by a computer.

ANALYSIS OF EXPRESSED GENE PRODUCTS

Complementary DNA (cDNA) corresponds in sequence to mRNA. It is synthesized *in vitro* by incubating mRNA with an RNA-dependent DNA polymerase (*reverse transcriptase* derived from a retrovirus) in the presence of deoxynucleotide triphosphates. It differs from *genomic* DNA in two important ways. Whereas genomic DNA is essentially identical in all cells in the body (excluding immunoglobulin and T-cell receptor gene rearrangements in cells of the immune system), the cDNA that is synthesized using mRNA from a particular cell type will mirror the abundance of the different mRNA transcripts in those cells. Thus, a different *library* of cDNA must be synthesized from each organ, tissue, or cell line of interest. Second, cDNA does not contain introns, because these were spliced out of mRNA before exportation from the nucleus. Hence, any efforts to express human proteins in bacterial cells must use cDNA (in a suitable expression vector) because bacteria lack the cellular machinery required to splice introns out of genes.

Screening

There are several ways to isolate a desired clone from a library of many clones of cDNA or genomic DNA. At present, cDNA libraries from many human and mouse tissues and genomic libraries from many species are commercially available.

Hybridization

Often, some sequence information is already available. This is the case if one is trying to use a cDNA clone (often containing less than the full sequence) to isolate a longer cDNA clone, a homologous cDNA in a different species, cDNAs encoding related proteins, or the corresponding genomic gene. The underlying principle is identical to that used for Southern or Northern blots. A nylon filter is dropped onto a culture plate containing bacterial colonies or bacteriophage plaques so that a replica of the plate is transferred to the filter. DNA in the bacteria on the filter is released, denatured by treatment with alkali, and hybridized with a labeled probe. Successful hybridization is detected as a spot on autoradiography film. When the film is aligned with the plate, the corresponding colony or plaque is identified.

Polymerase Chain Reaction

There are several variations of PCR screening; the following approach is used by large laboratories and commercial services. Robotic devices are used to pick individual bacterial colonies and transfer them to microtiter plates so that each clone has a unique three-dimensional *address* consisting of a particular plate and the column and row on that plate. For large libraries, a fourth dimension consisting of groups of plates can be used. Pools of DNA are generated robotically to identify each component of the address (e.g., *row* pools each consist of all clones in each row of every plate in the collection, and *column* pools each consist of all clones in each column of every plate). The PCRs are run using DNA from each pool and a primer pair derived from the desired sequence. Approximately 40 PCRs are required to screen a 10,000-clone library; if there is a single positive clone in the library, there will be four reactions that will yield a product, one corresponding to each dimension in the clone's address.

Immunological Screening

This may be feasible if an antiserum to the desired protein product is available. A cDNA library is constructed in a vector (usually a derivative of bacteriophage lambda) in which cDNA inserts are expressed as fusion proteins with a bacterial protein such as β-galactosidase. A filter is dropped onto each culture plate, as for hybridization screening, but it is processed differently and then incubated with antiserum. Replicas of plaques expressing the desired protein will bind the antibody, which is detected using a labeled second antibody.

The cDNA insert must be in the same orientation and reading frame as the gene for the fusion protein or it will not be translated correctly by the bacterial protein synthesis apparatus. This will occur by chance in only one-sixth of the clones (one-half chance of being in the correct orientation $\times$ one-third chance of being in the correct reading frame), but some methods of cDNA library construction force all clones into the correct orientation. In any case, this drawback is overcome by simply screening more clones.

Expression Screening

In some cases the desired protein has not been purified, and little structural information is available. In such cases the cDNA must be cloned based on some property that it confers on cells, such as a novel enzymatic activity.

A typical strategy is to transfect plates of mammalian cells with pools of 1000 clones and assay each plate for the desired activity. If such a plate is detected, the pool of 1000 clones is divided into 10 subpools of 100 clones, which are again transfected. If a subpool conferring the activity is detected, it is successively subdivided and rescreened until a single clone is isolated.

ANALYSIS OF GENOMES

The complement of DNA present in the nucleus of a single cell of an organism is termed the *genome;* the human genome consists of approximately 3 billion bp of genomic DNA in haploid cells (sperm and ova). This includes 30,000–40,000 genes, structural chromosome components such as centromeres and telomeres, and intergenic segments without apparent function.

Whole-Genome Sequencing

There are several different types of vectors that are used to clone segments of genomic DNA; the amount of DNA that can be cloned in each is to some extent inversely correlated with the ease of *in vitro* manipulation of the DNA and freedom from artifactual DNA rearrangements or chimerism (cloning of unrelated DNA segments in the same vector molecule). Those that can be grown in *E. coli* include *bacteriophage lambda*, which contains inserts of 15,000–20,000 bp (15–20 kb) of DNA; specialized plasmid vectors called *cosmids*; *bacteriophage P1*, with inserts of 100 kb (P1 artificial chromosomes, PACs), and *bacterial artificial chromosomes* (BACs) with inserts of a few hundred kilobases. *Yeast artificial chromosomes* (YACs) can carry far larger inserts of up to 2000 kb. After determination of their DNA sequences, PAC, BAC, and YAC clones of the human and mouse genomes have been conceptually assembled into long, overlapping *contigs* covering many megabases of DNA. Additional data have been obtained by *shotgun* sequencing of short (<1000 nucleotides) genomic DNA segments cloned in plasmid vectors.

The data obtained from whole-genome sequencing projects have been analyzed by computer to identify putative coding exons based on the presence of intron splice donor and acceptor sequences and possible open reading frames. The predicted amino acid sequence encoded by each exon is compared with sequences already in the database to see whether it represents the human homolog of a protein previously identified in some other species, or whether it is a member of a known gene family (such as cytochrome P450 enzymes or nuclear hormone receptors), or at least contains an amino acid motif (such as a nucleotide cofactor binding site) of known function.

Although much of the human and mouse genomes were characterized commercially, extensively annotated data from publicly funded studies are available through the Internet.

Expressed Sequence Tags

Whereas the Human Genome Project aimed to sequence the entire genome, a related project has partially sequenced thousands of cDNAs from each of many different cell types. At this time, over 50,000 such *expressed sequence tags* (ESTs) are available. As there are an estimated 30,000 genes, this implies that a great many genes have already been identified. This approach complements whole-genome sequencing because identification of an EST within a putative gene confirms that the gene is transcribed in a particular tissue. Conversely, ESTs are generally not full-length cDNA sequences and can usually be extended using the corresponding genomic sequence.

GENETIC DISEASES

Two general approaches have been used to determine the etiology of genetic diseases. In many cases, a *candidate gene* is immediately apparent. For example, a gene encoding an enzyme is likely to carry mutations in cases of deficiency of that enzyme. In such cases, the cDNA encoding the enzyme is usually isolated first (see the sections on screening of cDNA libraries) and used to identify the corresponding chromosomal gene. The gene is then analyzed as described below to detect mutations. These mutations are then re-created in cDNA, which is expressed in cultured cells to determine the effects of each mutation on the functioning of the encoded protein.

In diseases where a candidate gene is not available, the disease locus is mapped by linkage analysis (see the following section) and the affected gene identified by positional cloning approaches.

Linkage Analysis

Many diseases of interest to endocrinologists are inherited in a *Mendelian* manner; that is, the disease segregates in an affected kindred as a single locus with a well-defined mode of inheritance. If the gene causing a particular disease is unknown or if mutations in a candidate gene cannot be identified, it may be possible to determine the location of the affected gene by linkage studies. Consider an autosomal recessive disease such as congenital adrenal hyperplasia due to 21-hydroxylase deficiency, which was originally mapped by linkage analysis (however, the cDNA encoding the 21-hydroxylase enzyme was identified by immunological screening). All affected individuals in a given kindred should have identical alleles at the disease locus, and all unaffected individuals should differ from the affected individuals at that locus; thus testing of a few hundred markers will yield the approximate location of the disease gene. If a marker locus (e.g., for 21-hydroxylase deficiency, the gene encoding the transplantation antigen HLA-B) is a small genetic distance from the disease locus, affected individuals will likely still be identical at both the marker locus and the disease locus. However, there is a slight chance that they will not be identical at the marker locus because of a genetic recombination between the disease locus and the marker locus. Thus, if affected individuals in the same kindred are not identical at any particular locus, this might have occurred because the marker and disease loci are linked but were separated by a recombination, or it might mean that the marker locus was not linked at all to the disease (e.g., the marker might be on a different chromosome). The log of the ratio of the probabilities of either of these explanations being true is referred to as a *LOD score*. A LOD score of 3 (meaning that it is 1000 times more likely that two loci are linked than that they are not linked) is usually considered to confirm linkage.

The use of *microsatellite markers* has dramatically reduced the effort required for such an analysis. Such marker loci need not be within genes. They are anonymous segments of a few hundred base pairs that can be readily amplified by PCR. Each segment contains a region consisting of several (10–20) copies of a dinucleotide (such as CA), trinucleotide (such as CAG), or tetranucleotide sequence (Fig. 2-9). Many of these repeat sequences vary in copy number between individuals so that the length of the corresponding PCR-amplified segment also varies. Such length variations can be detected by electrophoresis using the same apparatus used for DNA sequence analysis. If there are a sufficient number of length variants (i.e., alleles) at a given locus, most individuals will be heterozygous for different alleles, permitting their two chromosomes to be distinguished in parents or offspring.

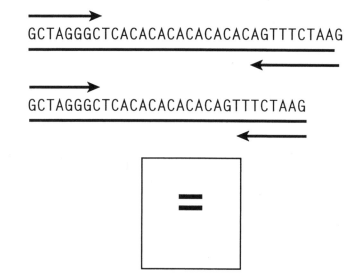

Fig. 2-9 Cytosine-adenine (CA) repeat polymorphisms. The CA repeat regions often vary in length between individuals. This can be detected by polymerase chain reaction (PCR) using primers (arrows) complementary to unique regions flanking the repeat. Bands of differing sizes containing different numbers of repeats are detected by electrophoresis, illustrated schematically at the *bottom*.

Positional Cloning

Once a disease locus has been genetically mapped, the DNA sequence between the closest linked marker loci is inspected. This is often an interval of at least a megabase of DNA corresponding to approximately a 1% chance of recombination between the disease gene and a marker locus. If a sufficient number of affected families is available, it may be useful to map additional polymorphic marker loci in the interval in the hope that some of the markers will be separated from the disease locus by genetic recombination in one or more affected individuals. If so, this can decrease the amount of DNA that must be analyzed.

Positional cloning was initially extremely laborious (the identification of the gene causing cystic fibrosis is an early example) because genomic clones spanning the entire interval between marker loci had to be isolated and sequenced, but the availability of the complete human genome sequence has dramatically decreased the effort required. Eventually, one or more candidate genes are identified based on their pattern of expression or likely functions based on the predicted amino acid sequences. Each such gene is then scanned for mutations in affected individuals (see the following section).

Detection of Point Mutations

To prove that mutations in a gene cause a disease, it is first necessary to identify such mutations. If the gene of interest is relatively small and the number of patients to be analyzed is small, it is usually most straightforward to sequence the gene in each patient. If larger numbers of samples need to be analyzed, scanning for mutations may save a great deal of time and labor. Scanning methods usually involve amplification of DNA segments using PCR. All work best on segments of a few hundred nucleotides.

The most commonly used methods make use of the fact that changes in nucleotide sequence may change the way in which DNA fragments migrate during electrophoresis (Fig. 2-10). For example, the conditions under which cDNA strands separate, or *melt*, may be affected. This is detected by subjecting the DNA to *denaturing gradient gel electrophoresis*, that is, electrophoresis under conditions in which the DNA becomes more likely to be denatured the farther it migrates in the gel, often by using a special apparatus that maintains the bottom of the gel at a higher temperature. As the DNA migrates down the gel, it eventually reaches a point at which the two strands begin to separate, or denature. Once a molecule is partially denatured, its mobility is drastically decreased. Thus, molecules with a mutation will stop at a different position in the gel from normal molecules, and this is detected by autoradiography. A related approach uses high-pressure liquid chromatography and has been highly automated.

In the related *single-stranded conformation polymorphism* technique, labeled double-stranded DNA is denatured by heating and quickly cooled so that the complementary strands cannot reanneal. Each single DNA strand will snap into its most energetically favorable conformation. This will include base pairing of nucleotides on the one strand, and thus the conformation may vary if the sequence has changed

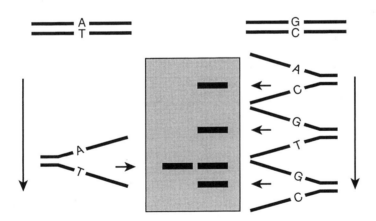

Fig. 2-10 Denaturing gradient gel electrophoresis. *Top,* two otherwise identical double-stranded DNA molecules differ at a single position (adenine-thymine [A-T] or guanine-cytosine [G-C]). If a homogeneous collection of such molecules (*left*) is subjected to electrophoresis through a denaturing gradient, they will all migrate (vertical arrows) to the same position in a gel (*center*). If a mixture of the two sequences is denatured to separate the strands and allowed to reanneal (*right*), four bands will be seen in the gel. The top two are *heteroduplexes* consisting of molecules with mismatched bases. These are relatively unstable and denature easily, so that they migrate slowly. The two molecules with fully complementary bases denature under slightly different conditions and thus migrate to slightly different positions in the gel.

due to a mutation. DNA strands in different conformations often migrate differently in the gel.

Detecting a Known Mutation

In many cases, previous work has identified mutations causing a particular disease, and an investigator wishes to determine the frequencies of these mutations in a different or larger population. This is often less difficult than identifying the mutations in the first place. Usually, segments of the gene of interest are amplified by PCR.

It may be possible to use single-stranded conformation polymorphisms or DNA sequencing on a routine basis. These may be the methods of choice for rare disease in which each family carries a different mutation. Other approaches are specifically useful for detecting limited numbers of known mutations; three are described.

Restriction Fragment Length Polymorphisms
Southern blots are a way to detect deletions or duplications of DNA, which will change the number or size of hybridizing fragments. They usually cannot detect smaller changes of DNA sequence. The exception to this is if a change in DNA sequence forms or destroys a recognition site for a restriction endonuclease, because this will change the size of a DNA fragment produced by digestion with that enzyme. This is referred to as a *restriction fragment length polymorphism* (RFLP) (Fig. 2-11). Because there are dozens of different restriction enzymes and recognition sequences, it is not unusual to find a suitable enzyme to detect a particular sequence change.. Since the advent of PCR, it has become common to detect restriction fragment polymorphisms by amplifying the appropriate segment of DNA,

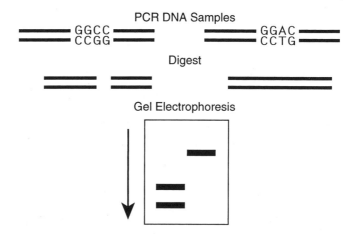

Fig. 2-11   Restriction fragment length polymorphism (RFLP). *Top,* two otherwise identical double-stranded DNA molecules differ at a single position (guanine cytosine [G-C] or adenine-thymine [A-T]). The former (*left*) is part of a GGCC sequence that is digested by a restriction endonuclease, whereas the latter (*right*) is part of a GGAC sequence that is not digested. Thus fragments of different sizes are produced (*center*); these are detected by electrophoresis (*bottom*).

digesting it with a restriction enzyme, and subjecting the fragments to electrophoresis. Because PCR produces relatively large quantities of DNA, the polymorphism can be detected by examination of gels stained with a DNA dye such as ethidium bromide, and radioactive labeling or hybridization are unnecessary.

Allele-Specific Oligonucleotide Hybridization
In this method, PCR-amplified DNA samples are denatured and blotted to a nylon membrane. The membrane is then hybridized with short (~20 nucleotides), single-stranded probes that are radioactively or chemically labeled. For each mutation, two probes are made, one corresponding to the normal sequence and the other to the mutant sequence. The probes are hybridized separately to duplicate samples under conditions in which only a perfectly matched probe will hybridize. Thus, homozygous normal, heterozygous mutant, and homozygous mutant samples will hybridize with only the normal probe, both probes, or only the mutant probe, respectively (Fig. 2-12).

This hybridization process can be reversed, with a fluorescently labeled PCR product hybridized to oligonucleotides immobilized on a solid substrate, or *gene chip*. This permits simultaneous detection of many different mutations. This technology is now being used on a large scale to scan hundreds of genes from dozens of individuals for *single nucleotide polymorphisms* (SNPs), with the idea that such polymorphisms can be used for association studies of common diseases (see below).

Allele-Specific Polymerase Chain Reaction
Two PCRs are run. They have one primer in common, but the *allele-specific* primers at the other end differ in the two reactions; one recognizes the normal sequence and the other the mutant sequence. Under appropriate PCR conditions, only a perfectly matched primer will work in the PCR. Thus, one or the other allele-specific reac-

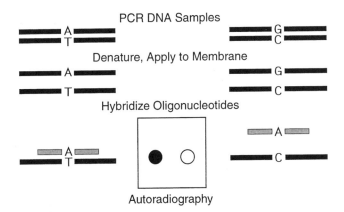

Fig. 2-12 Allele-specific oligonucleotide hybridization. *Top,* two otherwise identical double-stranded DNA molecules differ at a single position (adenine-thymine [A-T] or guanine-cytosine [G-C]). These are denatured and hybridized with a labeled single-stranded probe that is complementary to and will hybridize with one of these sequences; this is detected by autoradiography (*bottom*).

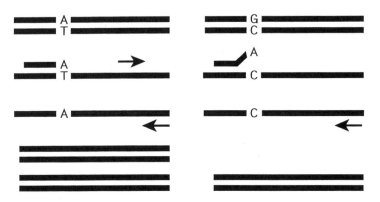

Fig. 2-13 Allele-specific polymerase chain reaction (PCR). *Top,* two otherwise identical double-stranded DNA molecules differ at a single position (adenine-thymine [A-
T] or guanine-cytosine [G-C]). They are subjected to PCR using one primer that is complementary to both molecules (arrow at the right of each molecule) and a second primer
(short strand ending in A) that is complementary only to one. Thus only the molecule
on the *left* can be amplified by PCR under these conditions.

tion (or both, if the sample is from a heterozygote) will yield a detectable product,
depending on the genotype of the sample (Fig. 2-13).

Categories of Disease-Causing Mutations

Mutations are usually classified by their effects on gene function. We give some
examples of frequently occurring types of mutations as they occur in the *CYP21*
gene encoding steroid 21-hydroxylase (Fig. 2-14). Such mutations cause congenital adrenal hyperplasia, a defect of cortisol biosynthesis (see Chapter 8).

Deletions and Other Rearrangements

Obviously, deletion of all or part of a gene prevents synthesis of a functional protein. Typically, such mutations are generated by recombinations between duplicated
gene segments. For example, CYP21 lies on a duplicated segment of 30 kb; the duplicate copy of CYP21 is a nonfunctional *pseudogene* containing several inactivating mutations. Approximately 20% of mutations involving CYP21 are deletions of
all or most of the normally active copy of the gene. Other mutations are *gene conversions*, which are transfers of segments containing deleterious mutations from the
pseudogene to the normally active gene.

Mutations in Coding Sequences

A *missense* mutation changes an amino acid incorporated into the protein. For example, the mutation of ATC to AAC in codon 172 of CYP21 changes the corresponding amino acid from isoleucine to asparagine; this reduces enzymatic activity
to 1% of normal and causes congenital adrenal hyperplasia.

A *nonsense* mutation generates a premature stop codon and prevents synthesis
of a functional protein. The mutation of CAG to TAG in codon 318 of CYP21 re-

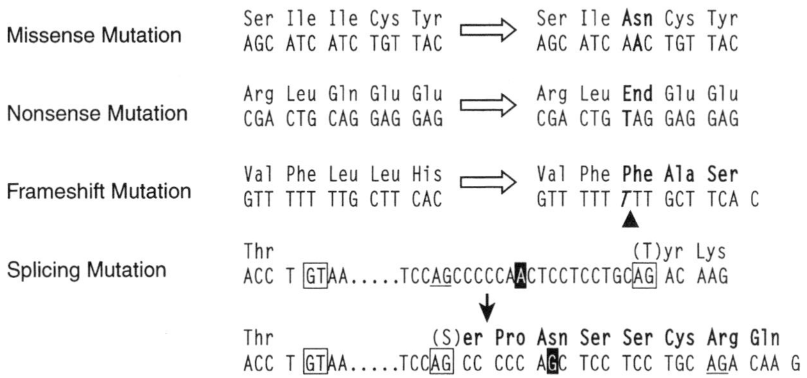

| Missense Mutation | Ser Ile Ile Cys Tyr
AGC ATC ATC TGT TAC | ⟹ | Ser Ile **Asn** Cys Tyr
AGC ATC AAC TGT TAC |

| Nonsense Mutation | Arg Leu Gln Glu Glu
CGA CTG CAG GAG GAG | ⟹ | Arg Leu **End** Glu Glu
CGA CTG TAG GAG GAG |

| Frameshift Mutation | Val Phe Leu Leu His
GTT TTT TTG CTT CAC | ⟹ | Val Phe **Phe Ala Ser**
GTT TTT *T*TT GCT TCA C
▲ |

Splicing Mutation

Thr   (T)yr Lys
ACC T GTAA.....TCCAGCCCCCA**A**CTCCTCCTGC AG AC AAG
                      ↓

Thr   (S)er Pro Asn Ser Ser Cys Arg Gln
ACC T GTAA.....TCC AG CC CCC A**G**C TCC TCC TGC AGA CAA G

Fig. 2-14 Examples of different mutations causing 21-hydroxylase deficiency. Nucleotide sequences with corresponding amino acid sequences are shown surrounding each mutation; coding sequences are grouped into triplet codons. Each normal sequence is on the *left,* with the mutant sequence on the *right.* Changed amino acids are in boldface. The insertion causing a frameshift mutation is a T marked by an arrowhead. The actual splicing mutation is shaded; this activates a cryptic splice acceptor site (boxed AG in the bottom sequence), causing retention of an extra 19 nucleotides of intron sequence in mRNA.

sults in synthesis of a truncated unstable enzyme leading to a severe form of adrenal hyperplasia.

A *frameshift* mutation inserts or deletes a number of nucleotides not divisible by 3. Because mRNA is translated in codons of three nucleotides without internal punctuation, this causes the ribosome to shift to an incorrect grouping of nucleotides (i.e., a shift in the reading frame), and thus the resulting protein sequence becomes completely abnormal at the point of the mutation. An insertion of a single extra T nucleotide in a run of seven T nucleotides beginning at codon 246 of CYP21 is an example of such a mutation.

Mutations Affecting Splicing
Mutations that affect the GT or AG sequences at the beginning or end of an intron prevent removal of the intron and result in its retention within mRNA. Attempts by the ribosome to translate the inserted sequence usually lead to a nonfunctional protein. Other mutations within the intron can activate a normally nonfunctional or *cryptic* splice site with the same result. For example, mutation of an A to a G 13 nucleotides before the end of the second intron of CYP21 leads to abnormal splicing and the retention of 19 extra nucleotides within CYP21 mRNA. This shifts the reading frame of translation and renders the resulting protein nonfunctional.

Genetics of Common Diseases

Many common diseases such as hypertension and obesity are presumed to have multiple genetic susceptibility traits as well as environmental or lifestyle etiologies. Genetic analysis of such disorders is consequently more difficult than for Mendelian traits. Two complementary strategies are used: linkage analysis and association studies. These methods have a number of difficulties in common, as well as some that are unique to each approach. First, traits such as blood pressure may result from the interplay of so many factors that it is difficult to identify any but those genetic loci with the strongest influence. This problem can be addressed by examining *intermediate phenotypes* that are presumed to influence the trait under study but are probably controlled by fewer genetic factors. For blood pressure, examples are levels of regulatory hormones such as renin and aldosterone. Second, some loci may influence the trait only at certain ages or in one sex or in a particular race. This can be addressed by stratifying the study population so that particular subsets of the population are analyzed individually. Third, some loci may have an effect only in combination with particular alleles at another locus, a phenomenon termed *epistasis*. This may require very large study populations to detect.

Affected Pedigree Member Analysis

It is difficult to study common multifactorial diseases by conventional linkage analysis of affected kindreds because these diseases do not segregate in simple ways. *Affected pedigree member* (affected sib pair) analysis is a powerful technique for addressing these problems. Two siblings will, on average, share 50% (one-half) of alleles at any given locus. If both sibs are affected by a disease and a gene near a particular locus contributes to the development of that disease, then the sibs will, on average, share >50% of alleles. Similar analyses apply to pedigree members who are not full siblings.

The power of this approach is limited in several ways. Most obviously, traits such as blood pressure are normally distributed, and thus division of a population into unaffected and affected individuals requires an arbitrary cutoff value. This problem can be obviated by use of quantitative trait locus analysis, which makes use of kindreds in which sibs differ widely for a trait and genetic differences between the sibs are sought. Second, linkage techniques have the greatest power when known candidate genes (e.g., components of the renin-angiotensin system for blood pressure) are analyzed. Although a *genome scan* may be carried out, analysis of (for example) 100 markers means that it is not unlikely that uncorrected p values of .001 (corresponding to a LOD score of 3) will occur by chance. Studies of quite large populations (or several independent populations) may be required to obtain significant p values after correction for multiple comparisons. In practice, this technique has adequate power to detect only those loci with relatively strong influence on a particular trait.

Association Studies

Simple (often single-nucleotide) polymorphisms are sometimes detected that might affect the function of a gene, perhaps because they change coding sequences or are reasonably supposed from their location in the promoter to influence gene expression. If a polymorphism is in a plausible candidate gene for a particular disease, one can determine whether the frequency of the polymorphism differs between unaffected controls and affected individuals. In the case of a continuously variable trait such as blood pressure, one can see whether levels of the trait differ in individuals who do or do not carry the polymorphism; if the polymorphism is frequent, those homozygous for the polymorphism can be compared to those who are heterozygous as well as to those who are not carriers.

A common problem with association studies is that the control and affected populations may not be strictly comparable. For example, whites tend to have lower blood pressure than blacks and may also differ from blacks in frequencies of many polymorphisms in various genes. Studies of blood pressure in American blacks may thus be easily confounded by the degree of white admixture in the black population. This problem can be obviated to some extent by population-based studies (e.g., examining blood pressure in all members of a single study population rather than comparing affected and control groups) or by studying relatively homogeneous populations (e.g., Africans from one tribe in a single locale). Other study designs might be useful; in *transmission disequilibrium* studies, for example, one examines the parents of an affected individual and compares alleles on the chromosomes inherited by the affected child with the parental chromosomes that were not inherited.

A second problem is the phenomenon of *linkage disequilibrium*; that is, particular alleles at polymorphic sites within a gene, or even within adjacent genes, may be nonrandomly associated with each other. Thus one cannot infer causation from a positive association between a polymorphism and a trait without careful studies of the functional effects of that polymorphism, because an unsuspected associated polymorphism may actually be responsible for the observed physiological effects.

ASSAYING GENE EXPRESSION

Because most hormones directly or indirectly influence patterns of gene expression, it is often useful to determine levels of expression of various genes under different circumstances in a particular tissue or cell type.

Northern Blots

In one of the oldest and most widely used methods for analyzing gene expression, mRNA is size-fractioned by electrophoresis through agarose and blotted to a nitrocellulose or nylon membrane. It is then hybridized with a radioactively labeled DNA or RNA probe corresponding to the gene of interest, washed, and exposed either to X-ray film or to a reusable charge-coupled imaging cassette that can be electronically scanned. The intensity of each hybridizing band is a measure of the level of gene expression, and the electrophoretic mobility of each band is proportional to its size.

Ribonuclease Protection Assays

Alternatively, a highly radioactive RNA probe complementary to the mRNA of interest can be hybridized in solution with a cell or tissue RNA sample and then digested with ribonucleases that destroy single-stranded but not double-stranded RNA.

Thus, probe molecules will remain intact only when they are bound to complementary mRNA molecules; they are detected by electrophoresis and autoradiography. This method is more sensitive but somewhat more technically demanding than Northern blots.

Reverse Transcriptase-Polymerase Chain Reaction

The PCR is able to amplify DNA with single-molecule sensitivity. Although it cannot directly use mRNA as a starting material, mRNA can be reverse-transcribed into cDNA and the cDNA molecules of interest amplified using specific primers. There are several ways in which reverse transcriptase-polymerase chain reaction (RT-PCR) can be used to quantitate mRNA.

Keep Amplification in the Exponential Phase of the Polymerase Chain Reaction

The intensity of an amplified fragment is directly proportional to the amount of starting DNA as long as the PCR has been run for few enough cycles that starting materials such as primers are not limiting and each cycle of PCR amplifies DNA with equal efficiency. The number of cycles for which this is the case varies with the abundance of the cDNA of interest, so it is often necessary to remove aliquots of the PCR every few cycles. After electrophoresis through agarose, the abundance of the amplified fragment is assayed by staining the DNA. To provide a basis for comparison, an unrelated cDNA of known constant abundance (a housekeeping gene) is usually amplified in the same PCR using a second set of primers. This approach is simple but only semiquantitative.

Competitive Polymerase Chain Reaction

To obtain more accurate quantitation, a competitive template is constructed that is identical in sequence to the cDNA of interest at both ends but different in length so that it can be resolved from the cDNA by electrophoresis. Different amounts of the competitor are added to duplicate RT-PCRs. When the competitor is present in amounts greatly in excess of the actual cDNA of interest, the competitor will be preferentially amplified, whereas the opposite will occur when the competitor is present in very small amounts compared to the actual cDNA. Equal amounts should be amplified when the molar amounts of the competitor and actual cDNA are equal.

Quantitative (Real-Time, Taqman) Polymerase Chain Reaction

This has become the method of choice for RNA quantitation, particularly for low-abundance transcripts or small samples. A *Taqman* probe is annealed to the cDNA of interest with each PCR cycle. This probe contains a fluorescent reporter tag at one end and a different fluorescent tag at the other end that acts to quench fluorescence of the first tag. The Taq DNA polymerase used for the reaction has exonuclease activity that digests the probe as the PCR proceeds, separating the reporter and quenching molecules and leading to increased fluorescence. The reaction is run in an apparatus that measures fluorescence in real time, and the rate at which fluorescence increases reflects abundance of the RNA of interest within the original sample.

DNA Arrays

It is now possible to bind covalently thousands of different cDNAs to a glass *chip*. An RT-PCR is run with fluorescent deoxynucleotide triphosphates, and the fluorescent cDNA is hybridized with the immobilized material on the chip. The intensity of fluorescence at each position is read by specialized equipment. Thus the abundance of thousands of different mRNAs in a sample can be determined simultaneously. As most genes have now been identified through whole-genome sequencing projects, most changes in gene expression occurring with (for example) treatment of a cell line with a particular hormone can be identified in a single experiment.

Analysis of Transcriptional Regulation

Whereas the preceding methods ascertain mRNA abundance, other approaches are required to identify sequences within a gene that regulate its expression. This process, colloquially known as *promoter bashing*, makes use of several complementary techniques.

Reporter Constructs

A *reporter gene* encodes a product the level of which can be easily and accurately measured. One of the most widely used is luciferase, an enzyme from fireflies. Luciferase levels are determined by lysing cells, adding luciferin and adenosine triphosphate (ATP) (the substrates for luciferase), and measuring light output with a luminometer. This gene has been cloned into vectors that have restriction enzyme sites immediately 5' of the gene into which fragments may be directionally cloned. To identify cis elements in the 5' flanking region of the gene, a series of constructs are made containing various portions of of interest (typically 100–2000 bp) in a reporter vector. Most often a *serial deletion* approach is used in which the constructs have inserts with a common 3' end (the normal transcriptional start site) but different 5' ends. As successively shorter segments of 5' flanking sequences are included, levels of transcription (measured by luciferase activity) are likely to change in a stepwise manner. A decrease in activity suggests that a positive regulatory (enhancer) element has been deleted, whereas an increase in activity implies deletion of a negative regulatory (silencer) element. These elements can be further characterized by *footprinting* and *gel mobility shift assays*.

Identification of trans-Acting Factors

Deoxyribonuclease I Footprinting. Once genetic regions that influence transcription have been identified by serial deletion or mutation of reporter constructs, proteins that interact with them are identified. One approach makes use of the fact that proteins bound to DNA can protect DNA from digestion by deoxyribonuclease I (DNase). A DNA segment of a few hundred base pairs is radioactively labeled at one end, incubated with an extract of nuclear proteins, and digested with DNAse I under conditions where each DNA molecule is cut an average of once. If no protein binds the DNA, a rather even distribution of fragment sizes is observed by autoradiography after the mixture is size-fractionated by electrophoresis through a poly-acrylamide gel. However, if a segment is protected from digestion because a protein is bound, there will be a corresponding region of reduced intensity on the gel, termed a *footprint*, because molecules of that size will be underrepresented in the DNAse I digestion reaction.

Electrophoretic Mobility Shift Assays. Double-stranded probes for each region of interest are synthesized and radioactively labeled. These probes can be complementary oligonucleotides each approximately 20 nucleotides long or somewhat longer (perhaps 100 bp) restriction fragments or PCR products. Probes are incubated with nuclear extracts. Protein–DNA interactions decrease mobility of the radioactive DNA upon electrophoresis under nondenaturing conditions, detected as slower-migrating bands on autoradiography. In some cases, multiple bands may be observed even with quite short probes, reflecting interactions of multiple factors with each other as well as with a particular DNA element.

Whereas footprinting analysis identifies regions of protein–DNA interaction with single-nucleotide resolution, it cannot detect complex interactions, as is possible with gel retardation assays. Thus, it is useful to carry out both types of analysis.

IN VITRO EXPRESSION OF PROTEINS

Methods exist for expressing recombinant polypeptides in bacteria, yeast, or cultured insect or mammalian cells (the latter three categories are examples of *eukaryotic* cells, meaning that they have a nucleus). These systems vary in their complexity and in the expected yield of protein. The system chosen to express a functional protein depends on the purpose of the experiment. A report of cloning of cDNA encoding a particular enzyme often includes a formal demonstration that the encoded enzyme indeed has the expected activity. If a detailed kinetic analysis is not desired, this requires only a relatively small amount of enzyme, and purification is not necessary. A technically simple system such as transfection of a plasmid into mammalian cells is often used. Large amounts of protein may be required for biochemical research (e.g., X-ray crystallography) or for the manufacturing of pharmaceuticals. If posttranslational modifications such as glycosylation are not required for activity, bacterial systems can be scaled up to yield large quantities of proteins. Certain eukaryotic expression systems, such as baculovirus-infecting insect cells, have also been employed for large-scale production.

Bacterial Expression Systems

The general advantages of such systems include a very high yield of protein, inexpensive culture media, and ease of purification. Lack of posttranslational modifications (e.g., glycosylation) can be either an advantage (if, for example, it is desired to crystallize the protein) or a disadvantage if such modifications are required for function. Some proteins are difficult to express in bacteria or they cannot be synthesized in the proper conformation. Bacterial systems cannot be used to express genomic DNA fragments containing introns because they lack the RNA-processing apparatus necessary to splice introns.

Bacteriophage lambda derivatives are used for construction of cDNA libraries that are to be screened by testing for expression of recombinant proteins (see above). Plasmids are used for most other purposes. If a particular recombinant protein is not deleterious to growth of E. coli, a host–vector combination may be used in which the vector's promoter is always active, recombinant mRNA is always being transcribed, and recombinant protein is always synthesized. However, in many cases bacteria do not tolerate the presence of large amounts of recombinant protein and it is impossible to grow bacteria while the protein is produced. Therefore, it is often desirable to *repress* transcription from the plasmid's promoter until large numbers of bacteria have been grown, following which the promoter is *induced* to allow high levels of transcription for a few hours. Different promoters are induced by changes in temperature, the absence of a nutrient (such as an amino acid), or the presence of a moderately toxic chemical.

Because foreign proteins are sometimes poorly tolerated by bacteria, many vectors contain all or part of a gene for a bacterial protein, followed by restriction enzyme sites into which DNA encoding the desired polypeptide may be inserted. If the translational reading frame of the DNA insert is the same as that of the bacterial gene, a *fusion protein* is synthesized consisting of the bacterial polypeptide at the N terminus followed by the foreign polypeptide. Such fusion proteins may be synthesized at higher levels and may be resistant to degradation by bacterial proteases.

Some vectors encode recognition sites for specific proteases such as the clotting factors Xa or thrombin, so that the bacterial portion of the fusion protein can be cleaved off from the recombinant portion, yielding the desired native protein. It is obviously necessary that the recombinant protein not itself contain sequences cleaved by the proteases.

Mammalian Cell Expression Systems

Expression of a mammalian protein in mammalian cells is the approach most likely to yield a functional protein with all necessary posttranslational modifications including appropriate protein folding. Genomic DNA containing introns may be expressed in mammalian cells. However, mammalian cells require much more expensive culture media than bacteria, grow much more slowly, require manipulation under strictly sterile conditions, and may carry human pathogens, particularly viruses. It is difficult to get the high levels of expression obtainable with optimized bacterial systems.

Transfection with Plasmids

This is technically the simplest method for introducing extraneous DNA into a cell. Plasmid vectors that can be used for eukaryotic expression are conceptually similar to those used for bacterial expression; indeed, they have the E. coli DNA replication origin and antibiotic resistance gene(s) necessary for growth in bacteria. In addition, they have a DNA replication origin for growth in mammalian cells and, instead of a bacterial promoter, a promoter that is effective in mammalian cells. The promoter and replication origin are usually of viral origin. All genetic manipulations (e.g., insertion of recombinant DNA, mutagenesis) of such vectors are carried out in bacteria, following which plasmid DNA is introduced into cells by one of several methods. DNA can be complexed with materials such as calcium phosphate precipitates or cationic liposomes, which are actively taken up by mammalian cells, or cells can be rendered permeable to DNA by exposure to electric current, a procedure termed *electroporation.*

Transient transfections are usually adequate for examining the activity of the protein encoded by a recombinant DNA. Plasmid DNA in the nucleus is transcribed, and mRNA is translated in the cytoplasm by the cell's ribosomes. Levels of protein or of the corresponding activity usually reach a maximum at about 48–72 hours, following which the plasmid is lost from the majority of cells as they divide. If it desired that the cell express transfected DNA for more than a few days, clones of permanently transfected cells can be selected in which the transfected DNA is integrated into chromosomal DNA. Unless the expressed DNA produces a change in phenotype that can be selected for, it is necessary to transfect simultaneously DNA that encodes a selectable characteristic, such as resistance to neomycin and related antibiotics that are toxic to mammalian cells.

Infection with Viruses

Viral vectors often permit higher rates of expression than plasmids because they infect almost all cells in a culture, whereas transfection protocols usually affect a minority of cells. However, many viruses require complex construction steps and/or packaging of DNA into intact virions prior to use, and many are actual or potential human pathogens that need to be handled with caution. Some useful viruses such as *vaccinia* and *adenovirus* have DNA genomes. *Retroviruses* have RNA genomes and copy their genome into DNA using a virally encoded reverse transcriptase. Because intact retroviruses infect a very high proportion of cells and retroviral genomes are efficiently integrated into mammalian chromosomes, this is a preferred method for trials of *in vivo* gene therapy.

Invertebrate Cell Expression Systems

Yeast

Saccharomyces cervesiae may be transformed with plasmids that have a yeast origin of DNA replication, a promoter that permits transcription in yeast, and a selectable marker gene. Because they are eukaryotic cells (and are thus structurally and metabolically closer to mammalian cells than to bacteria) but grow rapidly and in simple culture media, yeast combine many of the advantages of both bacterial and mammalian cell expression systems. However, not all mammalian proteins function the same way in yeast as in mammalian cells, so functional studies in yeast must be interpreted cautiously.

Baculovirus

This is a virus that infects *Spodoptera frugiperda* insect cells. Foreign DNA is inserted into the vector by homologous recombination using a shuttle plasmid, a relatively cumbersome method. Very high levels of expression can be achieved, and most required posttranslational modifications are made to expressed proteins. Baculovirus has the advantage of not being a pathogen for humans, and its host cells are more robust than most mammalian cells.

TRANSGENIC MICE AND KNOCKOUTS

Although studies of human genetic diseases have yielded great insights into the functions of many genes, the number of genes of interest far exceeds the number of known genetic diseases. Thus, techniques have been developed to introduce any desired genetic modification into mice. These fall into two categories. To make a *transgenic mouse*, DNA is injected into the male pronucleus of fertilized eggs; in some cases, DNA will be randomly integrated into mouse chromosomes. The eggs are then implanted in *pseudopregnant* female mice that have been hormonally treated to be receptive to implantation. If the procedure is successful, most cells in each resulting mouse, including at least some germ cells, will contain the transgenic DNA so that breeding of a founder mouse will establish a line in which all mice carry the transgene. This technique can be used to express particular proteins at higher levels or under different regulation than normal or to express proteins that are not normally carried by mice. For example, mice lacking a particular cell lineage (e.g., growth hormone–secreting cells in the pituitary) can be created by expressing a toxin under the control of a promoter specific for those cells (e.g., diphtheria toxin controlled by the growth hormone promoter).

Knockout mice, in which a particular gene is inactivated, are produced by a related but more complicated technique. Mouse embryonal stem cells are grown in culture and transfected with a targeting construct that contains several kilobases of a murine gene of interest with a portion replaced by a selectable marker (such as a gene coding for resistance to the toxic drug neomycin). Most of the time, this construct will integrate into random locations in the genome, but occasionally it will integrate into the corresponding gene by homologous recombination. Successfully transfected cells are selected by growth in the appropriate toxic drug, and cells in which one copy of the endogenous gene has been replaced by the targeting construct are identified using other selection techniques or genetic analysis by PCR. Such a cell line is grown, and cells are then injected into early mouse embryos at the blastocyst stage. The embryonic stem cells will grow and differentiate along with the other cells in the embryo so that the resulting mouse will be a chimera for the targeted cells. Again, breeding the founder should yield some mice carrying a single copy of the targeted gene in all cells including the germline. Breeding of two such heterozygous mice will produce mice (one-fourth of the total offspring) that are homozygous for the targeted, inactivated gene, and thus effects of loss of function of the gene can be assessed (of course, loss of some genes will be lethal and no homozygous offspring will be obtained).

SUGGESTED READING

Ausubel FM, Brent R, Kingston RE, Moore DD, Seidman JG, Smith JA, and Struhl K: *Current Protocols in Molecular Biology,* John Wiley, New York, 1994.

Dracopoli NC, Haines JL, Korf BR, Moir DT, Morton CC, Seidman CE, Seidman JG, and Smith DR: *Current Protocols in Human Genetics,* John Wiley, New York, 1994.

Lodish HF, Baltimore D, Berk A, Zipursky SL, Matsudaira P, and Darnell J: *Molecular Cell Biology,* Scientific American Books, New York, 1995.

Sambrook J, Russell DW, and Maniatis T: *Molecular Cloning: A Laboratory Manual,* 3rd ed., Cold Spring Harbor Laboratory Press, Cold Spring Harbor, NY, 2001.

3

Mechanisms of Hormone Action

CAROLE R. MENDELSON

The capacity of a cell to respond to a particular hormone depends on the presence of cellular receptors specific for that hormone. After binding hormone, the receptor is biochemically and structurally altered, resulting in its activation; the activated receptor then mediates all of the actions of the hormone on the cell. The steroid and thyroid hormones as well as retinoids and 1,25-dihydroxyvitamin D_3 diffuse freely through the lipophilic plasma membrane of the cell and interact with receptors that are primarily within the nucleus. On activation, the receptors alter the transcription of specific genes, resulting in changes in the levels of specific messenger RNAs (mRNAs), which are in turn translated into proteins. Hormones that are water soluble, such as the peptide and polypeptide hormones, catecholamines, and other neurotransmitters, as well as the relatively hydrophobic prostaglandins, interact with receptors in the plasma membrane. After hormone binding, the activated membrane receptors initiate signal transduction cascades that result in changes in enzyme activities and alterations in gene expression.

In this chapter, the properties of various classes of receptors that are localized within the plasma membranes of target cells and the signal transduction mechanisms that mediate interactions with their ligands will first be addressed. This will be followed by consideration of the structural properties of the nuclear hormone receptors, the events that result in their activation, and the mechanisms whereby the activated nuclear receptors alter the expression of specific genes. Finally, a number of endocrine disorders that are caused by alterations in the number and/or function of plasma membranes and nuclear receptors will be reviewed.

RECEPTOR PROPERTIES

The function of a receptor is to recognize a particular hormone among all the molecules in the environment of the cell at a given time and, after binding the hormone, to transmit a signal that ultimately results in a biological response. Hormones are normally present in the circulation in extremely low concentrations, ranging from 10^{-9} to 10^{-11} M. The receptor must therefore have an affinity for the hormone that is of a magnitude appropriate to the circulating levels. The receptor must also bind the hormone with high specificity, so that it has a greater affinity for a particular biologically active molecule rather than for a related but less biologically active species. The affinity of the receptor for a particular ligand in relation to its affinity for other related molecules determines the specificity of the hormone–receptor interaction.

The affinity of a hormone for its receptor results from noncovalent binding, primarily in the form of hydrophobic interactions that provide the driving force for the binding reaction, and from electrostatic interactions. The latter, which occur between oppositely charged groups on peptide hormones and their receptors, are important for hormone–receptor specificity. The affinity of a hormone–receptor interaction is defined in terms of the *equilibrium dissociation constant* (K_d). In a system in which there is a single class of binding sites with no interactions among receptors, the K_d is defined as the concentration of hormone, at equilibrium, that is required for binding to 50% of the receptor sites. The affinity can also be expressed as the *equilibrium association constant* (K_a), which is the reciprocal of the K_d.

The binding of hormone to receptor is a saturable process; there is a finite number of receptors for a given hormone on a target cell. In addition, the binding of hormone to receptor must either precede or accompany the biological response, and the magnitude of the biological response must be associated, in some manner, with receptor occupancy. Hormones or analogs that bind to receptors and elicit the same biological response as the naturally occurring hormone are termed *agonists*. Molecules that bind to receptors but fail to elicit the normal biological response are termed *competitive antagonists*, since they occupy the receptors and prevent the binding of the biologically active molecules. Molecules that bind to receptors but are less biologically active than the native hormone are termed *partial agonists*. The term *partial antagonist* also applies since partial agonists bind to receptors and prevent the binding of the fully biologically active native hormone.

RELATIONSHIP OF BINDING TO BIOLOGICAL RESPONSE

The biological response of a target cell to a hormone is determined by a number of factors, including the concentration of hormone, the concentration of receptors, and the affinity of the hormone–receptor interaction. Normally, the concentration of a particular hormone in the circulation is much lower than the K_d of the hormone–receptor interaction. Therefore, the receptors on a target cell are almost never saturated, and an increase in the concentration of circulating hormone results in an increase in the number of occupied receptors.

In a number of examples of peptide hormone binding to cell surface receptors, the response of the target cell to the hormone is directly proportional to the number of receptor sites that are occupied; that is, the binding and biological response curves are superimposable over the entire range of hormone concentrations, and a maximum biological response is achieved when 100% of the receptor sites are occupied (Fig. 3-1). If the number of cellular receptors is reduced without a change in the K_d, both the binding and biological response curves are reduced and remain superimposable.

In most cases, however, the maximum biological response of a target cell is achieved at concentrations of hormone lower than those required to fully occupy all

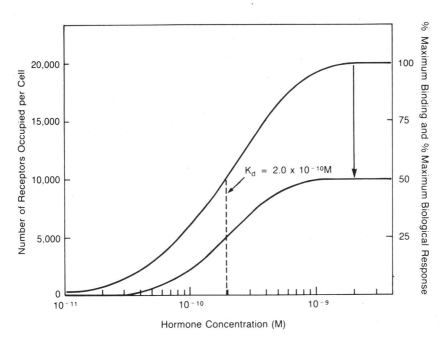

Fig. 3-1 Hormone binding and biological response curves when no spare receptors are present. In this example, the hormone binding and biological response curves are superimposed over the entire range of hormone concentrations. A 50% decrease in receptor number with no change in the K_d of the hormone–receptor interaction will result in an equivalent reduction in the maximum biological response.

of the receptors on that cell. For example, in isolated adipocytes, maximum stimulation of glucose oxidation is achieved at concentrations of insulin that occupy only 2%–3% of the cellular receptors. In Leydig cells, maximum stimulation of testosterone synthesis occurs at concentrations of gonadotropin that occupy only 1% of the cellular receptors. In these systems, >97% of the receptors are referred to as *spare receptors*. The term *spare receptors* does not imply that these receptors are not being utilized, but rather that a maximum biological response is achieved when all of the receptors on a target cell are occupied on average <3% of the time. The degree of spareness of receptors for a particular hormone on a target cell can vary from one cellular response to another, resulting in a different dose-response curve for each biological response of a cell to a given hormone.

Let us consider the hormone-binding (Fig. 3-2*A*) and biological response (Fig. 3-2*B*) curves for a hypothetical target cell that contains spare receptors for a particular biological response. The cell normally contains 20,000 receptors for the hormone. In this example, 75% of these receptors are considered to be spare receptors, since a maximum biological response is achieved at concentrations of hormone required to occupy only 5000 receptor sites per cell. When the number of cellular receptors is reduced by 50% and 75% without a change in receptor affinity, the maximum biological response remains unchanged; however, the maximum response is achieved at progressively increased concentrations of hormone. When the number

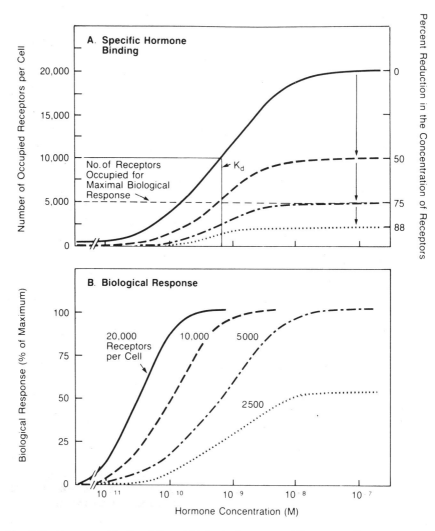

Fig. 3-2 Hormone binding (*A*) and biological response (*B*) curves when spare receptors are present. In this example, when the target cell contains its full complement of 20,000 receptors, a maximum biological response is achieved at concentrations of hormone required to occupy only 25% of the cellular receptors. When the number of cellular receptors is reduced to 10,000 or 5000 without a change in the K_d, a maximum biological response can still be achieved, albeit at progressively increased concentrations of hormone. When the number of cellular receptors is decreased by 88%, the maximum biological response is reduced by 50%.

of cellular receptors is reduced further, by 88%, the maximum biological response is reduced proportionately. From this example, one can see that the greater the proportion of spare receptors for a particular biological response, the more sensitive is the target cell to the hormone, that is, the lower the concentration of hormone required to achieve a half-maximum biological response. In addition to increasing the sensitivity of the target cell to the hormone, spare receptors serve to prolong the biological response of a cell to short bursts of circulating hormone. The hormone–receptor complexes in excess of those required for the maximum biological response will maintain the response for longer periods as the concentration of hormone in the circulation declines.

PEPTIDE AND POLYPEPTIDE HORMONES, NEUROTRANSMITTERS, AND PROSTAGLANDINS

Receptor Structure and Function

Receptors for peptide and polypeptide hormones, catecholamines, and other neurotransmitters and prostaglandins are integral membrane proteins that are interspersed within the phospholipid bilayer of the plasma membranes of target cells. Because these receptors are soluble in aqueous media only in the presence of detergents, they have proved difficult to purify and, until ~20 years ago, little was known of their structure. Most of the cellular components that are involved in the initial response of the target cell to such hormones are also present either within or associated with the inner leaflet of the plasma membrane.

Cell surface receptors for some nonhormonal ligands, such as low-density lipoprotein (LDL), transferrin, the asialoglycoproteins, immunoglobulin A/M (IgA/IgM), toxins, and viruses also are integral membrane proteins. The function of these receptors is to translocate the respective ligands to intracellular sites where the ligands themselves act to alter cellular function. For these systems, the information is contained within the ligand itself, and the receptor serves merely to facilitate the delivery of the ligand to its site of action within the cell. An example of a nonhormonal ligand that operates through such a system is cholera toxin, which binds to ganglioside G_{M1} receptors on the plasma membrane. The receptor serves to concentrate the toxin molecule and to facilitate its translocation to sites within the plasma membrane where the toxin causes the activation of adenylyl cyclase (see below).

By contrast, in the case of receptors for peptide and polypeptide hormones, prostaglandins, and neurotransmitters, the hormonal ligand merely activates the receptor, which in turn transmits various signals that result in altered cellular function. In fact, antibodies against the insulin and thyrotropin (thyroid-stimulating hormone, TSH) receptors can activate the respective receptors and mimic the actions of the hormones themselves. It is probable, therefore, that the hormone causes some conformational change in the receptor, which in turn transmits a signal that results in the generation of a biological response.

The primary structures of a large number of cell surface receptors for hormones and other bioactive molecules have been determined by the use of recombinant DNA techniques. Figure 3-3 diagrammatically shows the structures of representative members of different families of receptors that differ in structure and function. Shown are the β-adrenergic receptor, as a member of the large superfamily of G protein–linked receptors, receptors for epidermal growth factor (EGF), insulin, and platelet-derived growth factor (PDGF), which are members of the tyrosine kinase receptor superfamily; the growth hormone (GH) receptor, which associates with a

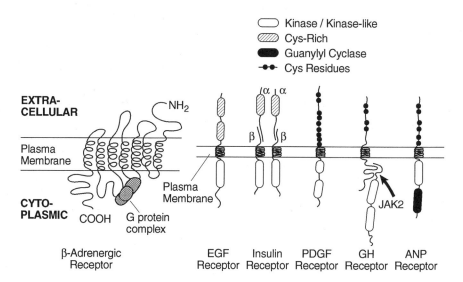

Fig. 3-3 Schematic representation of the proposed structures and plasma membrane orientations of the β-adrenergic, epidermal growth factor (EGF), insulin, platelet-derived growth factor (PDGF), growth hormone (GH), and atrial natriuretic peptide (ANP) receptors. All six receptors are transmembrane proteins oriented so that their carboxy termini are in the cytoplasm. The β-adrenergic receptor shown with its associated G protein complex crosses the plasma membrane seven times, whereas the other receptors cross the plasma membrane only once. The receptors for insulin and PDGF all contain intrinsic cytoplasmic tyrosine kinases, shown by the open areas. The hatched areas represent regions of the EGF and insulin receptors enriched in cysteine residues. The open areas represent domains with a high degree of sequence similarity to tyrosine kinases of the *src* gene family. The filled-in region of the ANP receptor has homology to soluble guanylyl cyclase. Solid circles represent individual cysteine residues. The cytoplasmic domain of the GH receptor is shown in association with the Janus kinase JAK2, a cytoplasmic tyrosine kinase that associates with the ligand-bound receptor and mediates signal transduction.

soluble tyrosine kinase and is a member of the cytokine receptor superfamily; and the atrial natriuretic peptide (ANP) receptor, a member of the family of receptor guanylyl cyclases. All of these receptors are glycoproteins that cross the plasma membrane either once (receptors for EGF, insulin, PDGF, ANP, and GH) or several times (β-adrenergic receptor).

Guanine Nucleotide-Binding Protein (G Protein)–Coupled Receptors

The β-adrenergic receptor, which mediates some of the actions of the catecholamines, epinephrine and norepinephrine, is a member of a large family of related receptor molecules, all containing seven hydrophobic regions, each of which forms an α-helix of sufficient length to span the plasma membrane. These receptor molecules cross the plasma membrane seven times (Fig. 3-3). This G protein–coupled receptor family includes the β- and α-adrenergic receptors, the muscarinic cholinergic receptors, receptors for vasopressin, angiotensin II, serotonin, substance

P, dopamine, luteinizing hormone (LH), follicle-stimulating hormone (FSH), TSH, platelet-activating factor, prostaglandins, the retinal rod outer segment protein rhodopsin, which serves as a *receptor* for light and mediates a complex signal transduction mechanism that culminates in the visual response, as well as sensory receptors for a variety of odorants and for sweet and bitter tastes. Each member of this receptor family interacts within the plasma membrane with a specific member of another family of proteins, the guanine nucleotide-binding proteins (G proteins). All of the G proteins are heterotrimers composed of α-, β-, and γ-subunits. The α-subunit is unique to each G protein, whereas the β- and γ-subunits are similar. Some 16 different α-subunit proteins have now been characterized, as well as 5 related β- and 12 γ-subunit proteins. The G protein family includes G_s (containing α_s), which mediates adenylyl cyclase stimulation; G_i (containing α_i), which mediates adenylyl cyclase inhibition; G_q (containing α_q), which mediates phospholipase C activation; and G_t (containing α_t, transducin), a protein of the rod outer segment that mediates activation of cyclic guanosine monophosphate (GMP) phosphodiesterase, resulting in the closure of Na^+ channels in the rod cell membranes to produce the visual response. The binding of the catecholamines epinephrine and norepinephrine to β-adrenergic receptors promotes interaction of the receptors with G_s, which results in activation of adenylyl cyclase (see below).

Nicotinic Acetylcholine Receptors

In higher vertebrates, there are two basic subtypes of acetylcholine receptors, *muscarinic* and *nicotinic*. As mentioned above, muscarinic receptors are members of the seven-transmembrane domain receptor family, are localized in cells throughout the body, and interact with G proteins. On the other hand, nicotinic receptors are members of a family of ligand-regulated ion channels that serve essential roles in transmission of nerve impulses. This family also includes receptors for γ-aminobutyric acid (GABA), glutamate, and glycine. Nicotinic receptors are present in the neuromuscular junctions. Acetylcholine, which is released from the presynaptic nerve endings on depolarization of the neuron, binds to such receptors clustered in the motor endplates of skeletal muscle. The acetylcholine receptors of electric eels and electric fish are structurally and functionally homologous to nicotinic acetylcholine receptors and are present in very high concentrations in the plasma membranes of electrocytes, which are specialized cells that develop from embryonic muscle cells and generate the electric potential that such species use to stun or kill their prey. The acetylcholine receptor is composed of five similar subunits, each of 50,000–65,000 molecular weight, which are the products of four different but homologous genes: the five subunits surround an ion-conducting channel. The binding of acetylcholine to the receptor results in the opening of the ion-conducting channel created by a conformational change in the subunits of the receptor, which form the walls of the ion channel. The channel predominantly transports sodium ions, resulting in a depolarization of the plasma membrane of the postsynaptic cell.

Receptors with Intrinsic Protein Tyrosine Kinase Activity

Receptors for EGF, PDGFs, fibroblast growth factors (FGFs), insulin, and insulin-like growth factor-I (IGF-1) contain intrinsic protein kinases that specifically stimulate phosphorylation of tyrosine residues on target proteins. Binding of the hormone to its receptor causes conformational changes involving receptor dimerization that lead to tyrosine kinase activation and subsequent stimulation of downstream signaling pathways mediating increased cell proliferation.

The Epidermal Growth Factor Receptor. The EGF receptor is a glycoprotein containing an intrinsic tyrosine kinase that is stimulated on the binding of EGF and is presumed to mediate some of its actions. The receptor is composed of a single polypeptide chain of 1186 amino acids. The protein can be divided into three domains: an N-terminal extracellular domain that contains the EGF-binding site, a short α-helical membrane-spanning domain of hydrophobic amino acids, and a C-terminal cytoplasmic domain that shares sequence homology with other tyrosine-specific protein kinases. The N-terminal region contains many cysteine residues, which are clustered into two regions that form an EGF-binding cleft. The EGF receptor is overproduced in a number of tumor cell lines, suggesting that overexpression of the EGF receptor gene may contribute to the phenotype of cellular transformation. It also is of interest that the transmembrane and the cytoplasmic portion of the EGF receptor, which encodes the tyrosine kinase, have a very high degree of sequence homology with one of the transforming proteins of the avian erythroblastosis virus, the *v-erb-B* oncogene product. Viral oncogenes are derived from host cellular genes that are acquired during the course of infection. Apparently, the progenitor of the avian erythroblastosis virus acquired from host cells is the portion of the EGF receptor gene that encodes the transmembrane and cytoplasmic domains, but not the part that encodes the extracellular EGF-binding region. It has been suggested that the *v-erb-B* gene product induces cellular transformation because of the constitutive expression of the tyrosine kinase domain in the absence of expression of the regulatory EGF-binding domain.

Insulin Receptor. The polypeptide hormone, insulin, exerts a variety of metabolic and growth-promoting effects on its target cells that are initiated by its interaction with specific plasma membrane receptors. The insulin receptor is a high-molecular-weight glycoprotein that exhibits insulin-dependent, tyrosine-specific protein kinase activity. The receptor probably exists in the plasma membrane as a tetramer consisting of two disulfide-linked heterodimers $(\alpha\beta)_2$ (Fig. 3-3). The α- and β-subunits of the insulin receptor are synthesized as part of a single precursor polypeptide chain, which is subsequently glycosylated, proteolytically cleaved, and inserted into the plasma membrane. The α-subunit contains the hormone-binding site of the receptor. The β-subunits contain the insulin-dependent tyrosine kinase activity. As previously discussed, tyrosine protein kinase activity also is associated with the EGF receptor and with other growth factor receptors, including those for IGF-I (closely related structurally to the insulin receptor), PDGFs, the colony-stimulating factor CSF-1, FGFs, HER-2/neu (closely related structurally to the EGF receptor), as well as a number of transforming retroviral oncogene products. Such findings are indicative of the role of tyrosine protein kinases in growth control (see Chapter 12). The α-subunit of the insulin receptor does not contain a hydrophobic membrane-spanning sequence and is localized on the outer face of the plasma membrane. Like the N-terminal extracellular domain of the EGF receptor, the α-chain is rich in cysteine residues.

Guanylyl Cyclase Receptors

Receptors for natriuretic peptides are transmembrane guanylyl cyclases that consist of an extracellular ligand-binding domain, a single α-helical transmembrane domain, and a cytosolic catalytic domain consisting of one region with homology to protein kinases and another with homology to soluble guanylyl cyclases (Fig. 3-3). Atrial natriuretic peptide, released from the atrium of the heart, binds to receptors on target cells, activates guanylyl cyclase, and promotes increased production of cyclic GMP. Members of this receptor family also include receptors for heat-stable enterotoxins from *Escherichia coli* (guanylins) and sea urchin sperm receptors for a number of chemoattractant peptides produced by sea urchin eggs.

Receptors for Growth Hormone, Prolactin, and Other Members of the Cytokine Receptor Superfamily

Receptors for GH and prolactin belong to a large superfamily that includes receptors for the hematopoietic growth factors, which control the proliferation, differentiation, and activity of eight lineages of blood cells that are generated from an ancestral pool of stem cells. Hematopoietic growth factors include the interleukin (IL) family, colony-stimulating factors G-CSF and GM-CSF, leukemia-inhibitory factor (LIF), oncostatin M (OSM), and erythropoietin, as well as ciliary neurotrophic factor (CNTF). The hematopoietic growth factors exert pleiotropic effects; that is, most of the factors act on cells of more than one lineage of blood cells, and more than one factor controls the growth and differentiation of cells in any one lineage. On the other hand, GH has a variety of metabolic effects and stimulates skeletal growth through induction of IGF-I. Prolactin has numerous biological effects; in mammals, its best-known action is the stimulation of growth and differentiation of the mammary gland, as well as lactogenesis. Interestingly, receptors for prolactin and GH also are present on cells of the immune system. In contrast, the CNTF receptor α-chain is restricted to the nervous system; CNTF supports the survival of chick embryonic ciliary ganglion cells and of sympathetic sensory and motor neurons.

The high-affinity binding forms of receptors in the cytokine superfamily consist of either a homodimeric complex of specific α-chains or a heterodimeric complex of the specific α-chains with one or more β-subunits that also are members of this superfamily. The extracellular domains of these receptors share a number of common structural features, including two pairs of disulfide-linked cysteine residues in conserved positions (usually near the aminoterminal end, that is, distal to the plasma membrane), and a WSXWS sequence (tryptophan, serine, and any amino acid, followed by another tryptophan, serine) proximal to the plasma membrane. Receptors for the interferons (IFN) α/β and IFNγ, as well as IL-10, are structurally related to the cytokine receptors described above but lack this WSXWS sequence in their extracellular domains.

Unlike the cytoplasmic domains of receptors for EGF, insulin, IGF-I, PDGF, and FGF, which have intrinsic protein tyrosine kinase activity, the cytoplasmic domains of members of the cytokine receptor superfamily lack homology to known protein kinases and have no intrinsic kinase activity. Despite this absence of a kinase domain, binding of cytokines, GH, and prolactin to their receptors is followed by a rapid increase in tyrosine phosphorylation of cellular proteins and of the receptor itself. Within the plasma membrane–proximal region of the cytoplasmic domain are two regions (box 1 and box 2) that are required for mediation of the growth-promoting effects of the cytokines. As will be discussed later in this chapter, signal transduction is mediated by the activation of soluble, cytoplasmic tyrosine kinases (Janus kinases, JAKs) that bind to the membrane-proximal cytoplasmic region. A schematic of the GH receptor and its associated kinase, JAK2, is shown in Figure 3-3.

As mentioned above, in the case of all members of the cytokine receptor superfamily, high-affinity binding requires either homodimerization of the receptor α-chains (prolactin, GH, G-CSF, and erythropoietin receptors) or heterodimerization with one or more β-subunits that also are members of this superfamily. The fact that some of these β-subunits are shared with different family members helps to explain the observed pleiotropic effects. As an example, the high-affinity binding forms of receptors for IL-3, IL-5, and GM-CSF consist of a heterodimeric complex of the specific α-chains with a common β-subunit. The α-chain receptors for IL-6, LIF/OSM, and CNTFR also share a β-subunit (gp130).

Signal Transduction Mechanisms

It is generally accepted that polypeptide hormones and catecholamines exert their effects on cellular metabolism by binding to receptors on the surface of target cells and activating a membrane-associated enzyme that in turn elaborates an intracellular second messenger. This second messenger subsequently mediates the various biological effects of the hormone. This so-called *second messenger hypothesis of hormone action* was proposed in the early 1960s, when it was discovered that the activation of glycogen phosphorylase by epinephrine and glucagon in liver slices was mediated by the formation of a heat-stable compound, which was identified as adenosine $3',5'$-monophosphate (cyclic adenosine monophosphate [AMP]). Cyclic AMP is formed from Mg·ATP by a membrane-associated enzyme, adenylyl cyclase. According to this concept, the hormone, or first messenger, carries information from its site of production to the target cell, where it binds to specific receptors on the cell surface. This results in the activation of a membrane-bound enzyme or effector (e.g., adenylyl cyclase), which generates a soluble intracellular second messenger (e.g., cyclic AMP), which then transmits the information to the cellular machinery, resulting in a biological response. In recent years, a number of other effector/second messenger systems have been discovered that mediate the actions of a variety of hormones on cellular metabolism and function.

G Protein–Coupled Signal Transduction

As discussed above, receptors for polypeptide hormones, prostaglandins, and neurotransmitters that cross the plasma membrane seven times are coupled to G proteins that are heterotrimers composed of unique α-subunits and common $\beta\gamma$-subunits. The α-subunit α_s mediates activation of adenylyl cyclase; the α-subunit α_i mediates inhibition of adenylyl cyclase, and the α-subunit α_q mediates activation of phospholipase Cβ (PLCβ), which ultimately results in an increase in cytosolic calcium and activation of protein kinase C. In the cases of all G protein–linked receptors, the binding of hormone to receptor causes the receptor to interact with a specific G protein heterotrimer. This interaction causes the release of bound guanosine diphosphate (GDP) from the α-subunit and the binding of GTP. The GTP-bound α-subunit, which now dissociates from $\beta\gamma$, is activated and binds to various effector molecules in the cell (e.g. adenylyl cyclase, PLCβ), resulting in changes in effector activity.

Hormone-Sensitive Adenylyl Cyclase. The hormone-sensitive adenylyl cyclase system has at least three components: the receptor (R_s or R_i), a form of guanine nucleotide-binding regulatory protein (G_s or G_i), and the catalytic component (C), which enzymatically converts Mg·ATP to cyclic AMP (Fig. 3-4). The guanine nucleotide–binding regulatory protein, G_s, mediates the actions of hormones that stimulate adenylyl cyclase activity, whereas G_i mediates the actions of hormones that inhibit adenylyl cyclase. All of these components can be independently isolated and recombined *in vitro* to reconstitute a functional hormone-sensitive adenylyl cyclase system. It is apparent that many different types of hormone receptors on a single cell can interact with the same pool of regulatory and catalytic components, and that these combined interactions result either in a net stimulation or inhibition of adenylyl cyclase activity. As discussed above, G_s and G_i are heterotrimers composed of a unique α-subunit (α_s or α_i) and a heterodimer of β- and γ-subunits. The $\beta\gamma$-subunits shared by G_s and G_i are essential for the integrated actions of stimulatory and inhibitory hormones on adenylyl cyclase activity. It has been proposed that the binding of hormone to receptor results in a conformational change that promotes the interaction or coupling of the hormone–receptor complex with the other components of hormone-sensitive adenylyl cyclase.

Receptor-Mediated Stimulation of Adenylyl Cyclase. The proposed mechanism for the hormonal activation of adenylyl cyclase, which is based on the studies from a

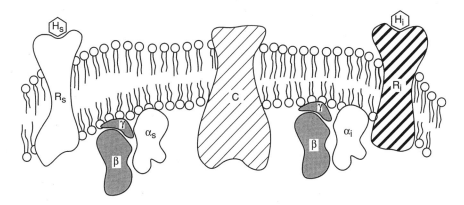

Fig. 3-4 Plasma membrane components of hormone-sensitive adenylyl cyclase. Hormone-sensitive adenylyl cyclase is composed of the following integral proteins of the plasma membrane: receptors for either stimulatory (R_s) or inhibitory (R_i) hormones (H_s and H_i), the guanine nucleotide-binding regulatory proteins G_s or G_i, and the catalytic component (C). G_s is composed of a unique α-subunit, $M_r \approx 45{,}000$, and β- and γ-subunits, $M_r \cong 35{,}000$ and $10{,}000$, respectively. G_i has a unique α-subunit, $M_r \approx 41{,}000$, and β- and γ-subunits that are similar to those of G_s.

number of laboratories, is presented in Figure 3-5. In the inactive state, the guanine nucleotide that is bound to the α_s-subunit of G_s is GDP. The binding of hormone (H) to receptor (R) promotes the formation of the ternary complex, H·R·G_s, which facilitates the dissociation of GDP and the binding of guanosine triphosphate (GTP) to the α_s-subunit. The binding of GTP to α_s results in its dissociation from the $\beta\gamma$-subunits. The α_s·GTP then associates with the catalytic subunit (C) of the adenylyl cyclase to form the active holoenzyme (α_s·GTP·C). The activated adenylyl cyclase then converts adenine triphosphate (ATP) to cyclic AMP. The activated α_s contains guanosine triphosphatase (GTPase) activity, which catalyzes the hydrolysis of GTP to GDP and terminates the cycle of adenylyl cyclase activation. Cholera toxin, which is produced by the bacterial organism *Vibrio cholera*, binds to G_{M1} gangliosides (complex glycolipids) on the cell surface and penetrates the cell membrane. Once within the cell membrane, the toxin catalyzes the ADP ribosylation of an arginine residue (Arg201) in α_s, causing inhibition of the GTPase activity (Fig. 3-5). This change results in a persistent activation of adenylyl cyclase. In intestinal mucosal cells, the binding of cholera toxin and subsequent activation of adenylyl cyclase re-

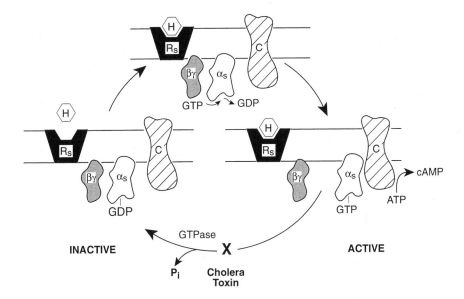

Fig. 3-5 Proposed mechanism for the hormonal activation of adenylyl cyclase, G_s, is composed of three subunits, α_s, β, and γ. In the absence of the binding of a stimulatory hormone to its receptor, the guanine nucleotide guanosine diphosphate (GDP) is bound to α_s and adenylyl cyclase is in the inactive state. The binding of hormone to receptor facilitates the dissociation of GDP and the association of guanosine triphosphate (GTP) with the α_s. This, in turn, results in the dissociation of α_s from the $\beta\gamma$-subunits and its association with the catalytic component (C), resulting in adenylyl cyclase activation. The activated α_s contains a guanosine triphosphatase (GTPase) that hydrolyzes the bound GTP to GDP, resulting in a return of adenylyl cyclase to an inactive state. Cholera toxin, which inhibits the GTPase activity, causes a persistent activation of adenylyl cyclase. ATP, adenosine triphosphate; cAMP, cyclic adenosine monophosphate.

sults in the stimulation of ion (primarily Cl^-) and water secretion across the intestinal brush border, causing massive diarrhea.

Receptor-Mediated Inhibition of Adenylyl Cyclase. A number of hormones inhibit adenylyl cyclase activity. They include catecholamines that bind to α_2-adrenergic receptors, muscarinic-cholinergic agonists, and opioids. These hormones bind to cell surface receptors that interact with the inhibitory guanine nucleotide-binding regulatory protein, G_i. G_i is similar in structure to G_s, having three subunits, α_i, β, and γ. The $\beta\gamma$-subunits of G_i are similar to those of G_s, whereas the α-subunit is distinct. $G\alpha_i$ contains a guanine nucleotide-binding site. The binding of these hormones to their receptors promotes the exchange of GTP for GDP on α_i. This results in the dissociation of α_i from $\beta\gamma$. The inhibition of adenylyl cyclase activity appears to be mediated primarily by the interaction of the free $\alpha_i \cdot$GTP with adenylyl cyclase. Inhibition of adenylyl cyclase also is mediated, in part, by the increased levels of free $\beta\gamma$, which by mass action reduce the concentration of free α_s. Islet-activating protein, one of the toxins of *Bordetella pertussis*, prevents the dissociation of $G_{i\alpha}$ from $\beta\gamma$, which results in adenylyl cyclase activation, since less free α_i is available to inhibit adenylyl cyclase and less $\beta\gamma$ is free to interact with α_s. Thus, cholera toxin activates adenylyl cyclase by promoting the dissociation of G_s, whereas islet-activating protein activates adenylyl cyclase by inhibiting the dissociation of G_i.

It should be noted that the free $\beta\gamma$-subunits can themselves regulate certain cellular effectors. For example, free $\beta\gamma$ directly binds and activates a K^+-selective ion channel in heart atrial cells, and binds to and activates PLCβ, resulting in its activation. The latter is an example of an enzyme that is activated both by an activated α-subunit (in this case $\alpha_q \cdot$GTP) and by free $\beta\gamma$.

Cyclic Adenosine Monophosphate Regulation of Cellular Function

The major mechanism by which cyclic AMP regulates cellular function is through its binding to cyclic AMP–dependent protein kinase A (PKA). The cyclic AMP–dependent protein kinase holoenzyme is composed of a regulatory subunit (R) dimer and two catalytic subunits (C). The R subunit is a cyclic AMP–binding protein, while the C subunit, when free of R, expresses protein kinase activity. Each molecule of R dimer binds four molecules of cyclic AMP. The binding of cyclic AMP to R causes dissociation of the inactive holoenzyme to yield two active catalytic subunits. The reaction is generally represented as

$$R_2C_2 + 4 \text{ cyclic AMP} \rightarrow R_2 \cdot 4 \text{ cyclic AMP} + 2 \text{ C}$$

The active free catalytic subunits can now catalyze the phosphorylation of a number of cellular proteins; protein kinase A (PKA) catalyzes the transfer of a high-energy phosphate from ATP to the hydroxyl groups of serine and, to a much lesser extent, threonine residues on cellular proteins. The phosphorylation of enzymes may result in changes in enzyme activity. For example, phosphorylation of hormone-sensitive lipase, cholesteryl esterase, or glycogen phosphorylase results in enzyme activation. On the other hand, phosphorylation of glycogen synthase decreases enzyme activity. The specific responses of various cell types to an increase in cyclic AMP and the activation of cyclic AMP–dependent protein kinase is determined by the cellular phenotype and, therefore, by the enzymes and substrates available for regulation. Thus, a major response of a liver cell to an increase in cyclic AMP is glycogenolysis, because the liver cell expresses the enzymes to synthesize and to metabolize glycogen. In a fat cell, on the other hand, the primary response to an increase in cyclic AMP is lipolysis, because the fat cell expresses the enzymes for uptake of triacylglycerol precursors from the circulation, and for the synthesis and metabolism of triacylglycerols.

In addition to its PKA-mediated actions to alter the activities of various metabolic enzymes, cyclic AMP through PKA-mediated phosphorylation also regulates the transcription of specific genes in eukaryotic cells. An effect of cyclic AMP at the level of gene transcription has been found for a number of eukaryotic genes, including those encoding phosphoenolpyruvate carboxykinase (PEPCK), tyrosine aminotransferase (TAT), the human glycoprotein hormone α-subunit gene, preprosomatostatin, vasoactive intestinal polypeptide (VIP), the surfactant protein, SP-A, and several forms of cytochrome P450 involved in steroid hydroxylation.

Our understanding of the molecular mechanisms whereby cyclic AMP activates gene transcription in mammalian cells was greatly advanced by the discovery of a DNA-binding protein or transcription factor, termed *cyclic AMP response element-binding protein* (CREB), which is activated by PKA-mediated phosphorylation to regulate the transcriptional activity of a number of specific genes. CREB is a member of a family of related DNA-binding proteins, the activating transcription factors (ATF proteins), that bind to a common sequence of DNA, TGACGTCA (the cyclic AMP response element, CRE), which is palindromic; that is, it possesses a twofold rotational axis of symmetry. Increased cellular levels of cyclic AMP result in activation of CREB through its phosphorylation on serine residues by PKA. The phosphorylated CREB homodimer bound to the CRE then recruits a family of coactivator proteins that stabilize binding of the basal transcription complex to the downstream promoter and facilitate the binding of RNA polymerase II, resulting in increased transcription of cyclic AMP–responsive genes. It should be noted, however, that the CRE does not appear to be present in the regulatory regions of all genes that are regulated by cyclic AMP. Therefore, additional cyclic AMP–responsive transcription factors and mechanisms mediate AMP regulation of eukaryotic gene transcription.

Cyclic AMP is rapidly metabolized in cells by the cyclic nucleotide phosphodiesterases, which hydrolyze cyclic AMP to form the inactive 5'-AMP.

$$\text{cyclic AMP} \rightarrow 5'\text{-AMP}$$

The actions of a number of hormones, including insulin and catecholamines binding to α_1-adrenergic receptors, are mediated in part by activation of phosphodiesterase and a subsequent decrease in cellular cyclic AMP levels.

Signal Transduction Mechanisms Independent of Cyclic Adenosine Monophosphate

A significant number of polypeptide hormones, which bind to G protein–linked receptors, exert their actions on cellular metabolism and function by mechanisms that do not involve adenylyl cyclase activation and cyclic AMP. Table 3-1 lists hor-

Table 3-1 Signal Transduction Mechanisms in Hormone Action

Receptors that mediate activation of adenylyl cyclase	Receptors that mediate inhibition of adenylyl cyclase	Receptors that mediate increased phosphoinositide turnover	Receptors that mediate tyrosine kinase activation
β-Adrenergic	α_2-Adrenergic	α_1-Adrenergic	Insulin
LH, FSH, TSH, hCG	Opioid	Angiotensin II	Growth factors (PDGF, EGF, FGF, IGF-I)
Glucagon	Muscarinic cholinergic—M2	Muscarinic cholinergic—M3	Growth hormone
PGE$_2$—EP$_2$, EP$_4$	PGE$_2$—EP$_3$	PGE$_2$—EP$_1$	Prolactin
Vasopressin—V$_2$		Vasopressin—V$_1$	
ACTH			

ACTH, adrenocorticotropic hormone; EGF, epidermal growth factor; FGF, fibroblast growth factor; FSH, follicle-stimulating hormone; hCG, human chorionic gonadotropin; IGF-I, insulin-like growth factor-I; LH, luteinizing hormone; PDGF, platelet-derived growth factor; PGE$_2$, prostaglandin E$_2$; TSH, thyroid-stimulating hormone.

mones that act by by activating adenylyl cyclase and increasing cyclic AMP, by inhibiting adenylyl cyclase, by increasing phosphoinositide turnover, and by activating intrinsic or associated tyrosine kinases. Hormones that act through cyclic AMP–mediated mechanisms include epinephrine and norepinephrine binding to β-adrenergic receptors, vasopressin, acting through V$_2$ receptors, prostaglandin E$_2$ (PGE$_2$) binding to the EP$_2$ and EP$_4$ subtypes of PGE$_2$ receptors, adrenocorticotropic hormone (ACTH), glucagon, and the pituitary glycoprotein hormones, luteinizing hormone (LH), follicle-stimulating hormone (FSH), and thyroid-stimulating hormone (TSH). The glycoprotein hormone of human placental origin, human chorionic gonadotropin (hCG), which is highly homologous to LH and binds to LH receptors, also increases cyclic AMP formation.

On the other hand, epinephrine and norepinephrine binding to α_2-adrenergic receptors, PGE$_2$ binding to EP$_3$ receptors, opioids binding to delta and mu receptors, and acetylcholine binding to M2 muscarinic receptors cause adenylyl cyclase inhibition. Furthermore, epinephrine and norepinephrine binding to α_1-adrenergic receptors, PGE$_2$ binding to EP$_1$ receptors, vasopressin binding to V$_1$ receptors, and acetylcholine binding to the M3 subtype of muscarinic cholinergic receptors act by signal transduction pathways initiated by increased phosphoinositide turnover. Other hormones, such as insulin, various growth factors, growth hormone, prolactin and other members of the cytokine receptor family act through signal transduction pathways initiated by activation of intrinsic or receptor-associated tyrosine kinases.

It is apparent that a number of G protein–linked receptors exist in different subtypes and interact with different heterotrimeric G proteins. Therefore, the same hormone may act through a cyclic AMP–mediated mechanism in one tissue and by a cyclic AMP–independent mechanism in another. As noted above, vasopressin binds to a specific subset of receptors (V$_2$) on cells of the kidney-collecting tubules and loop of Henle to promote sodium and water reabsorption. These actions of vasopressin are mediated by increased cyclic AMP formation and cyclic AMP–dependent protein kinase activation. On the other hand, in the liver, vasopressin acts through another subset of receptors (V$_1$) to enhance glycogenolysis, and this effect is mediated by increased phosphoinositide turnover. The catecholamines, epinephrine and norepinephrine, bind to several subsets of receptors that are present in different relative amounts in various tissues. In liver cells, norepinephrine binds both to β- and to α_1-adrenergic receptors to increase glycogenolysis. Binding to β-receptors results in adenylyl cyclase activation, an increase in cyclic AMP, and activation of cyclic AMP–dependent protein kinase, which in turn catalyzes the phosphorylation and activation of phosphorylase kinase. The activated phosphorylase kinase catalyzes the phosphorylation and activation of phosphorylase, resulting in enhanced glycogenolysis. Phosphorylase kinase also catalyzes the phosphorylation of glycogen synthase, resulting in its inactivation. Norepinephrine, acting through α_1-receptors, promotes an increase in the level of free cytosolic calcium ion, which causes, by mechanisms discussed below, the activation of phosphorylase kinase and the subsequent increase in glycogen breakdown. There are five different subtypes of muscarinic acetylcholine receptors (M1–M5) and four different subtypes of PGE_2 receptors that mediate different signal transduction pathways. For example, the EP_1 receptor subtype is linked to G_q and mediates increased phosphoinositide turnover; the EP_2 and EP_4 subtypes are linked to G_s and mediate adenylyl cyclase activation; and the EP_3 receptor is linked to G_i and mediates adenylyl cyclase inhibition.

Phosphoinositide Turnover. As previously mentioned, a number of hormone–receptor interactions increase free cytosolic calcium ion and activate protein kinase C, which play important roles in the regulation of cellular function. Hormone–receptor interactions that result in the formation of these second messengers include the binding of acetylcholine to the M3 subtype of muscarinic cholinergic receptors, epinephrine and norepinephrine, to α_1-adrenergic receptors, PGE_2 to EP_1 receptors, vasopressin to V_1 receptors, and angiotensin II to receptors on liver cells. The proposed mechanism of action of such hormones is presented in Figure 3-6. The binding of hormone to receptor results in its association with a heterotrimeric G protein that contains $\alpha_q\beta\gamma$. This, in turn, promotes dissociation of GDP from α_q and the subsequent binding of GTP. The $\alpha_q \cdot$GTP causes the activation of a plasma membrane–associated PLCβ, which catalyzes the hydrolysis of a specific inositol phospholipid within the plasma membrane, phosphatidylinositol 4,5-bisphosphate (PIP_2), to form the second messengers diacylglycerol (DAG) and inositol 1,4,5-trisphosphate (IP_3).

The hydrolysis of PIP_2 and the formation of IP_3 are specifically associated with an increase in the level of free cytosolic calcium ion and the subsequent physiological response. Incubation of permeabilized cells with IP_3 results in a profound increase in the release of calcium ion from intracellular stores, primarily the endoplasmic reticulum. An endoplasmic reticulum–associated receptor for IP_3 has been cloned and characterized. The IP_3 receptor is a high molecular weight protein that contains at least four membrane-spanning domains, which form the calcium channel. In addition to mediating IP_3-stimulated calcium release from the endoplasmic reticulum, this receptor may act in conjunction with the dihydropyridine (DHP)-gated calcium channels to facilitate the influx of extracellular calcium into the cell. Once formed, IP_3 is rapidly hydrolyzed to IP_2, IP, and inositol by the actions of specific phosphomonoesterases. The action of the esterase that hydrolyzes IP to inositol is inhibited by lithium ion.

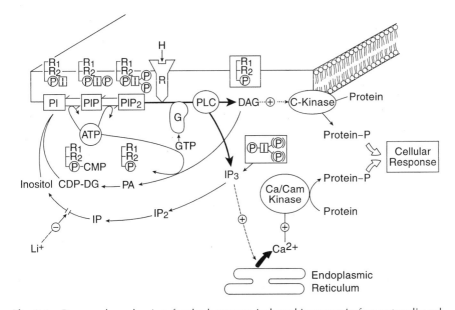

Fig. 3-6 Proposed mechanism for the hormone-induced increase in free cytosolic calcium and activation of protein kinase C. The polyphosphoinositides phosphatidylinositol 4-phosphate (PIP) and phosphatidylinositol 4,5-bisphosphate (PIP$_2$) are formed within the plasma membrane from phosphatidylinositol (PI) and adenosine triphosphate (ATP) in reactions catalyzed by kinases. The binding of hormone to receptor results in its association with a G protein heterotrimer containing $\alpha_q\beta\gamma$. This causes the dissociation of guanosine diphosphate (GDP) from α_q and the association of guanosine triphosphate (GTP). The α_q·GTP then dissociates from $\beta\gamma$ and activates a specific phospholipase C (PLC) within the plasma membrane, which catalyzes the hydrolysis of PIP$_2$ to form the putative second messengers, inositol trisphosphate (IP$_3$) and diacylglycerol (DAG). The water-soluble IP$_3$ diffuses into the cytoplasm and stimulates the release of calcium from storage sites, primarily within the endoplasmic reticulum. The increased free cytosolic calcium exerts most of its effects on cellular metabolism by binding to calmodulin (Cam). The calcium–calmodulin complex binds to various enzyme or effector proteins, causing changes in their activities. One such protein is phosphorylase kinase, which is activated by an increase in cytoplasmic calcium ion. The IP$_3$ is subsequently hydrolyzed by specific phosphatases to form the inactive IP$_2$, IP, and inositol. The DAG remains within the plasma membrane, where it facilitates the activation of protein kinase C (C-kinase) by calcium ion and phospholipid. The DAG and inositol are utilized for the resynthesis of PI. H, hormone; PA, phosphatidic acid; CDP-DG, cytidine diphosphate diacyl glycerol; R$_1$ and R$_2$, fatty acids in the sn-1 and sn-2 positions of the polyphosinositides.

CALCIUM. The levels of free calcium ion in the cytoplasm are normally quite low (10^{-7} M) as compared to the levels of calcium ion in the extracellular fluid (10^{-3} M). The influx of calcium into most cells at rest is minimal, despite a large electrochemical gradient, since the plasma membranes of most cells at rest are relatively impermeable to calcium ion. Within the cell, calcium is stored in high concentrations in the mitochondrial membrane, the endoplasmic reticulum (sarcoplasmic reticulum of muscle cells), and the plasma membrane. An increase in the levels of free cytosolic calcium ion can have a variety of effects on the cell, including changes in cell motility, contraction of muscle cells, increased release of secretory proteins, and activation of a number of regulatory enzymes. Calcium ion exerts most of these effects in cells by binding to specific calcium-binding proteins, such as calmodulin, in nonmuscle cells and troponin C in striated muscle cells. The binding of calcium results in the activation of these calcium-binding proteins. Calmodulin has no intrinsic activity of its own; after binding calcium ion (each molecule of calmodulin has four calcium-binding sites), it is activated and binds to various enzymes or effector molecules, causing a change in their activities. Two enzymes that are activated by the calcium-calmodulin complex are *phosphorylase kinase* and *cyclic AMP phosphodiesterase*. The activation of phosphorylase kinase by cyclic AMP–dependent protein kinase is dependent on calcium. Phosphorylase kinase has four subunits, α, β, γ, and δ. The δ-subunit is calmodulin, and the γ-subunit is the catalytic component of the enzyme. The α- and β-subunits are phosphorylated by cyclic AMP–dependent protein kinase. The phosphorylation of the α- and β-subunits in the presence of calcium ion activates the γ-subunit and increases the affinity of the δ-subunit (calmodulin) for calcium. In the presence of calcium ion, the enzyme binds a second molecule of calmodulin (δ'). This in turn activates the dephosphorylated form of the enzyme but has little effect in promoting the further activation of the phosphorylated enzyme.

Phosphorylase kinase is an example of an enzyme that is activated by an increase in intracellular calcium ion, cyclic AMP, or both. This provides an example of a system in which the actions of cyclic AMP and calcium occur in the same direction. There are other examples in which the actions of calcium antagonize those of cyclic AMP; cyclic AMP phosphodiesterase, the enzyme that catalyzes the metabolism of cyclic AMP to the inactive 5'-AMP, is activated by the calcium–calmodulin complex. An increase in free cytosolic calcium ion, therefore, can cause a decrease in the levels of cyclic AMP and of cyclic AMP–dependent protein kinase activity and a change in the activities of the enzymes that are substrates for this kinase.

PROTEIN KINASE C. The other product of the hydrolysis of inositol phospholipids, DAG, is also believed to serve as a second messenger by acting within the cell membrane to activate protein kinase C (PKC). Protein kinase C is a phospholipid- and calcium-dependent enzyme that catalyzes the phosphorylation of serine and threonine residues on a number of cellular proteins. Diacylglycerol dramatically increases the affinity of the enzyme for calcium ion and for phospholipid and therefore promotes an increase in enzyme activity at resting levels of intracellular calcium. The DAG-mediated hormonal activation of PKC can be mimicked by incubating cells with tumor-promoting phorbol esters, which interact with the enzyme at the same site as DAG. Since phorbol esters are not rapidly degraded, these agents cause long-term activation of PKC and promote the growth of tumors.

In addition to phosphorylating serine and threonine residues on a number of enzyme proteins, PKC can alter the expression of a number of specific genes. This action of PKC is mediated by the activation of a transcription factor known as

AP-1. AP-1 is a heterodimer of two related proteins, c-Fos and c-Jun, which are recognized as proto-oncogenes. AP-1 binds to a specific DNA sequence TGA$^C/_G$TCA, which is quite similar to that recognized by the cyclic AMP–activated transcription factor CREB. In contrast to CREB, which is activated by increased phosphorylation, AP-1 binding and transcriptional activity appear to be increased by dephosphorylation of constitutively phosphorylated amino acid residues near the carboxyterminus and phosphorylation of other residues near the aminoterminus of c-Jun. Thus, it is likely that activated PKC alters AP-1 transcriptional activity by activating both a specific phosphatase and a specific kinase.

It is therefore apparent that the hormonal activation of phosphatidylinositol turnover results in the elaboration of two important mediators, IP$_3$ and DAG, which in turn promote an increase in intracellular calcium and activation of PKC, respectively. The result is a variety of cellular responses that are dependent on cellular phenotype and include alterations in enzyme activity and in transcription factor activation.

Phosphatidylcholine Turnover. Although numerous hormones and neurotransmitters exert their effects through PIP$_2$ hydrolysis, a significant number have been found to stimulate the hydrolysis of phosphatidylcholine (PC). Phospholipase C–mediated hydrolysis of PC yields DAG and phosphorylcholine. The DAG that is formed has the capacity to activate PKC, as described above. Since PC is present in much greater abundance in cell membranes than is PIP$_2$, the former may serve as an important source of DAG for long-term activation of PKC. Another phospholipase, phospholipase D, has been implicated in the actions of a number of hormones that act through G protein–coupled receptors. In addition to stimulating phospholipase C–mediated PIP$_2$ hydrolysis, the binding of vasopressin to V$_1$ receptors on hepatocytes and of acetylcholine to muscarinic receptors in the brain promotes the activation of phospholipase D, which catalyzes the hydrolysis of PC to form choline and phosphatidate. Phosphatidate may serve as a calcium ionophore by promoting calcium entry into cells and the mobilization of intracellular calcium from membrane stores. The phosphatidate also may be hydrolyzed by phosphatidate phosphohydrolase to form diacylglycerol, which in turn can activate PKC.

The Sphingomyelin Cycle—Ceramide as a Second Messenger. Sphingomyelins are the only phospholipids in cell membranes that do not have a glycerol backbone. Rather, the backbone of sphingomyelin is sphingosine, an amino alcohol that contains an 18-carbon chain with one double bond. The amino group of sphingosine is linked to a long-chain fatty acid by an amide bond, and the primary hydroxyl group is in ester linkage with phosphocholine. Although it once was believed that sphingomyelin served merely as a structural component of plasma membranes and myelin sheaths of nerves, it recently has become apparent that sphingomyelin is actively metabolized by a cytoplasmic neutral sphingomyelinase and serves as a reservoir of second messengers in the action of a number of hormones and cytokines. Sphingomyelinase-induced hydrolysis of sphingomyelin to form ceramide and phosphocholine mediates the action of tumor necrosis factor-α (TNF-α) to stimulate apoptosis (programmed cell death) of lymphoid and myeloid cells. The ceramide that is formed causes the activation of a ceramide-activated protein phosphatase (CAPP), a serine-threonine phosphatase related to protein phosphatase 2A. Ceramide action also may be mediated in part by ceramide-activated protein kinases.

Signal Transduction through Guanylyl Cyclase Receptors. Cyclic GMP is formed from GTP in a reaction that is catalyzed by guanylyl cyclase. In contrast to adenylyl cyclase, which is exclusively localized to the plasma membrane, two forms of guanylyl cyclase have been characterized. One is a heme-containing soluble enzyme composed of two subunits, and the other is a plasma membrane-associated protein. A third form of guanylyl cyclase, which is associated with structural elements, is present in retinal rod cells and is involved in the synthesis of cyclic GMP involved in the visual cycle. The plasma membrane–associated form was intensively studied since atrial natriuretic peptides were found to activate guanylyl cyclase and promote increased synthesis of cyclic GMP in target cells. The actions of ANP, which include vasodilation, natriuresis, and diuresis (see also Chapter 7), appear to be mediated either entirely or in part by its binding to and activation of the ANP receptor, a membrane-bound guanylyl cyclase (Fig. 3-3), resulting in increased production of the second messenger, cyclic GMP. Homodimerization of the receptor appears to be required for ANP binding and guanylyl cyclase activation. Binding of natriuretic peptide induces a conformational change in the intracellular protein kinase homology domain of receptor that results in binding of ATP. This decreases the repressive effect of the kinase homology domain on the guanylyl cyclase, leading to increased cyclic GMP formation. The mechanism(s) whereby cyclic GMP mediates the actions of ANP have yet to be elucidated; however, it is apparent that cyclic GMP serves to maintain cation channels in an open conformation. This action may, in part, explain the natriuretic action of ANP. The natriuretic action of ANP may also be mediated by its effect to inhibit aldosterone biosynthesis by glomerulosa cells of the adrenal cortex, resulting in decreased sodium reabsorption. In addition, cyclic GMP may function to activate a phosphodiesterase, which, in turn, lowers cyclic AMP levels. In this manner, cyclic GMP may act to antagonize the actions of cyclic AMP in a number of cell types.

Signal Transduction by Receptors That Contain Tyrosine Kinase Domains. As discussed above, cell surface receptors for insulin and other growth factors are transmembrane proteins that contain a cytoplasmic domain that is a tyrosine kinase. More than 50 receptor tyrosine kinases have been identified that belong to 14 different families. Binding of ligands to these receptors and subsequent activation of the tyrosine kinases results in changes in cell proliferation, differentiation, shape, and migration. Listed below are four of the families of receptor tyrosine kinases.

1. THE EGF, HER-2/NEU FAMILY: the structure of the EGF receptor has already been described. HER-2/neu, which is homologous to the EGF receptor and to the *neu* oncogene, has been found to be amplified in many adenocarcinomas and is overexpressed in breast tumors of a significant number of breast cancer patients. The identification of a ligand for this receptor, produced by human breast cancer cells in culture, suggests a role of HER-2/neu in autocrine growth regulation of breast tumors.

2. THE INSULIN/IGF-I RECEPTOR FAMILY: like the insulin receptor, discussed above, the IGF-I receptor is a tetramer consisting of two disulfide-linked heterodimers $(\alpha\beta)_2$. The IGF-I receptor differs from the insulin receptor in its extracellular cysteine-rich region, which is believed to be responsible for ligand binding, and in the C terminus downstream of the tyrosine kinase domain.

3. THE PDGF, CSF-1, AND c-KIT RECEPTOR FAMILY: Platelet-derived growth factor is released from platelets when they adhere to injured vessels and acts to stimulate proliferation of mesenchymal cells. Colony-stimulating factor-1 acts on hematopoietic precursor cells and promotes their differentiation into monocytes and macrophages. The *c-kit* proto-oncogene appears to encode a receptor for a mast cell growth factor. The extracellular regions of these receptors contain five repeats of an immunoglobulin-like domain containing cysteine residues. In contrast to the EGF and insulin receptors, the tyrosine kinase domains of this group of receptors contain a 70–100 amino acid insertion (Fig. 3-3). Platelet-derived growth factor and CSF-1 are disulfide-linked heterodimers. Platelet-derived growth factor–induced activation of its receptor involves receptor dimerization and interaction with specific cytoplasmic effector molecules.

4. THE FGF RECEPTOR FAMILY: There are as many as 21 different FGFs that mediate cell proliferation, migration, and differentiation. Certain FGFs play an important role in organogenesis during embryonic development. In addition, FGFs appear to play an important role in wound healing and angiogenesis. The extracellular domain of these receptors contains three immunoglobulin-like domains with two cysteines in each, like the PDGF receptor family. The tyrosine kinase domain also is divided into two regions by an inserted stretch of only 14 amino acids.

Most, if not all, of the actions of the tyrosine kinase family of receptors are mediated by ligand-induced receptor dimerization/oligomerization, tyrosine kinase activation, and autophosphorylation. With the exception of the insulin receptor (which already exists as a dimer of two disulfide-linked α,β-heterodimers [see above]), all receptor tyrosine kinases undergo dimerization on ligand binding. Receptor dimerization plays an essential role in tyrosine kinase activation, autophosphorylation, and transmembrane signaling. The tyrosine kinase of one receptor polypeptide chain catalyzes the phosphorylation of tyrosines on the other receptor chain in the dimer. Autophosphorylation of the receptor on tyrosine residues increases tyrosine kinase activity and enhances its capacity to phosphorylate other cellular target proteins. This occurs because the phosphorylated tyrosines on the receptor serve as binding or docking sites for target proteins that contain a sequence of amino acids referred to as a *src-homology 2* (SH2) domain. The SH2 domain is so named because of its similarity to a region present in *src*, a cellular proto-oncogene product involved in cell growth control. Src, which lacks an extracellular ligand-binding domain, is activated by binding to receptor tyrosine kinases via its SH2 region. The binding of Src or other cellular target proteins to activated receptor tyrosine kinases through their SH2 domains orients these proteins for phosphorylation by the activated receptor tyrosine kinase.

Many of the SH2-containing cellular proteins that bind to activated receptor tyrosine kinases are components of downstream signaling pathways that involve other second messenger systems. In this manner, the tyrosine kinase receptor family interacts with other signal transduction systems. As an example, PDGF binding to its receptor results in an increase in phosphatidylinositol turnover and in cytosolic calcium. This action of PDGF appears to be mediated in part by the association and activation of a specific isoform of phospholipase C (PLC), PLC-γ, which interacts via its SH2 domain with the phosphotyrosines in the cytoplasmic domain of the activated PDGF receptor and, consequently, is phosphorylated on tyrosine residues. The activated PLC, in turn, catalyzes the hydrolysis of PIP_2, resulting in the elaboration of IP_3 with an associated increase in cytoplasmic calcium. The PDGF activation of PLC also catalyzes the hydrolysis of PC. It has been postulated that increased DAG formed through PC hydrolysis and the associated PKC activation provides an important component of the mitogenic action of PDGF. Autophosphorylation sites of the activated, PDGF receptor also interact with the adaptor protein, growth factor receptor–bound protein 2 (Grb2), which then recruits guanine nucleotide exchange factors that promote the binding of GTP to Ras, which in turn binds and activates the serine-threonine protein kinase Raf. This ultimately results in the activation of mitogen-activated protein kinases (MAPKs), which phosphorylate a number of cellular proteins, including the transcription factor AP-1.

It therefore is apparent that the tyrosine kinase family of cell surface receptors acts in parallel as well as in a cross-talking manner with other receptor-regulated effector systems that involve G proteins. Some of these interactions are additive or synergistic, whereas others are antagonistic. The net result is the integrated control of cellular function, homeostasis, and growth.

Signal Transduction by Members of the Cytokine Receptor Family. As discussed above, receptors for growth hormone, prolactin, and other members of the cytokine receptor superfamily do not have kinase domains. Furthermore, the cytoplasmic domains of superfamily members have only limited sequence similarity; this is confined to a membrane proximal region, which is functionally required for mitogenic responses. In spite of the absence of a kinase domain, ligand binding results in the rapid phosphorylation of cellular proteins, as well as of the receptor itself, on tyrosine residues. The membrane proximal region of the receptor is required for coupling of ligand binding to tyrosine phosphorylation. Tyrosine phosphorylation is mediated by a family of cytoplasmic tyrosine kinases, the Janus kinases (JAKs). These kinases associate physically with the membrane proximal region of the ligand-bound receptor, resulting in autophosphorylation of tyrosine residues and further activation of the JAK kinase, and phosphorylation of the receptor, as well as of other cellular proteins that bind to the receptor–kinase complex by their SH2 domains. The major cellular targets for JAK kinases are members of a family of transcription factors called *signal transducers and activators of transcription* (STATs), which bind to phosphorylated tyrosines on the activated receptor via their SH2 domains. Phosphorylation of STATs on tyrosine residues results in their dimerization and activation and subsequent binding to specific response elements within the regulatory regions of genes. It is apparent that receptor dimerization, which occurs as a result of ligand binding, is essential to initiation of the signal transduction cascade. The receptor dimerization causes an increased affinity for JAKs and facilitates cross-phosphorylation of their phosphorylation sites. A hypothetical model of the signal transduction pathway mediated by the binding of growth hormone to its receptor is presented in schematic form in Figure 3-7.

Four JAK kinase family members have been identified: JAK1, JAK2, JAK3, and tyk2; these have specificity for different ligand–receptor complexes. For example, JAK2 has been found to be associated with activated growth hormone, prolactin, and erythropoietin receptors; activated interferon-α/β receptors associate with JAK1 and tyk2; interferon-γ receptors associate with JAK1 and JAK2; and activated IL-2 receptors associate with JAK3. Further complexity results from the identification of at least four different STAT proteins, which appear to be substrates for the different JAKs. It should also be noted that binding of EGF and PDGF to their receptors, which have intrinsic tyrosine kinase activity and are autophosphorylated, promotes tyrosine phosphorylation of JAK1 and activation of a STAT1 transcription factor that binds as part of a complex to an enhancer in the c-*fos* promoter. Another family of proteins—the suppressor of cytokine signaling (SOCS) proteins—which contain an SH2 domain, suppress cytokine signaling by interacting with phosphorylated tyrosines on the receptors or on the JAKs. This blocks the interaction of signaling proteins (e.g., STATs) and inhibits the catalytic activity of the JAKs.

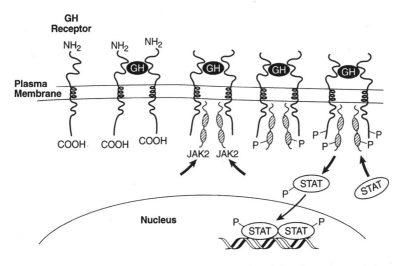

Fig. 3-7 Signal transduction mechanisms associated with binding of growth hormone (GH) to its receptor. The binding of a single molecule of GH promotes receptor dimerization. This in turn results in an increased affinity of the membrane-proximal region of the cytoplasmic domain of the receptor for the cytoplasmic tyrosine kinase, JAK2, a member of the Janus kinase family, which undergoes autophosphorylation and further activation. The activated JAK2 catalyzes phosphorylation of the recpetor. The phosphorylated tyrosines on the receptor now serve as docking sites for STAT (signal transducers and activators of transcription) transcription factors, which bind via an *src-homology* 2 (SH2) domain and are phosphorylated on tyrosine residues. The phosphorylated STATs form dimers and bind as a dimeric complex to a specific enhancer element in the regulatory region of a GH-inducible gene (i.e., insulin-like growth factor-I), resulting in increased transcription initiation.

STEROID HORMONES

Steroid hormones exert long-term effects on their target cells; they stimulate cell growth and differentiation and regulate the synthesis of specific proteins. Steroid hormones exert these actions on target cells after binding to specific receptors, which are ligand-inducible transcription factors that are localized primarily within the nucleus. The steroid–receptor complex regulates the synthesis of specific proteins primarily by altering the rate of transcription of specific genes. The first clear indication that steroid hormones could interact with specific genes and alter their activity was the finding in 1960 that the insect steroid ecdysone rapidly induced the formation of puffs in specific regions of the salivary gland polytene chromosomes of the midge *Chironomus*. It has subsequently been shown that the puffs correspond to active genes; several of these genes have been found to encode salivary proteins. Although the ecdysteroids were the first of the steroid hormones shown to regulate gene activity, studies of the receptors and mechanisms of action of steroid hormones in vertebrates rapidly progressed and outpaced those concerning the ecdysteroids. This was primarily due to the synthesis of radiolabeled vertebrate steroid hormones of high specific activity and the subsequent discovery of receptor proteins in cells of vertebrates.

Over the past two decades, studies in a large number of laboratories have led to a generally accepted hypothesis for the mechanism of action of steroid hormones (Fig. 3-8). Steroids travel in the circulation predominantly bound to several classes of serum proteins. Estrogens and androgens are transported in the circulation bound to sex hormone-binding globulin (SHBG), which binds estradiol-17β and testosterone with relatively high affinity ($K_d \approx 10^{-9}\ M$). These steroids are also weakly bound to serum albumin. Glucocorticoids and progesterone are bound in the circulation to corticosteroid-binding globulin (CBG), also referred to as *transcortin*. It is generally believed that only the free steroid can enter cells (see Chapter 5). Presumably, steroids can diffuse freely across the plasma membranes of all cells but are sequestered only within cells that contain specific intracellular receptors. The steroid binds to its receptor with an affinity ($K_d \approx 10^{-10}\ M$) that is at least 10-fold greater than the affinity with which it binds to the serum globulins.

Steroid Hormone Receptors

Cellular Localization

An issue that has been a source of controversy over the years is the subcellular localization of the unoccupied or so-called free steroid receptor. There has always been general agreement that the occupied or *bound* steroid receptor has increased affinity for chromatin and is localized to the nucleus. It was believed for some time, however, that the free steroid receptor was a cytoplasmic protein that moved to the nucleus only after binding hormone and undergoing an undefined process termed *transformation* or *activation*. This concept was derived from studies in which cells not previously exposed to a given steroid were homogenized and cytosolic and nuclear fractions were prepared by differential centrifugation. When these fractions were incubated with the radiolabeled steroid, the receptor was usually found to be present predominantly in the cytosol. On the other hand, if the cells were first in-

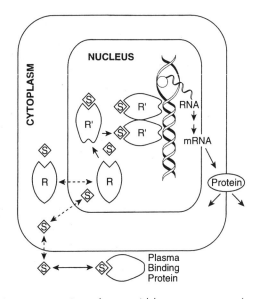

Fig. 3-8 Schematic representation of a steroid hormone–responsive cell. Steroid hormones (S) in the circulation are predominantly bound to specific proteins. Only a small proportion of the circulating steroid is free; it is the unbound steroid that has the capacity to enter cells by free diffusion. Within target cells, the steroids bind with high affinity to specific receptors that are primarily localized within the nucleus. After binding steroid, the receptor (R) undergoes a process of *activation,* which involves dissociation from heat shock proteins and formation of a receptor dimer. The receptor dimer binds to specific sequences of DNA proximate to steroid-regulated genes. The binding of the receptor as a dimer to these genomic regions can result in increases or decreases in the rates of gene expression. The steroid–receptor complex is believed to increase the rate of transcription of specific genes by causing the formation of a stable preinitiation complex and facilitating the binding of RNA polymerase II to the promoter regions of such genes. This results in the synthesis of RNA molecules that are processed within the nucleus to mRNAs that enter the cytoplasm and are translated into specific proteins.

cubated with the steroid hormone, then homogenized and subcellular fractions prepared, the receptor was found to be present almost exclusively in the nuclear fraction. With the availability of monoclonal antibodies specific for a number of steroid receptors and the technique of immunocytochemistry, it has generally been found that both the free and occupied steroid receptors are localized to the nucleus. Receptors for thyroid hormones, retinoic acid, and 1,25-dihydroxyvitamin D_3 are present within the nucleus, bound to their respective *hormone responsive elements* (HREs) in the absence or presence of bound hormone. By contrast, receptors for glucocorticoids (GR), progesterone (PR), estrogen (ER), androgens (AR), and mineralocorticoids (MR) in the absence of hormone binding are not bound to their respective HREs. Rather, these *free* receptors are present within the nucleus (PR, ER, AR, MR) or cytoplasm (GR) bound to a complex of heat shock proteins (hsps). On hormone binding, these receptors are released from the hsp complex and are activated to a DNA-binding, transcription-modulating state (see below). These activated receptors are now found within the nucleus bound to their respective HREs, which usually lie upstream of target genes.

Receptor Structure

The steroid hormone receptors belong to a superfamily of so-called *nuclear receptors* that also includes the receptor for 1,25-dihydroxyvitamin D_3, several tissue-specific forms of receptors for thyroid hormones and retinoic acid, as well as a large number of nuclear proteins for which ligands have not as yet been identified (*orphan receptors*). As mentioned above, these molecules are members of a large superfamily of ligand-activated transcription factors that bind to specific sequences of DNA and regulate the transcriptional activity of specific genes. The nuclear receptors comprise a superfamily of 48 transcription factors. The superfamily can be divided into three subfamilies: Type I receptors bind the steroid hormones. These include the GR, MR, AR, and ER. Type II receptors bind thyroid hormones (TR), all-*trans* retinoic acid (RAR), 9-*cis* retinoic acid (RXR), and 1,25 dihydroxyvitamin D_3 (VDR). Type III receptors, the orphan receptors, have no known ligands. Ligands for some of the orphan receptors have recently been found to be fatty acids and metabolites of cholesterol.

All of these receptors have the same general structure (Fig. 3-9) as well as a high degree of homology in their hormone-binding and DNA-binding regions. By comparison with the nucleotide sequences of the mRNAs as well as the deduced amino acid sequences of the receptor proteins, it has been found that there are specific domains that are highly conserved structurally and functionally among all members of this superfamily. The region of greatest homology is the DNA-binding domain (DBD), which is composed of 66–68 amino acids and contains nine perfectly conserved cysteine residues. This domain contains two repeated units enriched in the amino acids Cys, Lys, and Arg. Such repeated units have been identified in a number of nucleic acid–binding proteins. Each of these units is folded into a finger-

---

Fig. 3-9 *Upper panel:* Schematic representation of the zinc finger–containing DNA-binding domain of the glucocorticoid receptor. Amino acids in the P-box (important in recognition of the sequence of the DNA half-site) and the D-box (important in receptor dimerization and recognition of the spacing of the two half-sites in the response element) are highlighted. The amino acids of the P-box, which are important for half-site recognition of three different groups of receptors and the sequences of the half-sites to which they bind, are indicated. *Lower panel:* Domain structures of members of the nuclear receptor superfamily, including human receptors for glucocorticoid (hGR), mineralocorticoid (hMR), androgen (hAR), progesterone (hPR), estrogen (hER), retinoic acid (hRAR), thyroid hormone (hTR), 1,25-dihydroxyvitamin D_3 (hVDR), and the orphan receptor, hCOUP. Three highly conserved regions are indicated, the DNA-binding domain (DBD) and two regions involved in hormone binding (HBD_1 and HBD_2). The numbers within these regions indicate the percentage of amino acid similarity with hGR. The hypervariable region of the receptors extends from the amino terminus (indicated by the number 1) to the DBD. The number at the right end of each schematic indicates the number of amino acids in each receptor protein. The nuclear receptors can be divided into three subfamilies based on phylogenetic analysis, structure, and function: Type I—the classical steroid receptors; Type II—TR, RAR, VDR; Type III—COUP and other *orphan* receptors. RXR, retinoid-X receptor.

like structure containing four cysteines that coordinate one zinc ion. The loop of the so-called zinc finger is made up of 12–13 amino acids; a spacer region of 15–17 amino acids is present between the two fingers (Fig. 3-9). These DNA-binding fingers have the capacity to insert into a half-turn of DNA. Such repeated units have been identified in a number of nuclear proteins that are known to act as transcription factors.

Near the carboxyterminal end of the receptor molecules are two conserved regions (HBD$_1$ and HBD$_2$) of 42 and 22 hydrophobic amino acids, respectively, which comprise the hormone-binding domain (HBD). The HBD also contains a transcription activation domain, termed *activation function 2* (AF-2), which is essential for

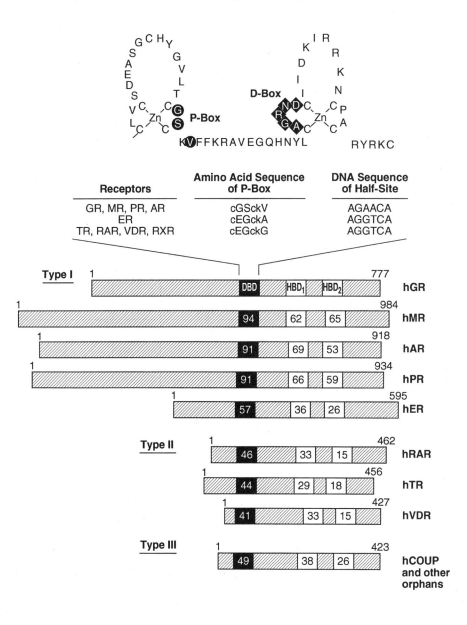

ligand-dependent activation of transcription by nuclear receptors. The carboxyter-minal regions of the members of this superfamily of receptors have a high degree of sequence similarity with the v-Erb-A protein of the oncogenic avian erythro-blastosis virus. The v-Erb-A protein, which is not oncogenic by itself, increases the oncogenic potential of another viral protein, v-Erb-B (which has a high degree of sequence homology with the tyrosine kinase domain of the EGF receptor, as previ-ously discussed). Estrogens stimulate the growth of estrogen receptor–positive mam-mary tumors and have been implicated as contributory factors in the pathogenesis of human breast cancer. These effects could be mediated through the induction of synthesis of growth factors or through a direct action on growth factor receptors. It has been postulated that the estrogen receptor may potentiate the action of an onco-gene in breast cancer in much the same way that *v-erb-A* potentiates the oncogenic potential of *v-erb-B*.

The region of these receptors between the aminoterminus and the DBD is hy-pervariable (HV) both in size and in amino acid sequence (Fig. 3-9). For example, the HV region of the glucocorticoid receptor is 421 amino acids in size, whereas the HV region of the receptor for VDR consists of only 24 amino acids. This re-gion contains a ligand-independent transcriptional activation domain (AF-1). The transcription factor COUP, which is involved in the transcriptional activation of a number of genes, including those for chicken ovalbumin, mammalian insulin, and pro-opiomelanocortin, is a member of the nuclear receptor superfamily of proteins based on structural homology. Like the thyroid hormone (TR), retinoic acid (RAR), and VDR receptors, COUP binds to DNA as a heterodimer with the retinoid-X re-ceptor (RXR); however, the existence of a ligand for COUP remains to be deter-mined. The finding that the carboxyterminal region of COUP has significant se-quence similarity to other members of the steroid receptor superfamily, and that this region of COUP is evolutionarily conserved, is suggestive of the existence of such a ligand. It has been suggested that COUP may be activated by a ligand produced within the same cell in which it is synthesized. It is postulated that the steroid re-ceptor superfamily originated from a primordial receptor gene in primitive organ-isms in which it may have served as a receptor for environmental nutrients and other factors. The different classes of receptors for steroids and other regulatory mole-cules within the present superfamily of receptors and related molecules evolved in response to the increasing regulatory requirements imposed by cellular specializa-tion of higher eukaryotes.

Molecular Forms and Receptor Transformation (Activation)

Free GR, MR, AR, PR, and ER are believed to exist in the cell as monomers that are associated with a complex of proteins that includes two molecules of a 90,000 dalton phosphoprotein, hsp90, one molecule of hsp70, and a number of other pro-teins (Fig. 3-10). In this conformation the receptor is incapable of binding DNA or regulating gene transcription. The binding of hormone to the receptor results in the dissociation of receptor from this complex, which forms a homodimer with another receptor molecule. This receptor homodimer has a greatly increased affinity for bind-ing to HREs in DNA. On binding to DNA, the receptor homodimer recruits pro-teins termed *coactivators*, which facilitate transcription initiation by mechanisms to be described below. By contrast, *free* TR, RAR, and VDR are not bound to hsps.

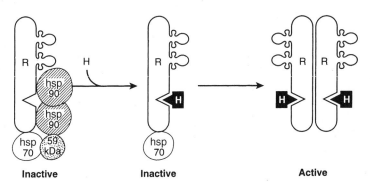

Fig. 3-10 Proposed mechanism for hormone-induced activation of the glucocorticoid receptor. The inactive *free* glucocorticoid receptor (R) exists in the cytoplasm as a monomer in association with a protein complex composed of two molecules of heat shock protein (hsp)90, one molecule of hsp70, and a number of other proteins. After hormone (H) binding, the receptor dissociates from the hsp complex and forms a homodimer with another molecule of glucocorticoid receptor. This process is required for transformation of the receptor to a DNA-binding, transcription-modulating state.

Rather, they are bound to their HREs either as homodimers or as heterodimers with a molecule of a member of the retinoic acid receptor subfamily, termed *retinoid-X receptor*. In their free state, receptors in this subgroup recruit proteins termed *corepressors* and inhibit transcription of their respective target genes by mechanisms to be described below. On hormone binding, the corepressors are released and replaced by *coactivators*, which facilitate transcription initiation, as above.

Regulation of Gene Expression by Members of the Nuclear Receptor Superfamily

The primary action of steroid, retinoid, and thyroid hormones is to regulate the rate of transcription of specific genes and thus to alter the synthesis of specific proteins. As discussed above, certain members of the nuclear receptor superfamily (Types I and II) are ligand-activated transcription factors that increase gene transcription on hormone binding. This group of transcription factors interacts with specific genomic sequences, the so-called HREs, which are predominantly localized in the 5′-flanking regions of target genes, usually within several hundred base pairs upstream of the transcription initiation sites. The activated forms of these receptors bind to their HREs as homodimers (GR, MR, AR, PR, ER) or as heterodimers with RXR (TR, VDR, RAR).

Hormone-Response Elements and Regulation of Gene Transcription

After hormone binding and receptor activation, the GR, PR, MR, AR, and ER bind as homodimers to their respective HREs. The GR, PR, MR, and AR bind to an identical core HRE, which consists of a double-stranded inverted repeat or palindrome of six nucleotides (half-site) separated by a three-nucleotide spacer:

AGAACAnnnTGTTCT

TCTTGTnnnACAAGA

The fact that more than one hormone receptor binds to the same sequence of DNA implies that specificity is dependent on the type of hormone receptor(s) present in the target cell. Additionally, DNA sequences outside of the core HRE, as well as interaction with other transcription factors bound to other *cis*-acting enhancer elements, may be responsible for differential activation of target genes by structurally related hormone receptors.

The ER does not bind to HRE recognized by GR, MR, AR, and PR. Rather, the ER binds specifically to an HRE that consists of a double-stranded inverted repeat of similar sequence, also with a three-nucleotide spacer:

AGGTCAnnnTGACCT

TCCAGTnnnACTGGA

Specificity for the primary sequence of the DNA half-site (e.g., AGAACA vs. AG-GTCA) is determined by three amino acids in the shoulder of the first zinc finger of the receptors, the so-called P-box (Fig. 3-9). In the GR, MR, PR, and AR, these amino acids are glycine, serine, and valine. By contrast, in the ER, these amino acids are glutamate, glycine, and alanine. Within the shoulder of the second zinc finger is the *dimerization* box (D-box) (Fig. 3-9). This region of the receptor is important for dimerization of the two receptor monomers and establishes orientation of the monomers for appropriate binding to differentially spaced half-sites.

Receptors for TH, retinoids, and 1,25-dihydroxyvitamin D_3 usually bind as heterodimers with RXR to a double-stranded, direct hexameric repeat separated by a spacer of one to five nucleotides. Although the sequence of the half-site is the same as that of the estrogen-responsive element ([ERE] AGGTCA/TGACCT), binding specificity is determined by the presence of a direct repeat, rather than a palindrome (as is the case for the ERE), and by the number of nucleotides in the spacer. As an example, the VDR-RXR heterodimer preferentially binds to a direct repeat with a three-nucleotide spacer, the TR-RXR heterodimer binds preferentially to a direct repeat with a four-nucleotide spacer, and the RAR-RXR heterodimer binds preferentially to a direct repeat with a five-nucleotide spacer, as shown below.

AGGTCAn$_{1-5}$AGGTCA

TCCAGTn$_{1-5}$TCCAGT

Glucocorticoid, Mineralocorticoid, Progesterone, and Androgen Receptor Regulation of Gene Expression. A model of the proposed mechanism whereby steroid hormones such as glucocorticoids, mineralocorticoids, progesterone, and androgens regulate eukaryotic gene expression is shown in Figure 3-11. After binding a molecule of hormone, the receptor undergoes a conformational change, is released from the complex with hsp90 and other hsps, and forms a homodimer with another receptor molecule. The receptor dimer now binds with high affinity to an HRE, which usually exists within several hundred base pairs upstream of the target gene. The receptor dimer, which may be phosphorylated, can now recruit a complex of coactivators containing histone acetyltransferase (histone acetylase) activities. Histone acetylation causes destabilization of the nucleosomal structure and a local opening

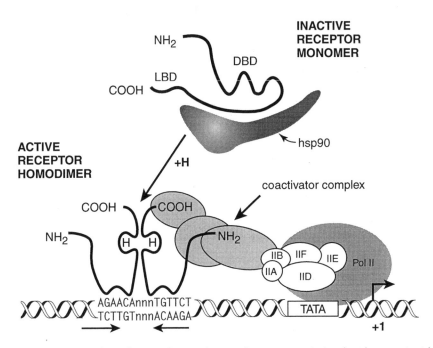

Fig. 3-11 Proposed mechanism for regulation of gene transcription by glucocorticoid, progesterone, mineralocorticoid, and androgen receptors. After binding hormone (H), the receptor dissociates from a complex with heat shock protein 90 (hsp90) and other proteins and binds to its hormone response element upstream of the target gene as a homodimer. The activated receptor dimer can now recruit a complex of coactivators containing histone acetyltransferase activity. This results in an opening of chromatin structure, which facilitates assembly of the preinitiation complex, the binding of RNA polymerase II, and activation of transcription initiation. DBD, DNA-binding domain; LBD, ligand-binding domain.

of chromatin into a transcriptionally permissive state. This results in recruitment of general (i.e., basal) transcription factors to form a stable preinitiation complex at the TATA box. Coactivators (which do not bind to DNA directly) also serve to bridge transcription factors with the basal transcription complex, resulting in further stabilization, the recruitment of RNA polymerase II (Pol II) and initiation of gene transcription. The formation of the preinitiation complex may be a sequential process; the binding of transcription factor IIB (TFIIB) is the rate-limiting step. It has been found that a number of receptors in the nuclear receptor superfamily can bind directly to TFIIB. This suggests that the nuclear receptors also may facilitate the interaction of TFIIB with the preinitiation complex.

Thyroid, Retinoid, and Vitamin D_3 Receptor Regulation of Gene Expression. As discussed above, receptors for retinoids, THs, and 1,25-dihydroxyvitamin D_3, when bound to their HREs in the absence of ligand binding, cause silencing of their target genes. The proposed mechanism whereby the active thyroid hormone tri-iodothyronine (T_3) regulates gene expression is shown in Figure 3-12. In the ab-

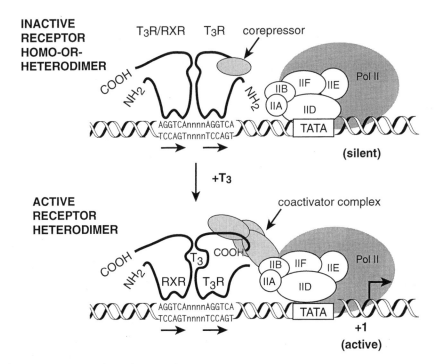

Fig. 3-12 Proposed mechanism for regulation of gene transcription by thyroid hormones, retinoids, and 1,25-dihydroxyvitamin D_3. In its *free* state, the thyroid hormone receptor (T_3R) binds to its hormone response element as homodimer (shown), or as a heterodimer with a molecule of retinoid-X receptor (RXR). The free T_3R interacts with a complex of corepressors containing histone deacetylase activity, which silence transcription by promoting a closed chromation structure and preventing formation of a stable preinitiation complex. On binding of triiodothyronine (T_3), the receptor undergoes a conformational change resulting in the dissociation of the corepressor and association of a complex of coactivators containing histone acetyltransferase. This in turn facilitates transcription initiation by mechanisms described in the legend to Figure 3-11.

sence of hormone binding, the thyroid hormone receptor (T_3R) is bound to its response element (a direct repeat of the sequence AGGTCA with a four-nucleotide spacer) as a homodimer or heterodimer with RXR. The *free* receptor dimer interacts with a co-repressor complex containing histone deacetylases, which keep chromatin in a *closed* conformation and silence transcription. The binding of T_3 to T_3R stabilizes formation of a heterodimer with RXR, and causes dissociation of the corepressor complex and recruitment of a coactivator complex containing histone acetyltransferases. As described above, histone acetylation causes destabilization of the nucleosomal structure, resulting in an opening of the local chromatin structure into a transcriptionally permissive state that allows assembly of the preinitiation complex. Coactivators also facilitate interaction of transcription factors with the basal transcription complex, resulting in its stabilization, the recruitment of Pol II and initiation of transcription of thyroid hormone–responsive genes.

Tissue-Specific Expression of Hormonally Regulated Genes

The phenotype of a given cell is the result of the complement of genes that are expressed; the expression of a number of these cellular genes is subject to hormonal regulation. A hormone acting through its cellular receptors can regulate the expression of different genes in different tissues. For example, estrogen regulates the expression of the ovalbumin gene in the chick oviduct and the vitellogenin gene in chick liver. Since the ERs in oviduct and liver tissues are apparently identical, and since the DNA sequences within and surrounding eukaryotic genes should be essentially the same in all cell types of a given organism, there must be other structural features that determine which genes are expressible and available to hormonal regulation. The complement of genes that are expressed in a given cell type is determined at the time of cellular differentiation. It is apparent that such expressible genes exist in so-called DNase I–sensitive regions; that is, they reside in *open* regions of the chromatin that are more readily digested *in vitro* by DNase I than is the bulk of chromosomal DNA. The DNase I–sensitive regions define the structural framework in a given cell for the genes that are available for expression. Most of the cellular genes are not expressed and are tightly packaged with histone proteins in higher-order chromosomal structures, rendering them DNase I resistant.

Steroid Receptor Effects Mediated by Protein–Protein Interactions

Some of the actions of steroid hormones are mediated by direct interaction of the steroid receptor with another transcription factor rather than a response element in DNA. This frequently represses that transcription factor's capacity to activate its target genes. An example of this mode of action involves the anti-inflammatory effects of glucocorticoids. The ligand-activated GR exerts its anti-inflammatory effects in part by direct interaction with the transcription factor nuclear factor κB (NF-κB). This, in turn, represses NF-κB–mediated transcription of genes encoding a number of inflammatory cytokines, as well as cyclooxygenase-2 (COX-2), which catalyzes the rate-limiting step in synthesis of inflammatory prostaglandins (see Chapter 4).

Nongenomic Actions of Steroid Hormones

The actions of steroid hormones to activate or inhibit transcription of specific genes—*genomic actions*—occur within the nucleus and typically take one or more hours or even days. However, numerous effects of steroid hormones have been reported that occur within seconds to minutes after exposure to the hormone. These rapid effects do not involve direct binding of steroid receptors to response elements in DNA, but rather are mediated by interaction either with *classical* steroid receptors or with G protein–coupled receptors localized within the plasma membrane. Such rapid nongenomic effects have been described for all of the steroid receptors, as well as the VDR and TR.

Steroid Hormone Actions via Classical Steroid Receptors within the Plasma Membrane

Rapid effects of estrogen to activate the MAPK pathway have been reported to occur through interactions with classical ER within the plasma membrane. These effects are typically inhibited by ER antagonists. The ER has been found to activate MAPK through its interaction with either the IGF-I receptor or with c-Src or its downstream targets. The interaction of ER with c-Src occurs through the c-Src SH2 domain and results in activation of c-Src kinase activity. These events likely mediate some of the actions of estradiol-17β to stimulate cell proliferation in the breast and uterus. The transport of the ER to the plasma membrane has been suggested to be facilitated by *caveolin*, a major structural protein of *caveolae*, which are plasmalemmal vesicles of the plasma membrane. Caveolin serves as a scaffold for assembly of various signaling molecules. One of the rapid actions of estrogen that is believed to occur in caveolae is the activation of *endothelial nitric oxide synthase* (eNOS). This effect of estrogen appears to be mediated by direct ER activation of phosphatidylinositol-3 kinase, which in turn catalyzes the phosphorylation of another kinase (Akt or protein kinase B), which subsequently catalyzes phosphorylation of eNOS, leading to its activation. The activated eNOS promotes the synthesis of nitric oxide in vascular endothelial cells, leading to vasodilation and increased blood flow.

Steroid Hormone Actions via Other Membrane-Associated Receptors

Rapid effects of estrogens, androgens, and mineralocorticoids to alter rates of phosphatidylinositol turnover, concentrations of cytosolic calcium, MAPK pathways, and adenylyl cyclase activity are reported to occur via interaction of the steroids with a number of G protein–coupled receptors. These effects are not inhibited by steroid receptor antagonists. Progesterone has also been found to inhibit the function of the nicotinic acetylcholine receptor in *Xenopus* oocytes by direct interaction with the nictonic receptor extracellular domain and to alter reproductive behavior by direct interaction with a membrane-associated binding protein in brain. Progesterone or one of its metabolites also has been found to bind with relatively high affinity to the G protein–coupled oxytocin receptor and block its function to increase uterine contractility associated with labor.

ENDOCRINE DISORDERS DUE TO ALTERATIONS IN RECEPTOR NUMBER AND FUNCTION

As discussed above, changes in the concentration of cellular receptors for a specific hormone can markedly alter the sensitivity of the target cell to that hormone; a decrease in the concentration of receptors can decrease sensitivity to the hormone, whereas an increase in receptor concentration can increase the sensitivity of the target cell to the hormone. It is apparent that the concentration of cellular receptors for a specific hormone can vary considerably with the physiological state and that the concentration of the hormone itself can regulate the concentration of its own receptors on target cells. Most commonly, an increase in the level of a specific hormone will cause a decrease in the available number of its cellular receptors. This decrease in available receptors can be due either to receptor phosphorylation by a specific kinase and sequestration of receptors away from the cell surface or to an actual disappearance or loss of receptors from the cell. This hormonally induced negative regulation of receptors is termed *homologous down-regulation* or *desensi-*

tization. Studies of the down-regulation of receptors for insulin and EGF by the homologous hormones indicate that down-regulation is caused, at least in part, by a clustering of hormone–receptor complexes in coated pits on the cell surface, internalization within coated vesicles, and degradation by lysosomal enzymes. Coated pits and coated vesicles are so named because they contain a single protein, clathrin, that forms a *coat* on their cytoplasmic surfaces. There is little doubt that receptor internalization provides an important homeostatic mechanism that serves to protect the organism from the potential toxic effects of hormone excess.

Desensitization is defined as a decrease in the responsiveness of a cell to a constant level of hormone or factor on prolonged exposure. Homologous desensitization also can result from a hormone-induced alteration in the receptor (e.g., phosphorylation), which uncouples it from some component of the signal transduction pathway. Another form of desensitization, *heterologous desensitization*, occurs when incubation with one agonist reduces the responsiveness of a cell to a number of other agonists that act through different receptors. This phenomenon is most commonly observed with receptors that act through the adenylyl cyclase system. Heterologous desensitization reflects a broad pattern of refractoriness that has a slower onset than homologous desensitization.

In certain instances, endocrine dysfunction arises from pathological alterations in receptor levels and/or function. Specific examples of such endocrine dysfunction are discussed below.

Endocrine Dysfunction Caused by Homologous and Heterologous Receptor Regulation

The process of homologous down-regulation of receptors may be a contributing factor to a number of clinical states. Probably the most common receptor defect in humans is the down-regulation of insulin receptors that is caused by the chronic hyperinsulinemia of obesity. Obesity is generally characterized by hyperinsulinemia, variable degrees of glucose intolerance, and resistance to both endogenous and exogenously administered insulin. The insulin resistance associated with obesity is caused, at least in part, by a decrease in the concentration of available insulin receptors on target cells because of increased insulin receptor endocytosis and degradation; postreceptor defects may play some role in the reduced sensitivity to insulin. When obese individuals are maintained on calorie-restricted diets for several weeks, there is a marked reduction in the circulating insulin concentration, an increase in the concentration of insulin receptors on target cells, and a decline in the insulin resistance.

Another example of endocrine dysfunction resulting from homologous desensitization is the reduced sensitivity to both endogenous and exogenous catecholamines that results from the use of β-adrenergic agonists as bronchodilators in the treatment of asthma. This reduced sensitivity to catecholamines is caused by a β-adrenergic agonist–induced reduction in the concentration of β-adrenergic receptors on the cell surface and by reduced coupling of receptors to adenylyl cyclase. Homologous desensitization of β-adrenergic receptors is associated with phosphorylation of the receptors by a G protein–coupled receptor kinase. The phosphorylation of the receptors promotes the binding of an *arrestin* molecule, which prevents further interaction between the receptor and the G protein by steric hindrance. The sequestered receptors are then either recycled to the cell surface or targeted for degradation within lysosomes.

There are a number of examples of one hormone acting through its own receptors to alter the sensitivity of target cells to another hormone. Thyroid hormones can enhance the sensitivity of cardiac muscle cells to catecholamines by increasing the number of β-adrenergic receptors. This can result in an increased heart rate, atrial fibrillation, and congestive failure. Frequently, an alteration in cardiac function is the only manifestation of an otherwise masked hyperthyroidism.

Endocrine Dysfunction Caused by Autoimmune Disease Involving Antireceptor Antibodies

The presence of antibodies to receptors appears to be of central importance in several disease states.

Acetylcholine Receptors
In myasthenia gravis, a disease characterized by muscle weakness and flaccid paralysis, there are circulating antibodies to the nicotinic acetylcholine receptors localized in the neuromuscular junctions. These antibodies do not block the binding of acetylcholine to the receptor; however, they enhance the rate of receptor degradation and thus render the skeletal muscle cells less sensitive to endogenous acetylcholine.

Thyroid-Stimulating Hormone
Individuals with hyperthyroidism associated with diffuse goiter (Graves' disease) have circulating antibodies to the receptor for TSH, a polypeptide hormone produced by the anterior pituitary that acts on the thyroid gland to stimulate the production of the thyroid hormones (see Chapter 13). One of the effects of the thyroid hormones is to act on the hypothalamus and pituitary to inhibit the production of TSH. These autoantibodies bind to the TSH receptors on thyroid cells and mimic the actions of TSH itself. Since such antibodies are not regulated by negative feedback of the thyroid hormones, as is TSH, the thyroid gland is persistently stimulated to produce elevated levels of circulating thyroid hormones (see Chapter 13).

Insulin Receptors
In patients who have an unusual form of diabetes associated with insulin resistance, there are circulating autoantibodies to the insulin receptor. The antibodies bind to insulin receptors, block insulin binding, and mimic insulin action. This usually results in desensitization to endogenous insulin with associated hyperinsulinemia and extreme insulin resistance. In rare instances, receptor desensitization does not occur and the patient manifests severe hypoglycemia.

Disorders Due to Receptor and Postreceptor Defects

Disorders Due to Defects in G Protein–Coupled Signal Transduction
As previously mentioned, the family of guanine nucleotide-binding (G) proteins mediate the actions of a wide variety of hormones and factors in tissues throughout the body. The massive secretory diarrhea associated with *Vibrio cholerae* infection was

the first disorder found to be caused by the modification of a G protein. As discussed above, the cholera exotoxin catalyzes ADP-ribosylation of arginine 201 of $G\alpha_s$ in intestinal epithelial cells. This causes a marked inactivation of the GTPase activity associated with this subunit, resulting in persistent activation of adenylyl cyclase and of cyclic AMP formation. It now is apparent that there are a variety of somatic mutations of G proteins that result in their activation or inactivation. Two endocrine disorders associated with activation and inhibition of G_s function are described below.

McCune-Albright Syndrome. This disorder is caused by a missense mutation of arginine 201 of $G\alpha_s$ resulting in decreased GTPase activity and constitutive activation of adenylyl cyclase in one or more endocrine glands, including the adrenal cortex, gonads, thyroid, and pituitary thyrotrophs. This results in elevated levels of cyclic AMP formation, abnormal cell proliferation, and hyperfunction of the affected endocrine tissues. The symptoms can include acromegaly, precocious puberty, hyperthyroidism, hyperparathyroidism, Cushing's syndrome, fibrous dysplasia of bone that is polyostotic (involving more than one bone), and café au lait skin pigmentation.

Parathyroid Hormone–Resistant Hypoparathyroidism. Subjects with this disorder manifest a variety of missense mutations in the gene encoding $G\alpha_s$ that include loss-of-function mutations and mutations that prevent coupling of $G\alpha_s$ with activating receptors. Most affected individuals manifest a 50% decrease in $G\alpha_s$ activity. This results in pseudohypoparathyroidism (see Chapter 15) accompanied by variable resistance to a variety of hormones that act through adenylyl cyclase activation, including TSH, gonadotropins, and other hormones that act through G_s-coupled receptors.

Endocrine Tumors—Multiple Endocrine Neoplasia Type 1 (MEN1)

This collection of hereditary endocrinopathies involves benign and occasionally malignant neoplasms of endocrine glands, including the parathyroids, anterior pituitary, and enteropancreatic neuroendocrine tissues that result from a somatic mutation of the *MEN1* gene. Tumor recurrence postoperatively is a common sequela. The *MEN1* gene appears to be a tumor suppressor gene. As with other tumor suppressor genes, in the case of *MEN1*, one copy of the mutated gene is inherited from one parent. Tumors arise when the second gene copy is subsequently mutated by a so-called second hit. Acquired mutations of the *MEN1* gene also appear to be involved in sporadic parathyroid adenomas, insulinomas, gastrinomas, and bronchial carcinoids.

Androgen Resistance

Testosterone, the major steroid product of the Leydig cells of the testis and the principal circulating androgen, serves as a prohormone in most androgen target tissues for dihydrotestosterone, which is formed from testosterone in these tissues by the action of the enzyme 5α-reductase (see Chapter 10). During embryogenesis, androgens produced by the fetal testis play a critical role in the differentiation of the male internal and external genitalia (see Chapter 8).

Androgen resistance can be caused by (*1*) complete absence, diminished amounts, or qualitative abnormalities of AR in target tissues or (*2*) defects in the signal transduction pathway despite apparently normal androgen binding. The gene that encodes the androgen receptor is X linked; therefore, mutations are expressed in the hemizygous 46,XY state. A syndrome of complete androgen resistance in humans, *termed testicular feminization* (see Chapter 8), is commonly due to decreased amounts of functional AR. Testicular feminization has been found to be associated with a variety of point mutations scattered throughout the AR gene. Such mutations can result either in the insertion of a premature translational *stop codon,* so that a truncated nonfunctional protein is synthesized, or in a loss of functional activity of the hormone-binding or DNA-binding domains. Affected genotypic males are born with female external genitalia and a blind vaginal pouch. Wolffian duct structures are absent or vestigial; müllerian duct structures are absent, and the external genitalia are female. Testes are present in the labia, inguinal canals, or abdomen. At puberty, these individuals develop female secondary sex characteristics. Since the negative feedback of testosterone at the hypothalamic-pituitary level is defective, circulating levels of LH and testosterone are elevated. Increased levels of LH cause enhanced secretion of estrogen by the testis, and the increased estrogen production contributes to the development of female secondary sex characteristics at puberty.

Vitamin D Resistance

Vitamin D–dependent rickets types I and II are inherited disorders in the pathway of vitamin D action. Both are inherited as autosomal recessive traits and are associated with childhood rickets and adult abnormalities of bone mineralization termed *osteomalacia.* Vitamin D–dependent rickets type I appears to arise from a deficiency in the activity of renal 1α-hydroxylase, the enzyme that converts 25-(OH)D$_3$ into 1,25-(OH)$_2$D$_3$, the active form of the vitamin. The defect can be treated by administering physiological amounts of 1,25-(OH)$_2$D$_3$. On the other hand, vitamin D–dependent rickets type II appears to be due to a defect in the VDR, or at the postreceptor level. Children suffering from vitamin D–dependent rickets type II in two unrelated families were found to have single point mutations in the tip of one of the zinc fingers of the DBD of the VDR. These mutant receptors are apparently defective in their ability to interact with and transcriptionally regulate vitamin D–responsive genes. Almost all individuals afflicted with this disorder present within the first year of life with hypocalcemia, osteomalacia, or rickets and secondary hyperparathyroidism. An unexplained phenomenon that is frequently associated with this disorder is total alopecia. Almost all afflicted individuals are resistant to pharmacological doses of vitamin D and its metabolites in the healing of bone lesions and normalization of serum calcium levels.

SUGGESTED READING

Berridge MJ: Inositol trisphosphate and calcium signalling. Nature 361:315–325, 1993.
Berridge MJ, Lipp P, and Bootman MD: The versatility and universality of calcium signalling. Nat Rev Mol Cell Biol 1:11–21, 2000.

Cato AC, Nestl A, and Mink S: Rapid actions of steroid receptors in cellular signaling pathways. Sci STKE 138:RE9, 1–11, 2002.

Clapham DE and Neer EJ: G protein $\beta\gamma$ subunits. Annu Rev Pharmacol Toxicol 37:167–203, 1997

Cobb MH and Goldsmith EJ: How MAP kinases are regulated. J Biol Chem 270:14843–14846, 1995.

Exton JH: New developments in phospholipase D. J Biol Chem 272:15579–15582, 1997.

Garbers DL and Lowe DG: Guanylyl cyclase receptors. J Biol Chem 269:30741–30744, 1994.

Gether U and Kobilka BK: G protein–coupled receptors. II. Mechanism of agonist activation. J Biol Chem 273:17979–17982, 1998.

Glass CK: Differential recognition of target genes by nuclear receptor monomers, dimers, and heterodimers. Endocr Rev 15:391–407, 1994.

Griffin JE, McPhaul MJ, Russell DW, and Wilson JD: The androgen resistance syndromes: Steroid 5α-reductase 2 deficiency, testicular feminization, and related disorders. In: *The Metabolic and Molecular Bases of Inherited Disease*, 7th ed., Vol. 2, CR Scriver, AL Beaudet, WS Sly, and D Valle, eds., McGraw-Hill, New York, pp. 2967–2998, 1995.

Hannun YA: The ceramide-centric universe of lipid-mediated cell regulation: stress encounters of the lipid kind. J Biol Chem 277:25847–25850, 2002.

Ihle JN, Witthuhn BA, Quelle FW, Yamamoto K, Thierfelder WE, Kreider B, and Silvennoinen O: Signaling by the cytokine receptor superfamily: JAKs and STATs. Trends Biochem Sci 19:222–227, 1994.

Kitamura T, Ogorochi T, and Miyajima A: Multimeric cytokine receptors. Trends Endocrinol Metab 5:8–14, 1994.

Lefkowitz RJ: The superfamily of heptahelical receptors. Nature Cell Biol 2:E133–E136, 2000.

Lösel RM, Falkenstein E, Feuring M, Schultz A, Tillmann H-C, Rossol-Haseroth K, and Wehling M: Nongenomic steroid action: controversies, questions and answers. Physiol Rev 83:965–1016, 2003.

Marx S, Spiegel AM, Skarulis MC, Doppman JL, Collins FS, Liotta LA: Multiple endocrine neoplasia type 1: clinical and genetic topics. Ann Intern Med 129:484–494, 1998.

McKenna NJ, Lanz R, and O'Malley BW: Nuclear receptor coregulators: cellular and molecular biology. Endocr Rev 20:321–344, 1999.

McKenna NJ and O'Malley BW: Combinatorial control of gene expression by nuclear receptors and coregulators. Cell 108:465–474, 2002.

Meyer TE and Habener JF: Cyclic adenosine 3′,5′-monophosphate response element binding protein (CREB) and related transcription-activating deoxyribonucleic acid-binding proteins. Endocr Rev 14:269–290, 1993.

Nishizuka Y: Intracellular signaling by hydrolysis of phospholipids and activation of protein kinase C. Science 258:607–614, 1992.

O'Malley BW: The steroid receptor superfamily: more excitement predicted for the future. Mol Endocrinol 4:363–369, 1990.

Pierce KL, Premont RT, and Lefkowitz RJ: Seven-transmembrane receptors. Nat Rev Mol Cell Biol 3:639–650, 2002.

Pratt WB and Toft DO: Steroid receptor interactions with heat shock protein and immunophilin chaperones. Endocr Rev 18:306–360, 1997.

Quigley CA, De Bellis A, Marschke KB, El-Awady MK, Wilson EM, and French F: Androgen receptor defects: historical, clinical and molecular perspectives. Endocr Rev 16:271–321, 1995.

Rhee SG and Choi KD: Regulation of inositol phospholipid-specific phospholipase C enzymes. J Biol Chem 267:12393–12396, 1992.

Schlessinger J: Cell signaling by receptor tyrosine kinases. Cell 103:211–225, 2000.

Schussheim DH, Skarulis MC, Agarwal SK, Simonds WF, Burns AL, Spiegel AM, and Marks SJ: Multiple endocrine neoplasia type 1: new clinical and basic findings. Trends Endocrinol Metab 12:173–178, 2001.

Spiegel AM: G protein defects in signal transduction. Horm Res 53(Suppl 3):17–22, 2000.

Spiegel AM, Weinstein LS, and Shenker A: Abnormalities in G protein–coupled signal transduction pathways in human disease. J Clin Invest 92:1119–1125, 1993.

Tsai M-J and O'Malley BW: Molecular mechanisms of action of steroid/thyroid receptor superfamily members. Annu Rev Biochem 63:451–486, 1994.

4

Immune–Endocrine Interactions

ROBERT S. MUNFORD

Animals react to dangerous situations by mounting a *flight or fight* response. Mediated largely by the hypothalamic–pituitary–adrenal axis (HPA) and the autonomic nervous system, the visceral elements of this response are familiar to everyone: rapid heart rate, sweating, apprehension, and an automatic impulse to escape. In a remarkably similar way, animals react to microscopic danger—invading microbes—by developing tachycardia, sweating, fever, and withdrawal. The body's reactions to macroscopic and microscopic threats are activated differently, however. Whereas reactions to macroscopic harm are initiated by the central nervous system (CNS) in response to visual or auditory inputs, the CNS receives neural and bloodborne signals from peripheral tissues that trigger its responses to microscopic *non-self* invaders. Before describing some of these signals, this chapter will give a little background information on immunity.

Immunity is the name given to the body's ability to prevent invasion by microorganisms (bacteria, viruses, protozoa and other parasites, fungi). It is convenient to think of two general kinds of immunity, innate and acquired. *Innate immune* mechanisms are *hard-wired* in the genome (they have been shaped by evolution and do not change during the life of the individual), and they respond within minutes to confront invaders. Another key feature of innate immunity is its ability to defend the host from invasion by a wide range of microorganisms. This is accomplished, in part, by a family of *pattern recognition proteins* that bind to highly conserved microbial carbohydrate or lipid molecules (e.g., the lipopolysaccharides [LPSs] of gram-negative bacteria). Some of these pattern recognition proteins promote microbial killing by activating complement, which can produce pores in microbial membranes, while others deliver the microbial molecules, or the microbes that bear them, to cells that bear *pattern recognition receptors* on their surfaces. These cells include the dendritic cells and macrophages that populate submucosal and subepidermal sites throughout the body; they respond to engagement of pattern recognition receptors by secreting mediators that (*1*) dilate local blood vessels, increasing blood flow to the infected site; (*2*) activate nociceptive (pain) fibers, prompting withdrawal; and (*3*) increase local capillary permeability, allowing transudation of plasma constituents, including several anti-infective molecules, into the tissue. These responses produce the cardinal signs of local inflammation: redness (rubor), swelling (tumor), heat (calor), and pain (dolor). In addition, some of the mediators attract circulating neutrophils and other leukocytes to the infected tissue, while others enhance the ability of these cells to stick to local vascular endothelium and move across the vessel wall to enter the injured tissue. Together these responses increase the ability of these blood cells to *home* to the infected site, where they are needed to kill the invaders.

The body's systemic responses to infection and injury have also been highly conserved during evolution. There are mechanisms that rapidly increase the number of neutrophils that circulate in the blood (leukocytosis), increase blood flow to an infected site (tachycardia, regional vasoconstriction), and raise body temperature (fever). The liver increases the production and secretion of proteins that can neutralize the proteases and oxidants that diffuse from an infected site into the blood. The circulating concentrations of numerous anti-infective and anti-inflammatory molecules also increase. In essence, the systemic response to acute injury or infection seems to support local host defenses while preventing inflammation in uninvolved tissues.

In striking contrast to innate immunity, *adaptive immunity* takes many days to develop, requires rearrangements within immunoglobulin and T-cell receptor genes, and achieves exquisite molecular specificity. Vaccines induce adaptive immunity, as does infection with most pathogenic microbes. In essence, innate immune mechanisms may be viewed as protecting animals from the microbes that live on or within them throughout their lives—from each individual's *normal flora*. Adaptive immunity is needed to survive infection with microbial *pathogens*—the unusual microbes that have evolved one or more mechanisms (e.g., specific toxins) that allow them to survive our innate immune defenses.

Successful immune defenses require both short- and long-distance communication, both between the cells within an infected local site and from those cells to others throughout the rest of the body. In return, signals must reach the immune cells from the brain, liver, adrenal glands, and other organs.

Although many kinds of molecules are involved in transmitting signals from immune cells, some of the most important are proteins called *cytokines*. The term *cytokine* is used to describe proteins that influence immune responses in various ways (Fig. 4-1). In general, there are inflammatory cytokines (tumor necrosis factor [TNF]-α, interleukin [IL]-1, IL-12, IL-18, interferon-γ) and anti-inflammatory ones (IL-4, IL-6, IL-10, IL-13, transforming growth factor [TGF]-β). Some cytokines have natural antagonists—for example, IL-1 receptor antagonist and soluble TNF receptors—while others have *partner* molecules that prolong or enhance their actions (e.g., soluble IL-6 receptors). The various cytokines differ in their cells of origin and biological activities. Some cytokines are growth factors, for example; these include TGF-β, interferons, and colony-stimulating factors ([CSF]: macrophage CSF, granulocyte CSF, granulocyte-macrophage CSF).

The name *chemokine* is used for a subset of cytokines that are *chemotactic*; they attract specific cells of the immune system. They provide directional cues by forming concentration gradients that migrating cells can sense. They also stimulate various leukocyte responses. The most prominent example is IL-8.

Cytokines often have the following properties:

- Rapid synthesis and/or release in response to stimuli.
- Action by inducing intracellular signaling downstream of specific receptors on responding cells.

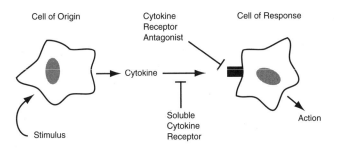

Fig. 4-1   Cells of many types can produce cytokines and/or chemokines. In most cases, synthesis and release of these proteins occurs in response to discrete stimuli (infection, injury, exercise, stress). Some cytokines may also be produced constitutively by immune or nonimmune cells (e.g., adipocytes). Cytokines and chemokines interact with specific receptors on responding cells. Engagement of these receptors triggers intracellular signaling events that induce specific responses. Soluble receptors bind circulating cytokines and may either inhibit (e.g., soluble tumor necrosis factor-R [TNF-R]) or enhance (soluble interleukin [IL]-6R) their ability to stimulate responding cells. Another mechanism for inhibition is illustrated by the IL-1 receptor antagonist, which competes with IL-1 for receptor binding and does not activate the signaling apparatus of the responding cell.

- Pleiotropic actions. Like many classical endocrine hormones, these proteins can often have multiple effects, depending upon the cell target and other variables.
- Context-dependent actions. The biological effects of some cytokines differ, depending on the physiological context.
- Nonlinear dose–response relationships *in vivo*.
- Diverse interactions with cells (Fig. 4-2)
  - Autocrine—with the same cell that makes the cytokine
  - Juxtacrine—with a close neighbor (contact dependence)
  - Paracrine—with other cells in the same tissue
  - Endocrine—with cells in other tissues via the blood. When cytokines act in this way, they are called *hormones.*
- Redundancy. Different cytokines may have similar effects. For example, there are over 50 chemokines and 20 chemokine receptors. Many of these receptors can bind several different chemokines, and many chemokines can bind different receptors. Similarly, some transmembrane proteins are components of multiple cytokine receptors.
- Synergy. When they act together, some cytokines may have a greater-than-additive effect.
- Antagonism. The actions of different cytokines on target cells may be antagonistic.
- The ability of some cytokines to initiate signal transduction in target cells is influenced by soluble proteins that either bind the cytokine or compete with it for receptor occupancy.

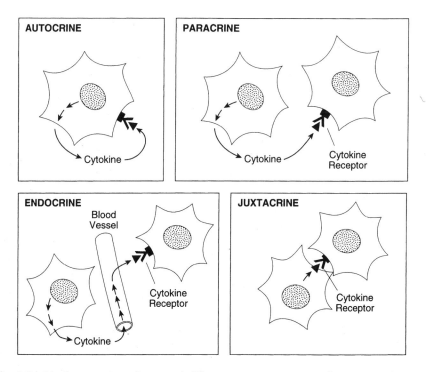

Fig. 4-2 Mediators can act in several different ways. *Autocrine* refers to a mechanism by which a mediator, such as a cytokine, acts on its cell of origin. *Paracrine* refers to a mechanism by which a mediator produced in one cell acts on a neighboring cell, diffusing through intercellular spaces rather than through the blood. In *endocrine* communication, the mediator enters the blood and reaches its target cell through the circulation. *Juxtacrine* refers to the ability of a cell-bound mediator to interact with a specific receptor in a juxtaposed cell.

THREE IMPORTANT CYTOKINES

To illustrate many of the properties of cytokines, three important cytokines will now be described briefly.

Tumor Necrosis Factor

Tumor necrosis factor, also known as *TNF-α*, is a major pro-inflammatory cytokine; the others are IL-1, IL-12, and interferon-γ. Tumor necrosis factor is produced by a variety of hematopoietic cells, especially monocytes and macrophages, as well as by cells such as astrocytes, epidermal cells, hepatocytes, adipocytes, and smooth muscle cells.

    Tumor necrosis factor plays a central role in the mobilization of antimicrobial host defenses. Animals that cannot make TNF are more susceptible to tuberculosis, listeriosis, and other infections. Further, TNF stimulates vascular endothelial cells to increase their expression of molecules that allow circulating neutrophils to bind to, and move through, a vessel wall in order to seek and destroy invading microbes in the adjacent tissue spaces. It is also one of the most important inducers of shock in the setting of uncontrolled infection and/or inflammation (*septic shock*). When TNF is injected into animals (including humans), it induces the production of numerous other cytokines, including IL-1, IL-6, and IL-10, as well as cortisol and prostaglandin E_2. Tumor necrosis factor can induce mature T cells, tumor cells, and other cells to undergo programmed cell death (apoptosis). By suppressing lipoprotein lipase and other anabolic enzymes in fat, it contributes to infection-associated wasting; in fact, at one time TNF was also called *cachectin,* for its ability to induce cachexia.

Tumor necrosis factor is a 157-amino acid (17 kDa)–soluble peptide that is processed from a transmembrane 226-amino acid (26 kDa) precursor and assembled into a homotrimeric complex. A metalloproteinase is responsible for cleaving the transmembrane form to release soluble TNF. There are two major TNF receptors, TNFR p55 and TNFR p75, both of which are expressed on the surfaces of most cells. The two receptors have different cytosolic domains, and each activates a distinct signaling pathway. p55 is the receptor primarily responsible for TNF's proinflammatory properties. Both receptors are released from cell surfaces during the acute phase response (see below) and travel in plasma, where they can neutralize the TNF that they encounter in the blood (see Fig. 4-1).

Interleukin-10

Interleukin-10 is perhaps the most important anti-inflammatory cytokine. Others include IL-4, IL-6, IL-11, and IL-13. Interleukin-10 inhibits the synthesis of IL-1 and TNF, IL-12 (limiting T-cell activation), IL-2 (reducing T-cell expansion), and IL-5 (limiting mast cell proliferation). On the other hand, it promotes the synthesis of cytokine inhibitors (IL-1Ra and soluble TNF receptors), and it diminishes the expression of antigen-presenting molecules by macrophages and dendritic cells (these molecules allow full development of acquired immunity). Its actions on phagocytes include inhibition of nitric oxide (NO) formation (NO is microbicidal), metalloproteinase activity, and procoagulant activity. Excess IL-10 may impair host defenses.

In addition, IL-10 is immunostimulatory. In other words, it promotes the proliferation and maturation of of B cells (which produce antibodies) as well as the expression of Fc receptors (Fc receptors bind the Fc region of an antibody molecule to a cell's surface and allow the cell to internalize the particle bound to the other end of the antibody).

Mice that cannot make IL-10 develop severe enterocolitis, suggesting that IL-10 normally prevents the body from developing inflammatory reactions to the bacteria in the bowel. They are also highly susceptible to lethal inflammation following challenge with endotoxin or other inflammatory stimuli.

Interleukin-10 is a 160-amino acid (18.5 kDa) peptide that exists extracellularly as a noncovalently linked homodimer. It is produced by many cell types, including monocytes, CD4$^+$ lymphocytes, B cells, and keratinocytes. It has a single high-affinity receptor that is expressed principally in hematopoietic tissues, including the thymus and spleen. Interleukin-10 binding to its receptor activates a Janus kinase/signal transducer and activator of transcription-3 (JAK/STAT-3) tyrosine kinase signaling pathway.

Interleukin-6

Interleukin-6 can be produced by most (if not all) cells in the body in response to injury, infection, and/or stress. It has been called an *SOS* cytokine because it seems to mobilize many of the body's protective responses to stress.

Interleukin-6 is a major stimulus for a*cute phase protein* synthesis. Many of the human body's responses to injury and infection also occur in very primitive animals (e.g., horseshoe crabs). In particular, there is a highly programmed set of changes known as the *acute phase response.* Although this term has been used most often to describe changes that occur in response to trauma or infection, many of the same changes may be induced by strenuous exercise, cold exposure, and even psychological stress; elevated blood IL-6 levels have been noted in each of these conditions. When hepatocytes sense IL-6 (or TNF or IL-1β, although IL-6 is most important), they increase their production of several proteins that seem to serve important host defense functions. In particular, the molecules have anti-infective or anti-inflammatory actions. They include (*1*) protease inhibitors and antioxidants. These may help neutralize the proteases and oxidants that leach into the circulation from sites of injury or infection. (*2*) Microbial pattern recognition molecules. There are several of these; they bind to conserved microbial molecules and facilitate the ingestion of the microbes by phagocytes (cells that eat particulate matter). The most dynamic and easily measured of these molecules, C-reactive protein, is used by clinicians as an index of ongoing inflammation. (*3*) Cytokine antagonists. In particular, IL-1 receptor antagonist and soluble TNF receptors are acute phase proteins; the blood concentrations of these inhibitors increase substantially during the acute phase response. (*4*) Activation of lipolysis. Another feature of the acute phase response is an increase in circulating free fatty acids and triglycerides. Recent evidence indicates that IL-6 can promote lipolysis from adipose tissue in humans. In fact, adipocytes make and release IL-6; blood IL-6 levels are higher in obese humans.

Another major function of IL-6 is *activation of the HPA axis.* In humans, infusion of IL-6 activates the HPA axis and thus increases adrenal cortisol release. Studies in IL-6-deficient mice have shown that IL-6 is as important as corticotropin-releasing hormone (CRH) for stimulating adrenocorticotropin (ACTH) release from the pituitary under stressful conditions. In keeping with this notion, glucocorticoids inhibit IL-6 production. High doses of IL-6 also increase plasma levels of vasopressin, which has important effects on vascular contractility and water metabolism.

In addition, IL-6 has important *cell growth–promoting and procoagulant activity.* Interleukin-6–deficient mice have reduced numbers of cells in all of the hematopoietic lines (red cells, lymphocytes, platelets, granulocytes). There is also evidence that excess IL-6 may be harmful: in humans, IL-6 produced within the bone marrow may help drive the production of B cells in patients with multiple myeloma, a plasma cell dyscrasia. Interleukin-6 also may be the major pro-coagulant cytokine. Although the molecular mechanism is not fully understood, IL-6 can increase the expression of tissue factor, which initiates clotting by monocytes and increases blood fibrinogen levels. (Clotting is thought to be a host defense mechanism; when a *wall* is formed around an infected tissue, spread of infection to other tissues may be avoided.)

Administration of IL-6 or IL-1 produces changes in thyroid hormone physiology that resemble those seen in the *euthyroid sick* syndrome (see Chapter 13). This seems to be partly due to a decrease in 5′ deiodinase activity but also to diminished thyroid-stimulating hormone (TSH) secretion. In experimental animals, hypothyroidism increases survival from some infections.

Interleukin-6 is a 19 to 30 kDa protein, depending on its state of glycosylation and phosphorylation. It binds to an 80 kDa receptor (IL-6Rα) that, in turn, interacts with a second protein, gp130, and initiates tyrosine phosphorylation. gp130 is a common receptor component that also can complex with receptors for four other molecules; specificity is determined in part by the cellular distribution of the primary (α) component. Interleukin-6Rα is found in monocytes, T cells, and some B cells, as well as in hepatocytes. Interleukin-6Rα also exists as a soluble form in plasma and other body fluids; it binds IL-6, prolongs its half-life in plasma, and preserves its ability to signal various cells.

The Stress (Acute Phase) Response Paradox

Animals' systemic responses to stress and injury have been so highly conserved through evolution that their important role in human physiology is not disputed. On the other hand, there is evidence that prolonged activation of these responses, even at very low levels, may be harmful. For instance, almost all of the biochemical measurements that have been found to predict the risk of coronary artery disease are stress reactants (e.g., low blood high-density lipoprotein [HDL] concentrations, high blood levels of C-reactive protein, secretory phospholipase A_2, fibrinogen, etc.). There is currently controversy over whether the cytokines that trigger these responses arise in the atheromatous blood vessel or elsewhere (such as at sites of local infection/inflammation or within adipose tissue). It is also not certain that these changes, many of which theoretically should promote atherosclerosis and/or thrombosis, actually do so in humans. Cytokines may also play a role in the pathogenesis of type II diabetes mellitus, whereas maximal activation of systemic stress responses, as occurs during many critical illnesses, may reduce innate immune defenses and allow nonpathogenic microbes to cause disease. Interleukin-6, which is present in above-normal concentrations in the blood of patients with metastatic prostate cancer, can activate the androgen receptor in human prostate cancer cells in an androgen-independent fashion. It is intriguing to think that this may be a mechanism by which IL-6 might contribute to the progression of malignancy.

These potentially harmful effects of the systemic stress response have become more apparent as humans have been able to live well beyond reproductive age and, with modern technology, survive many conditions that previously would have been fatal.

COMMUNICATION BETWEEN IMMUNE CELLS AND THE CENTRAL NERVOUS SYSTEM: AFFERENT SIGNALS

Afferent signals that arise in peripheral tissues (such as an infected foot) can reach the brain in two general ways, via peripheral nerves and via the bloodstream (Fig. 4-3). Recent evidence suggests that the neural route may be important. In rodents,

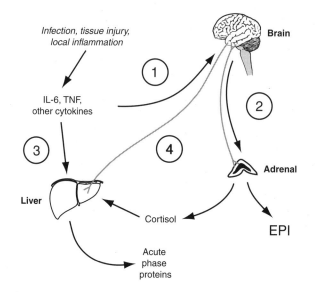

Fig. 4-3 Cytokine-mediated communication pathways between peripheral cells, the liver, the hypothalamic–pituitary–adrenal (HPA) and the autonomic nervous system. (*1*) Following injury or in response to infection, cells in local tissues release cytokines that travel via the bloodstream to the liver and central nervous system (CNS) (hypothalamus and brain stem). Similar information may also be transmitted to the CNS via afferent neural pathways, including the vagus nerve and nociceptive fibers. (*2*) Activation of the HPA by interleukin (IL)-6 increases the secretion of adrenocorticotropin (ACTH), which in turn increases cortisol release from the adrenal cortex. Increased activity along sympathetic nerves enhances the release of epinephrine from the adrenal medulla. Both cortisol and epinephrine (EPI) have important anti-inflammatory actions within the bloodstream (see text). (*3*) Interleukin-6 and other cytokines also stimulate the production of acute phase proteins and activate the other features of the acute phase response (see text). (*4*) Efferent activity along the vagus nerve releases acetylcholine, which inhibits the production of tumor necrosis factor (TNF) and other pro-inflammatory molecules by Kupffer cells and other tissue-resident macrophages.

for instance, the ability of low doses of bacterial agonists (such as bacterial lipopolysaccharide) or cytokines (IL-1β) to elicit fever can be blocked by cutting the hepatic branches of the vagus nerve. Stimulation of the vagal fibers may involve prostaglandin E_2 that is released into the blood by cells that respond to the inciting agonist. On the other hand, the same agonists are also able to interact directly with the hypothalamus and brain stem to raise body temperature and activate the HPA. Of the various cytokines, TNF and IL-1 are probably the most potent pyrogens and IL-6 and IL-1 are the most important stimuli to secretion of ACTH.

Other investigators have reported that stimulation of pain fibers in one hind limb of a rat can block inflammation in the opposite extremity; the signal travels along a path that involves the spinal cord and activation of the HPA. As with the aforementioned role for the vagus nerve in the febrile response, however, at this time there is no evidence that this pathway is operative in humans.

COMMUNICATION BETWEEN THE CENTRAL NERVOUS SYSTEM AND IMMUNE CELLS: EFFERENT SIGNALS

The CNS exerts regulatory control over circulating immune cells through at least three mechanisms (Fig. 4-3):

1. The HPA axis. Activation of the HPA axis induces the production of three anti-inflammatory molecules: α-melanocyte-stimulating hormone (α-MSH), ACTH itself, and cortisol. Alpha-MSH inhibits pro-inflammatory cytokine synthesis, in part by stimulating production of IL-10. Cortisol inhibits the production of pro-inflammatory molecules by macrophages and other cells. It is also needed (permissive) for maximal acute phase protein production.
2. The sympathetic nervous system. Both epinephrine and norepinephrine can modulate the production of cytokines by immune cells. Monocytes have β_2-adrenergic receptors. Epinephrine stimulates cyclic adenosine monophosphate (AMP) production in these cells, inhibiting LPS-stimulated TNF and IL-12 synthesis while augmenting the production of IL-10. Epinephrine's likely importance as a modulator of inflammation is suggested by the experiment shown in Figure 4-4.
3. The parasympathetic nervous system. The *cholinergic anti-inflammatory pathway* diminishes TNF production by the liver and heart. Cutting the vagus nerve renders rats much more sensitive to the lethal reaction to bacterial LPS, at least in part by allowing greater TNF production to occur. Acetylcholine inhibits TNF production by macrophages *in vitro*.

In addition, the nervous system contributes to local inflammatory reactions. Peripheral nerve endings release numerous molecules that influence local inflammation. These include substance P, CRH, β-endorphin, and vasoactive intestinal polypeptide.

ENDOCRINE CONTROL OF INFLAMMATION: CORTISOL AND EPINEPHRINE AS IMMUNOMODULATORY MOLECULES

The CNS controls inflammation by using molecules that regulate other essential functions such as metabolism and blood pressure. Cortisol and epinephrine are important immunomodulatory molecules.

Cortisol is produced by the adrenal cortex in response to stimulation by ACTH. It is the predominant glucocorticoid in humans. It contributes to stress-induced leukocytosis by inhibiting leukocyte-endothelium adhesion. It inhibits the synthesis of numerous cytokines. In physiological concentrations, however, cortisol inhibits the production of TNF, but not of IL-6 or IL-10, in response to LPS stimulation. It acts, in part, by inhibiting nuclear factor kappa B (NF-κB), a transcription factor that plays a prominent role in the synthesis of many mediators of inflammation.

Epinephrine has important actions on the heart (increasing the heart rate as well as myocardial contractility) and on the liver (increasing gluconeogenesis), and it also modulates inflammatory responses by stimulating IL-6 production, inhibiting leukocyte adhesion to vascular endothelium, and inhibiting stimulus-induced TNF

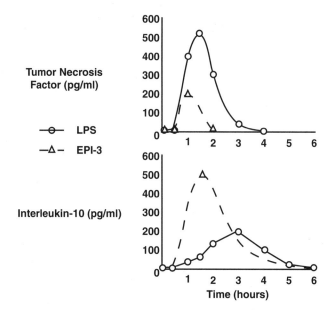

Fig. 4-4 Effect of epinephrine (EPI) on the responses of humans to an intravenous bolus of bacterial lipopolysaccharide (LPS). Healthy human volunteers were infused with a standardized dose of bacterial endotoxin. Over the next 2–6 hours, they developed fever, muscle aches and headache, and transient hypotension. Assays of their blood revealed a peak of immunoreactive tumor necrosis factor (TNF) at 1.5–2 hours and a lower peak of interleukin (IL)-10 at 3 hours (circles, LPS). Another group of volunteers was administered a constant infusion of EPI for 3 hours, then given the same dose of endotoxin (triangles, EPI-3). Now the TNF response was much smaller, while blood levels of IL-10 peaked much higher and earlier than before. In other words, increasing the circulating concentration of EPI converted the response to endotoxin from proinflammatory (TNF dominant) to anti-inflammatory (IL-10 dominant). A similar shift in the body's responses to bacterial agonists has been noted following strenuous exercise and during major trauma (such as major surgery). Propranolol, a β-adrenergic receptor antagonist, inhibits this shift, confirming that it is due to catecholamines. *In vitro*, prostaglandin E_2 and other agents that raise cyclic adenosine monophosphate (cyclic AMP) levels in monocytes can also change the production of TNF and IL-10 so that less TNF and more IL-10 is made in response to LPS. (Adapted from van der Poll et al., p. 715, 1996.)

production. Epinephrine is thus an important immunomodulatory mediator within the blood compartment. The clinical investigation by van der Poll and colleagues illustrates this point (Fig. 4-4).

Note that epinephrine has this effect only on cells that have been stimulated by agonists such as LPS. Neither *in vitro* nor *in vivo* administration of epinephrine increases IL-10 production. On the other hand, there is evidence that epinephrine can induce IL-6 release from cells, in keeping with Il-6's role as a mediator of many stress responses.

It is well known that supraphysiological concentrations of glucocorticoids are immunosuppressive; they prevent the body from responding normally to microbial invasion. Recent evidence suggests that concentrations of cortisol and epinephrine that are in the high physiological range can also be immunosuppressive, at least when accompanied by the other elements of the acute phase response. These changes may be an important reason that individuals who sustain major trauma have an increased risk of infection during the posttrauma recovery period.

IMMUNE CELLS AS SOURCES OF ENDOCRINE HORMONES

During the 1980s, scientists made a remarkable discovery: lymphocytes and other immune cells can make numerous neurohormones. For example, pro-opiomelanocortin (p mRNA is present in lymphocytes, which can produce ACTH and endorphins in response to CRH, arginine vasopressin, or certain microbial agonist molecules. Other neurohormones for which there is evidence of production by immune cells include TSH, luteinizing hormone (LH), follicle-stimulating hormone (FSH), growth hormone (GH), and CRH. Hypothalamic releasing hormones (CRH, growth hormone-releasing hormone [GHRH]) may also be made by lymphocytes. Immune cells may have receptors for prolactin, GH, ACTH, and other neurohormones.

Although there is strong evidence that the immune cell–produced hormones are bioactive, the role(s) that they play *in vivo* are still uncertain. They seem to exert their effects locally, in sites of inflammation or immune reactivity, where even small amounts may reach high concentrations. Since immune cells do not store the neuropeptides, they release them more slowly than does the pituitary gland. The degree to which they contribute to the blood levels of the neurohormones is also not known.

After CRH is produced in the hypothalamus and arrives in the pituitary, it triggers pro-opiomelanocortin (POMC) production. Then ACTH and α-MSH are released into the blood, where they and (ACTH-induced) cortisol have anti-inflammatory actions on circulating immune cells. In contrast, when it is released into local tissue beds, from either peripheral nerve endings or immune cells, CRH is pro-inflammatory; it stimulates the production of IL-1, TNF-α, and other pro-inflammatory cytokines, promotes neutrophil influx, and so on. Corticotropin-releasing hormone–stimulated IL-1 induces B cells to produce POMC; β-endorphin derived from this POMC can enhance natural killer cell activity and, by acting on nociceptive nerve terminals, reduce pain. The distinctive actions of CRH in different body compartments provide one example of a phenomenon that seems to be common among cytokines and neurohormones: *context-dependent* action.

SUMMARY

- The classical endocrine hormones play important roles in regulating immune responses. In addition to the hormones that are produced by the HPA and autonomic nervous system and circulate in the blood, acting on immune cells through specific receptors, numerous peptide hormones can be made by immune cells and act locally to modulate inflammation.
- Conversely, cytokines produced by immune and nonimmune cells may influence the functions of several endocrine organs, including the HPA, thy-

roid, and reproductive organs. Many authors have noted that there is a *bidirectional* communication between the CNS and the immune system.

- Just as immune cells can make endocrine hormones, endocrine organs can make and release cytokines.
- The body's reactions to stressful stimuli require effective communication between cells in the initiating tissue (e.g., an infected or injured extremity) and the cells in the hypothalamus, brain stem, adrenal gland, liver, and other tissues that mediate systemic responses. The communication network involves both cytokines and hormones and both neural and bloodborne pathways. Since chronic or excessive activation of this network may contribute to various disease states in humans, immune–endocrine communication is a major focus of current biomedical research.

SUGGESTED READING

Besedovsky HO, del Rey AE, and Sorkin E: Immune-neuroendocrine interactions. J Immunol 135:750s–754s, 1985.

Blalock JE: The syntax of immune–neuroendocrine communication. Immunol Today 15: 504–511, 1999.

Blalock JE, Harbour-McMenamin D, and Smith EM: Peptide hormones shared by the neuroendocrine and immunologic systems. J Immunol 135:858s–861s, 1985.

Borovikova LV, Ivanova S, Zhang M, Yang H, Botchkina GI, Watkins LR, Wang H, Abumrad N, Eaton JW, and Tracey KJ: Vagus nerve stimulation attenuates the systemic inflammatory response to endotoxin. Nature 405:458–462, 2000.

Elenkov IJ, Wilder RL, Chrousos GP, and Vizi ES: The sympathetic nerve—an integrative interface between two supersystems: the brain and the immune system. Pharmacol Rev 52:595–638, 2000.

Green PG, Miao FJP, Levine JD, and Levine J: Negative feedback neuroendocrine control of the inflammatory response in rats. J Neurosci 15:4678–4686, 1995.

Munford RS: Statins and the acute phase response. N Engl J Med 344:2016–2018, 2001.

Munford RS and Pugin J: Normal responses to injury prevent systemic inflammation and can be immunosuppressive. Am J Respir Crit Care Med 163:316–321, 2001.

Ozaki K and Leonard WJ: Cytokine and cytokine receptor pleiotropy and redundancy. J Biol Chem 277:29355–29358, 2002.

Ueda T, Bruchovsky N, and Sadar MD: Activation of the androgen receptor N-terminal domain by interleukin-6 via MAPK and STAT3 signal transduction pathways. J Biol Chem 277:7076–7085, 2002.

van der Poll T, Coyle SM, Barbosa K, Braxton CC, and Lowry SF: Epinephrine inhibits tumor necrosis factor-α and potentiates interleukin 10 production during human endotoxemia. J Clin Invest 97:713–719, 1996.

Webster EL, Barrientos RM, Contoreggi C, Isaac MG, Ligier S, Gabry KE, Chrousos GP, McCarthy EF, Rice KC, Gold PW, and Sternberg EM: Corticotropin releasing hormone (CRH) antagonist attenuates adjuvant induced arthritis: role of CRH in peripheral inflammation. J Rheumatol 29:1252–1261, 2002.

5

Assessment of Endocrine Function

JAMES E. GRIFFIN
RICHARD J. AUCHUS

The first step in the laboratory assessment of endocrine function is usually to determine if hormone production is within the normal range. The ability to measure hormone concentrations accurately in plasma, urine, and saliva has allowed us to define normal endocrine function and to diagnose abnormalities in hormone production. Perhaps the single most important advance in modern endocrinology has been the development of immunoassays to measure the small quantities of hormones that circulate in the blood. Static hormone measurements, however, may not provide conclusive evidence of dysfunction in a given endocrine system. Therefore, dynamic or provocative endocrine tests have been developed to stimulate or suppress production of a particular hormone. As our understanding of the role of receptors in mediating hormone action has grown, assays that assess target tissue responsiveness to hormones have been developed. Advances in chromatographic and analytical chemistry techniques have also allowed more precise measurements of some hormones for which good immunoassays have not yet been developed. This chapter describes the various methods for quantifying hormone concentrations and thus assessing endocrine function.

PLASMA HORMONE CONCENTRATIONS

Types of Assays

Hormones circulating in the plasma were first detected by *in vivo* bioassays, in which plasma or extracts of plasma were injected into animals and biological responses were measured. Unfortunately, most *in vivo* bioassays lack the precision, sensitivity, and specificity required to measure the low concentrations of many hormones in plasma, and the assays are cumbersome and impractical for routine use in clinical chemistry laboratories. Great progress in measuring plasma hormone concentrations came with the development of competitive binding assays and radioimmunoassays (RIAs). In both of these assays, the unknown concentration of a hormone in plasma is estimated by allowing that hormone to compete with a labeled hormone or hormone analog for specific binding sites on a protein, which is

101

an antibody in the case of the RIAs. By measuring the amount of labeled compound that remains bound in the presence of an aliquot of plasma and comparing that quantity to the amount displaced by known amounts of hormone in a series of reference standards, the amount of hormone in the plasma can be estimated.

While RIAs provide information about the concentration of immunoreactive hormone in plasma, these assays do not quantify the biological activity of the hormone. Moreover, the site in the hormone to which the antibodies used in the assay are directed may not be the site(s) involved in receptor binding (see Chapter 3); therefore, some forms of the hormone assayed may not be functional. This caveat is particularly important for peptide hormones such as growth hormone (GH), which exists in a variety of forms due to differences in the extent of glycosylation, proteolysis, and other modifications. Therefore, radioreceptor assays and *in vitro* bioassays were developed to determine the biological activity attributable to a specific hormone in plasma.

In a radioreceptor assay, the specific receptor sites on cells or cellular components are substituted for the antibody as a binding protein for the hormone (or ligand). Thus, the specificity of binding is determined not by the antibody determinants but by the biologically relevant receptor site that mediates hormone action. Such radioreceptor assays can add to the information obtained from RIAs by assessing the quantity of *bioactive* hormone, particularly for polypeptide hormones that ordinarily exist in multiple forms and whose amino acid sequence may be modified by genetic mutations. The radioreceptor assay is also useful in assessing the total activity in plasma attributed to a class of compounds interacting with one type of receptor, such as competition of all plasma glucocorticoids (cortisol, corticosterone, etc.) for binding to the glucocorticoid receptor. Analogously, drugs that interfere with androgen binding have been assessed by competition of these compounds with labeled androgen for binding to the androgen receptor. Radioreceptor assays are also useful in assessing the presence of autoantibodies to hormone receptors in the plasma of some subjects with endocrine disorders—for example, antibodies to the thyrotropin or insulin receptors.

Although radioreceptor assays give some clue to the biological activity of a hormone, they measure only the first step in hormone action, the binding of hormone to its receptor. They do not assess the effects of hormone–receptor interactions in generating second messenger(s) or in stimulating a specific response. Thus, the assessment of plasma hormone levels has come full circle with the development of modern *in vitro* bioassays. These assays involve the incubation of plasma or plasma extracts with responsive tissues, membrane preparations, or cultured cells. The cells may be genetically engineered to express the specific hormone receptor and an easily measured response to active hormone, usually a colorimetric, immunometric, or chemiluminometric signal. Conversely, these assays may be used to evaluate the functional capacity of a mutant receptor from a patient with a genetic disorder of hormone action rather than of hormone production. For example, rat Leydig cells have been used to assay the ability of luteinizing hormone (LH) and human chorionic gonadotropin (hCG) to stimulate testosterone production. This bioassay has greater analytical sensitivity for LH and hCG than the RIA and radioreceptor assays and can detect bioactive LH when immunoreactive LH is undetectable by other methods.

Additional technologies are employed, separately or in conjunction with immunoassays, to further evaluate endocrine function. Electrophoretic techniques, including electrofocusing and immunoblotting, can detect alterations in the net charge or size of a protein hormone. Chromatographic techniques to separate the desired hormone from interfering substances are used in conjunction with various detection methods including immunoassays. Finally, molecular biology techniques are used to assess the gene for a polypeptide hormone, receptor, or enzyme in hormone biosynthesis, as described in Chapter 2.

Principle of Radioimmunoassays

The principle underlying RIAs is the competitive inhibition of binding of a radio-labeled antigen or ligand (the hormone or a hormone analog, L*) to the antibody (Ab) by unlabeled antigen (hormone H) present in a reference standard or in a plasma sample (the unknown):

$$L^* + Ab \underset{k_d}{\overset{k_a}{\longleftrightarrow}} L^* \cdot Ab$$

$$H + Ab \underset{k_d}{\overset{k_a}{\longleftrightarrow}} H \cdot Ab$$

The antigen-antibody reaction is reversible, as shown above by the arrows, with an association rate constant of k_a and a dissociation rate constant of k_d. The rate of dissociation is slower than the rate of association, and at equilibrium the amount of antigen bound to antibody is a function of the ratio of the rates of association and dissociation. Following an appropriate period of incubation, the antibody-bound antigen (B) is separated from the unbound or free antigen (F) by one of several different methods. Because a fixed amount of antibody and labeled antigen (L*) is present in each assay tube, the amount of L* bound to antibody (the measured radioactivity) depends principally on the concentration of unlabeled hormone H in either the standard or the unknown sample. The higher the concentration of unlabeled hormone, the more L* is displaced from the Ab and the lower the quantity of radioactivity that remains bound to the fixed amount of Ab. A standard curve is generated first by plotting the ratio of the amount of L* bound in the presence of the standard (B) to the amount bound in the absence of any unlabeled hormone (B_0) as a function of amount of standard (H). This plot is nonlinear, but semilogarithmic transformation of the data usually results in a linear relationship between B/B_0 and H in the midportion of the curve, which usually spans two to three orders of magnitude (Fig. 5-1). To determine the amount of hormone present in an unknown sample, the quantity B/B_0 for that assay is located on the y-axis and interpolated on the standard curve, and the quantity of hormone in the sample (H) is read from the x-axis (follow the solid or dashed lines in Fig. 5-1). The calculation can be automated

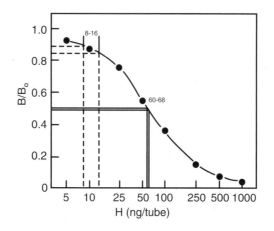

Fig. 5-1 Standard curve for radioimmunoassay of plasma testosterone. The ratio of the amount of radioactive testosterone bound in the presence of standard (B) to the amount bound in the absence of any unlabeled hormone (B_0) is plotted as a function of the amount of standard (unlabeled hormone H) in each assay tube. Note that the semilogarithmic plot is roughly linear in the midportion of the curve, where the assay is most reliable. Given a 5% error in determination of B/B_0 near the middle of the curve, the uncertainty in estimating H is near 10% (64 ± 4 ng, solid lines); however, a 5% error in B/B_0 in the flat portions at the extreme ends of the curve translates into an uncertainty of over 50% (12 ± 4 ng, dashed lines).

by fitting the linear portion of the curve to an equation ($y = mx + b$). Note that, in the linear portion, a small error in B/B_0 will not change H significantly, making the assay reliable in this range of H values.

However, inspection of Figure 5-1 shows that at the extreme high and low values of B/B_0, the curve flattens considerably. Thus, locating the exact point on the curve corresponding to a given value of B/B_0 becomes less precise, and small errors in B/B_0 are magnified in attempting to determine H (compare the solid and dashed lines in Fig. 5-1). Assays yielding B/B_0 values below the linear portion must be repeated with dilution of the sample, and samples with high values of B/B_0 reflect H values that are below the limits of reliable measurement by the assay. Furthermore, curves generated by dilution of the standards or the samples should yield parallel lines on the B/B_0 versus H plots as evidence of similar interaction of L^* and H with the antibody and absence of interfering substances.

Protein hormones (like prolactin) can be used as antigens themselves for raising antibodies; small molecules and peptides must be modified and coupled to a protein carrier first to raise specific antibodies. Antibodies suitable for RIAs are usually of the IgG class of immunoglobulins, obtained by injecting a protein hormone or a small hormone coupled to an immunogenic protein into a rabbit or other suitable animal. Antisera produced in this manner are polyclonal, containing a repertoire of antibody molecules directed to different epitopes of the antigen. Polyclonal antisera tend to have high affinity and thus high sensitivity, but the quantities are limited, and polyclonal sera alone cannot be used for immunometric assays. It is also possible to produce monoclonal antibodies to hormones using immortalized hybridoma cells derived from spleen cells of immunized mice. Monoclonal antibodies may be regenerated indefinitely from the hybridoma cell line and are ideally suited for immunometric assays; hence monoclonal antibodies are the dominant forms in commercial hormone assays today.

Labeled peptides and thyroid hormones (L*) are generated by incorporating ^{125}I into the molecules; ^{125}I emits gamma radiation and is detected with a gamma counter. For peptide hormones, iodination is performed using reagents to incorporate $Na^{125}I$ label into tyrosine, lysine, or histidine residues in the hormone. With small polypeptides lacking tyrosine or histidine in their structure, it may be necessary to engineer a tyrosine residue into the hormone in a manner that minimally alters the immunoreactivity of the polypeptide. Alternatively, small peptides may be labeled with an amino acid containing ^{3}H by solid-phase chemical synthesis, and the ^{3}H (which emits beta particles) is detected by liquid scintillation counting. For optimal stability and immunoreactivity, only one atom of ^{125}I is incorporated per molecule of hormone. With steroid hormones, one or more ^{3}H atoms are incorporated into the molecule to achieve high specific activity, which lowers the background noise and improves sensitivity without changing immunoreactivity.

In earlier immunoassays, the hormone was always labeled with a radioactive isotope (RIA). Immunoassays that use fluorescent labels and avoid radioisotopes have become popular because they avoid risks of radiation exposure/contamination and because many of these assays are quite sensitive and convenient. To achieve optimal sensitivity in all immunoassays, the concentration of the labeled ligand must be critically adjusted, the antibody must be quite dilute, and the incubation must often be conducted for many hours to achieve equilibrium. For many hormones, the traditional competitive immunoassay has been replaced by another form of immunoassay termed the *immunometric assay*, which lacks these drawbacks (see below). Immunoassays have been developed for all polypeptide, steroid, and thyroid hormones.

The method used to separate antibody-bound and free hormone depends on the physical properties of the radioligand and the nature of the antibody. The most widely used method for polypeptide hormone assays is the precipitation of the antigen—antibody complex with a second antibody coupled to a heavy particle, such as *Staphylococcus aureas* protein A (that binds the Fc portion of IgG) affixed to sepharose beads. Thus, if the first antibody (to the hormone) was generated in a rabbit, an antibody to rabbit IgG is generated in another species (e.g., goat). The secondary antibody is bound to protein A–sepharose beads, and the complex is used to precipitate the original antigen–antibody complex. The beads are washed to remove trapped free L*, and the radioactivity bound to the beads is measured. The most common means of separating antibody-bound and free hormone in steroid radioimmunoassays is by using an excess of dextran-coated charcoal. The unbound steroid (L*) is adsorbed to the surface of the charcoal and centrifuged to the bottom of the tube. The soluble antigen–antibody complex, containing the L* · Ab complexes, remains in the supernatant, and the radioactivity in an aliquot is measured.

Problems in the Interpretation of Radioimmunoassays

In selecting antisera for use in immunoassays, one must consider the affinity and specificity of each antiserum. A plethora of steroid molecules circulate in human plasma, and the structures may differ subtly, by one hydroxyl group or by two hydrogen atoms. An antibody suitable for measuring estradiol concentrations in girls starting puberty must have exquisite affinity to detect ~30 pM concentrations of the hormone without cross-reacting with other steroids, which can be present at 100,000-fold higher concentrations. Hence, it is important to establish cross-reactivity of related compounds in each specific immunoassay to avoid spuriously high values due to other substances rather than the intended hormone. Sometimes, immunoassays with even the best antisera available cannot be directly performed on whole plasma, and the assay procedure must incorporate extraction (i.e., to distinguish pregnenolone from its sulfate) and/or chromatographic separation of steroid mixtures prior to immunoassay. The glycoprotein hormones luteinizing hormone (LH), follicle-stimulating hormone (FSH), thyroid-stimulating hormone (thyrotropin, TSH), and hCG are examples of a group of closely related peptide hormones that also present problems in assay specificity. These four hormones contain a common α-subunit, so polyclonal antisera generated to intact hormones will cross-react with the other members of the group. Because the β-subunit of each of these hormones confers immunological and biological specificity, it is necessary to select antisera that recognize this component of the molecule for an assay to have appropriate specificity.

Furthermore, peptide hormones do not exist as single, discrete molecular entities in the circulation but as mixtures of species with different sizes and posttranslational modifications (glycosylation, sulfation, etc.) due to variable processing and degradation. Growth hormone exists in multiple different forms in human plasma, and each molecular species has its own unique bioactivity and immunoreactivity. Consequently, GH immunoassays from two patients can yield identical numerical results but correspond to different amounts of bioactivity. In addition, many peptide hormones have glandular precursors with different biological activities (see Chapter 2) that circulate at higher or lower concentrations than the hormone itself, depending on the clinical situation. Thus, proinsulin may at times be present in the circulation with full immunoreactivity but less biological activity than insulin itself. Likewise, some peptide hormones have inactive metabolites that normally circulate at modest concentrations but may accumulate in disease states, such as the C terminal portion of the parathyroid hormone (PTH) molecule that rises in states of diminished renal function. Antisera directed to the C terminus can yield falsely elevated PTH values in renal failure, but current antisera for PTH assays recognize the N-terminal portion of the intact molecule to avoid such pitfalls (see Chapter 15). As assays become more specific and correlate better with bioactive hormone species, normal ranges must be redefined, especially for provocative tests.

Some peptide hormones are quite vulnerable to proteases present in serum, so sample collection methods can be very important. The degradation of hormone before assay will result in artifactually low values if the structures of the hormone fragments are sufficiently different from those of the parent polypeptide that the fragments do not react with the antibody. In such instances, protease inhibitors (disodium ethylenediaminetetraacetic acid [EDTA]) are added to the tubes in which the blood sample is collected, and the specimens should be quickly refrigerated to inhibit proteolytic degradation. Corticotropin (ACTH), for example, requires such special attention to avoid degradation. Small peptides like ACTH also stick to glass, and ACTH assays require collection in siliconized tubes. Conversely, prorenin is cleaved to renin at 4°C, so renin samples for immunoassay should be centrifuged at room temperature and quickly frozen.

Circulating endogenous antibodies (autoantibodies) to hormones provide an additional problem in the interpretation of RIAs. Antibodies to insulin are common in diabetic patients who take subcutaneous insulin injections, and antibodies to thyroglobulin are common in patients with autoimmune thyroid diseases. The effect of an autoantibody to the hormone in double antibody immunoassays (see below) is normally a spuriously high estimated concentration of the hormone in the plasma sample. Both the autoantibody and the assay antibody will bind the labeled hormone L* added to the sample. However, the second antibody will only precipitate the labeled hormone bound to the assay antibody, because it derives from the appropriate species (i.e., rabbit) targeted by the second antibody (i.e., goat anti-rabbit IgG). If the autoantibody is present in excess of the assay antibody, it will bind most of the L*, and little radioactivity will be precipitated by the second antibody, which will be interpreted as high concentrations of unlabeled hormone in the sample. When circulating autoantibodies are suspected, their presence can be detected by omitting the assay antibody, incubating the labeled hormone L* with the patient's plasma, and then using nonspecific agents such as ammonium sulfate to precipitate all hormone–antibody complexes.

Characteristics and Advantages of Immunometric Assays

In the early to mid-1980s, two advances revolutionized the immunoassays: the advent of hybridoma technology for monoclonal antibody production and the introduction of the immunometric assay. Monoclonal antibodies are generated by fusing spleen cells from immunized mice, which carry the genetic information to produce a specific antibody, with a selectable myeloma cell to create hybrid cells (hybridomas) capable of producing large quantities of homogeneous (monoclonal) antibody with a definable affinity for a single antigenic determinant. This technology overcame many of the problems associated with the use of heterogeneous (polyclonal) antibody preparations. Moreover, the introduction of a new type of immunoassay that used a labeled antibody, in lieu of a labeled antigen, (i.e., an *immunometric* assay) and incorporated the use of a second antibody bound to a solid phase provided an assay for the measurement of hormones with exquisite analytical sensitivity and specificity (Fig. 5-2). In addition, a nonisotopic chemical label could be attached to the second antibody, thus obviating the need for a gamma counter, a Nuclear Regulatory Commission license, and the time and effort required to comply with isotope safety procedures. In Figure 5-2, the antigen (e.g., protein hormone) of interest is *captured* by the first antibody (capture antibody), which is attached to a solid phase with a large surface area that permits many antibodies to be bound to its surface. Moreover, the capture antibody recognizes an epitope on the antigen of interest that is different from the antigenic determinant recognized by the labeled or *signal* antibody containing the chemical molecule whose signal is used to quantify the amount of antigen in the patient's sample.

The signal antibodies can be modified with a variety of agents to yield different physical signals and hence different types of assays. When the molecule bound

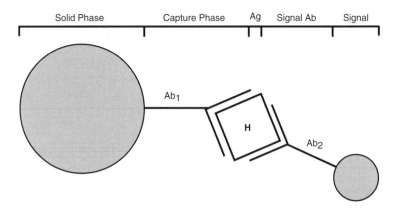

Fig. 5-2 Principles of immunometric assays. In the prototypic immunometric assay, the capture monoclonal antibody (Ab$_1$) bound to a solid phase (e.g., a plastic bead, a paramagnetic particle, the surface of a plastic tube or microtiter plate, etc.) recognizes a certain epitope on the antigen (hormone) and *captures* all of the hormone molecules in the sample. A second, labeled monoclonal (or polyclonal) antibody (Ab$_2$) recognizes a different epitope on the antigen (Ag) of interest than Ab$_1$. The nature of the label (or signal) attached to the second antibody describes the type of immunometric assay. Because the analyte being measured (e.g., thyrotropin [TSH] in this example) is *sandwiched* between the capture and signal antibodies and because both of these antibodies may be monoclonal, this type of immunometric assay is referred to as a *dual-monoclonal sandwich immunoassay*.

to the signal antibody is a radioisotope, the assay is referred to as an *immunoradiometric assay* (IRMA). Similarly, when the molecule bound to the signal antibody is capable of chemiluminescence, fluorescence, or enzyme activity on addition of an appropriate substrate or conditions, the assay is referred to as an *immunochemiluminometric* (ICMA), *immunofluorometric* (IFMA), or *immunoenzymetric* (IEMA) assay, respectively. Each of these different labels provide a signal-to-noise level that considerably improves the analytical sensitivity of these assays over RIAs, and the underlying principle of the assay is identical regardless of the type of signal.

Immunometric assays do not rely on the competition of hormone with labeled ligand L* for a limited amount of antibody, so the antibodies are generally used in excess to ensure that the antibody binds all of the hormone in the sample. This condition of antibody excess expedites hormone binding and allows the assay to be completed in only a few hours. Third, the working range of immunometric assays is expanded without the limitations imposed by antibody competition between hormone and L*, and the assay may be capable of measuring all anticipated values without requiring serial dilution and repeat assays. Finally, because there is no labeled L* in the assays, the problem of circulating autoantibodies to hormones (see above) is minimized.

Immunometric assays have greatly enhanced the sensitivity of hormone assays, decreasing the lower limit of detection of peptide hormones such as TSH by one to two orders of magnitude (see Chapter 13). When comparing the performance characteristics of immunometric assays, however, it is important to distinguish functional from analytical sensitivity. *Analytical sensitivity* refers to the smallest amount of analyte (antigen) that an assay can reliably distinguish from *zero* antigen with 95% confidence. A more practical sensitivity limit is *functional sensitivity*, defined as the 20% interassay coefficient of variation. For example, manufacturers of several immunometric TSH assays report an analytical sensitivity of 0.03 μU/ml. However, only those assays with a functional sensitivity of $\leq$0.2 μU/ml can reliably distinguish the truly suppressed TSH values of hyperthyroid patients from low-normal values in euthyroid subjects (see Chapter 13).

In addition, the antigenic specificity of the two antibodies used in immunometric assays markedly improved the analytical specificity of these assays over RIAs. *Analytical specificity* refers to the assay's freedom from interference from other molecules, which requires cross-reactivity to both antibodies in the immunometric assays. Lastly, the availability of fully automated instruments for performing nonisotopic immunometric assays enabled simple, rapid, and less costly measurement of endocrine hormones than RIAs.

While immunometric assays have obviated problems due to autoantibodies, the use of excess murine monoclonal antibodies renders these assays vulnerable to confounding effects of heterophilic antibodies. Some patients, such as laboratory workers constantly exposed to mice or patients treated with other monoclonal antibodies, harbor nonspecific anti-mouse IgG antibodies in their serum. For example, in assays using murine-derived signal and capture molecules, divalent human anti-mouse antibodies (HAMA) in a patient's serum could link the signal and capture molecules and cause a spuriously high value. A little over 3% of unselected serum samples contain sufficient HAMA to give falsely elevated readings in the TSH assay. As a result, manufacturers have added small quantities of mouse serum or nonspecific immunoglobulins to absorb potential HAMA that could interfere with the assay. Even with these additions of mouse immunoglobulins, rare patients have such elevated HAMA in their serum that the assay still yields falsely high readings.

Chromatography and Spectrometry

Although antibodies can be very specific for a single structural unit on a protein or small molecule, human plasma contains a multitude of different compounds, many of which may share similar if not identical structural elements that can bind to antibodies intended for a specific hormone. If cross-reactivity in an assay is sufficient to invalidate the method, then additional means of distinguishing the desired hormone from the interfering substances are required. One approach used to separate the target molecule from related compounds is chromatography, most commonly high-performance liquid chromatography (HPLC). In HPLC, a sample of plasma or urine is applied to a column filled with fine particles of some material (the stationary phase) and forced along the column with a solvent (the mobile phase) under high pressure. The different compounds each interact with both the stationary and mobile phases, and the relative strengths of these interactions determine how rapidly each compound passes along the column. Molecules that interact weakly with the stationary phase but strongly with the mobile phase elute relatively quickly, whereas molecules that bind tightly to the stationary phase elute slowly. The time required to pass through the column, the elution time, is characteristic for each compound under a given system of stationary and mobile phases, allowing separation of mixtures based on their elution times.

The stationary phase can be a polar material like silica gel, which is used with organic solvents. The more polar the compound, the tighter it binds to the silica and the longer it takes to elute; this is called *straight-phase* or *standard* HPLC. For steroids and peptides, most of these molecules are so hydrophobic (nonpolar) that the interaction with silica is uniformly weak, such that minimal separation is achieved by standard HPLC. Instead, a hydrophobic column material containing hydrocarbon chains 4 to 18 carbon atoms in length (C4 to C18 columns) is used with mixtures of alcohol (typically methanol) or acetonitrile and water. In the latter systems, the more polar compounds bind poorly to the stationary phase and elute quickly. Since the order of elution of polar and nonpolar compounds is reversed from that of standard HPLC, this method is called *reverse-phase* HPLC. Subtle structural differences can be exploited by HPLC, particularly reverse-phase HPLC, to separate very similar compounds.

The compounds eluting from the column must be detected, characterized, and quantitated. Many peptides and steroids absorb ultraviolet (UV) light, so absorbance detectors are commonly plumbed into the system directly. Electrochemical and refractive index detectors may detect compounds that do not absorb UV light, but their sensitivities are poor. The column is also calibrated with known reference compounds or *standards* to ascertain when the desired compounds are expected to elute. Small amounts of *internal standards*—readily detected compounds that elute characteristically at different times than the target compounds—are often added to each specimen to ensure that the instrument is operating properly and that the elution times are reliable. If the abundance of the compound and its UV absorbance are sufficient, the analyte can be quantitated simply by integrating the UV absorbance of the *peak* generated in the absorbance tracing as the compound elutes from the column. Otherwise, small aliquots of eluate or fractions are collected over time, and the fractions containing the desired analyte(s) are analyzed by immunoassay. The effluent of the column can also be sent directly to an instrument that performs mass spectrometry (MS) to accurately determine the molecular mass of the compound. Addition of a known amount of deuterium-labeled standard to the specimen allows direct measurement of the quantity of analyte present by the tandem HPLC/MS system. Other compounds, such as fatty acids, require chemical derivitization prior to HPLC analysis. Gas chromatography (GC) is similar to HPLC except that an inert gas is used for the mobile phase and the column, which is often simply a long, thin capillary tube, is warmed to keep small samples of hormones or chemical derivates of hormones in the gas phase. Particularly when coupled to MS (GC/MS), GC is an even more powerful tool for separating complex mixtures, but GC requires great technical expertise.

Sampling the Plasma

For hormones whose plasma concentrations are relatively stable (e.g., thyroxine), the use of a single random plasma sample provides a reliable estimate of hormonal status in most circumstances. In contrast, circulating concentrations of many hormones vary substantially during the day and in response to physiological conditions. To assess hormone levels accurately for hormones secreted in short pulses (e.g., LH and testosterone), it is preferable to draw three or more samples at 20- to 30-minute intervals and pool aliquots of each for a single determination. For hormones with a significant diurnal or sleep-related secretion pattern, the result must be interpreted relative to the time of sampling. Plasma concentrations of ACTH and cortisol are normally high only in the early morning hours, and GH secretion rises soon after an individual falls asleep. Normal ranges and patterns of secretion also vary with age: diurnal cortisol secretion is not entrained in newborns, and LH pulsation occurs only during sleep in early and midpuberty. In women, the plasma concentrations of gonadotropins, estradiol, and progesterone must be interpreted in light of the phase of the menstrual cycle. Finally, the stress of a venipuncture itself can elevate concentrations of many hormones, from catecholamines to prolactin.

Effect of Plasma-Binding Proteins

Whereas most polypeptide hormones circulate in the plasma unbound to other plasma constituents, steroid and thyroid hormones circulate largely bound to albumin and to specific binding proteins (Fig. 5-3). Less than 1% of thyroxine (T_4) and

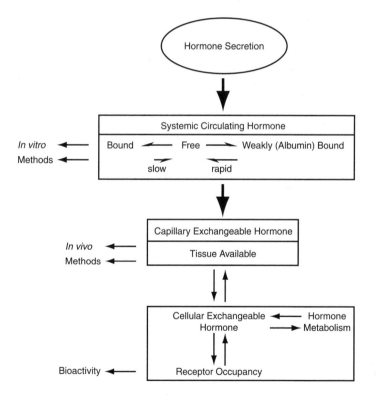

Fig. 5-3 Conceptual diagram depicting hormone distribution, disposition, and compartmentation. *In vitro* assays measure bound, free, and/or weakly bound hormones in the circulation. *In vivo* methods measure the capillary exchangeable fraction, which is often much greater than the systemic free hormone fraction. It is the capillary exchangeable fraction that is available to tissues as the bioactive cellular exchangeable hormone that, in turn, binds to and activates receptors.

triiodothyroxine (T_3) and only about 1%–3% of androgens, estrogens, and gluco-corticoids in the plasma are in the unbound or free form. The free hormone concentrations of these hormones can be determined *in vitro* by a tedious procedure termed *equilibrium dialysis*. For some time, the free fraction was regarded as the biologically active portion of the circulating hormone concentration, as it was thought to be the only fraction available for entry into cells and thus for interaction with receptors.

It is now clear that the process of steroid and thyroid hormone transport into cells is more complicated, and more than just the free fraction estimated *in vitro* is available to enter cells. Protein-bound hormones can dissociate more readily within a capillary bed than under equilibrium conditions *in vitro*, such that the active fraction can be larger than estimated in the assay. *In vivo* methods (Fig. 5-3) are needed to estimate the *capillary exchangeable hormone* because binding proteins, including albumin, thyroid hormone-binding globulin (TBG), and sex hormone-binding globulin (SHBG), may interact with the components on the microcirculation surface (e.g., endothelial glycocalyx). These interactions may elicit conformational changes at the hormone-binding site on the plasma protein, which may markedly increase the rate of hormone dissociation from that protein in the microcirculation, freeing more hormone than is measured *in vitro*. These *in vivo* assays are cumbersome and generally used for research purposes only; alternative tests that approximate the biologically active hormone are used routinely.

Although there are differences for specific hormones, albumin, which is the most abundant protein in plasma, binds many hormones weakly; hence the fraction bound to albumin is called the *weakly bound* hormone. Because hormones bind to and dissociate from albumin readily, the free and the albumin-bound hormone pools exchange rapidly, and both components appear to be available for entry into most tissues. In the case of plasma testosterone, this free plus albumin-bound component constitutes about half of the total circulating hormone (because albumin is so abundant), and this amount is referred to as the *bioavailable testosterone*. In general, it is the free plus weakly bound or bioavailable component of the hormone that is precisely regulated by feedback mechanisms.

The laboratory measurement or estimation of free plus albumin-bound steroid and thyroid hormones is technically easier than the measurement of free hormone by equilibrium dialysis. The free plus albumin-bound fraction of testosterone is measured by precipitating the SHBG (and its bound testosterone) with ammonium sulfate and measuring the testosterone that remains in the supernatant. More commonly, the total steroid and T_4 concentrations are measured as a surrogate for the bioavailable hormone if the binding protein concentrations are relatively normal. The free T_4 concentration can be estimated by immunometric methods that employ short incubation times to sample only the unbound T_4. However, when the concentrations of specific binding proteins are likely to be significantly increased (TBG and SHBG in pregnancy) or decreased (TBG in debilitating illness, SHBG in thyrotoxicosis), some assessment of the amount of binding protein is required to interpret the total hormone concentrations. Both TBG and SHBG may be measured directly, and the amount of TBG sites may be inferred by the T_3 resin uptake test (see Chapter 13). Equilibrium dialysis is used when more convenient methods yield insufficient information.

Interpretation of *Normal Ranges*

Stated normal ranges are often quite broad, extending over a two- to threefold range for T_4 and testosterone, and more narrow and appropriate normal ranges are obtained if reference populations are properly matched. Whereas the normal range for free T_4 is rather invariant, normal plasma testosterone concentrations vary with age, sex, and pubertal stage. As almost all hormone systems are under some regulatory feedback control, measuring both members of a *hormone pair* (e.g., T_4 and TSH, testosterone and LH) may provide insights not available from measuring only one hormone (Fig. 5-4). The interpretation of laboratory results in the context of feedback and homeostatis originated from the study of pituitary trophic hormones and the hormones secreted by their target endocrine glands (Fig. 5-4); however, the concept applies broadly to pairs of hormones and analytes such as calcium and PTH, insulin and glucose, and plasma osmolality and vasopressin.

This paradigm of feedback regulation is central to the assessment of endocrine status. For example, because the normal range of plasma T_4 is broad, a low-normal T_4 level coupled with an elevated TSH level indicates early, compensated thyroid failure. Conversely, a normal TSH level in the face of a very low free thyroxine is not the normal homeostatic response and suggests pituitary failure. Likewise, a normal plasma PTH level in a patient with a simultaneously elevated serum calcium level is inappropriate and suggests primary hyperparathyroidism. The measurement of hormone pairs permits the analysis of hormone concentrations in the context of their regulatory control mechanisms. Other possible outcomes of measuring both members of a hormone pair are also indicated in Figure 5-4.

In general, low concentrations of both members of a hormone pair implicate trophic hormone deficiency (often pituitary failure) as the primary disorder (Fig. 5-4). High concentrations of a target gland hormone coupled with low concentra-

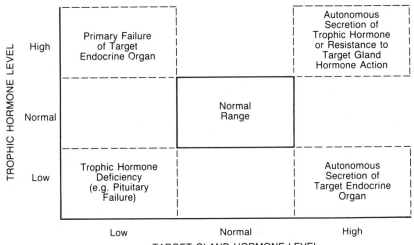

Fig. 5-4 Diagram depicting the possible interpretations of alterations in trophic and target gland hormone pairs (e.g., T_4 and thyrotropin). (Redrawn with modification from Griffin, 1992, p. 1664.)

tions of the corresponding trophic hormone suggest autonomous secretion by the target endocrine organ, as is typical in primary hyperthyroidism (high T_4, suppressed TSH). Elevated concentrations of both members of a hormone pair usually indicate autonomous secretion of the trophic hormone, either from the normal site or from a tumor in an ectopic location. For example, excess cortisol production driven by a high plasma ACTH level may be due to the secretion of pituitary ACTH or secretion of ACTH by lung tumors. Alternatively, the combined elevation of trophic and target endocrine gland hormones can result from resistance to the action of the target endocrine gland hormone (e.g., elevated LH and testosterone in androgen resistance). Autonomous hypersecretion of the trophic hormone typically results in clinical evidence of target gland hormone excess, whereas resistance to the target gland hormone leads to manifestations of hormone deficiency. Hence clinical assessment and knowledge of the relative frequency of various endocrine disorders is always applied in the interpretation of the laboratory results.

URINARY HORMONE EXCRETION

Documenting excess hormone production using plasma measurements of a hormone pair that fluctuates markedly over the course of a day is problematic, as values at any one point in time may be normal yet overall production is elevated. In order to obtain an integrated measure of hormone production and/or mean plasma concentrations, one may measure the urinary excretion of a hormone or hormone metabolite over a defined period. Thus, the 24-hour urinary 17-hydroxycorticosteroids represent a summation of all glucocorticoid metabolites produced during the day. The urinary free cortisol sums or integrates the plasma cortisol concentrations that exceed the saturation of binding proteins. Urinary excretion of cortisol and its metabolites is often elevated in patients with Cushing's disease due to sustained, moderate plasma cortisol concentrations throughout the evening, whereas the plasma cortisol level may not be frankly elevated at any time during the day. Likewise, measurement of urinary metabolites of catecholamines may provide a useful clue to their sustained or episodic excess in the plasma.

To ensure a complete urine collection, total creatinine should be measured on all specimens. Men excrete about 1.5 g of creatinine each day, and women excrete about 1.0 g. Urine creatinine values are reduced in patients with malnutrition, renal insufficiency, and advanced age. To account for variably complete collections, hormone excretion values should be explicitly or qualitatively adjusted for urinary creatinine content. Urine aldosterone excretion must be related to urine sodium content, because aldosterone production should be suppressed in sodium surfeit and elevated in sodium restriction. Urine collection containers may require a preservative such as various acids for specific hormone measurements. Many urinary hormone measurements involve determination of a metabolite rather than of the hormones themselves, and drugs or disease states that alter hormone metabolism may thus alter the urinary measurement without producing an abnormality of hormone secretion. Because of these inherent limitations, difficulties, and caveats, urinary hormone measurements have been largely supplanted by reliable plasma immunoassays, but urinary excretion of aldosterone, cortisol, and catecholamine metabolites is still widely used.

SALIVARY HORMONE MEASUREMENTS

Measurement of hormone concentrations in saliva is appealing because such tests are noninvasive, reflect the concentrations of free hormone in the plasma, and may be performed at any time of day in the patient's own home without added stress. The disadvantages are that larger polypeptides do not pass into saliva, salivary hormone concentrations are influenced by saliva production rates, and hormone concentrations in saliva are much lower than concentrations in the plasma. An excellent use of salivary hormone assays is in measuring midnight cortisol values in patients suspected of having Cushing's disease. Elevated saliva cortisol concentrations obtained at midnight in the patient's home reflect sustained cortisol production at night and a loss of the diurnal cortisol rhythm that characterizes Cushing's disease.

HORMONE PRODUCTION RATES

Measuring the actual secretion or production rate of a hormone should overcome most of the problems inherent in plasma and urinary hormone measurements for assessing endocrine function. However, such measurements are technically difficult and usually involve the administration of hormone labeled with a radioisotope or stable isotope to track its dilution over time by endogenous hormone production. Alternatively, the metabolic clearance rate (MCR) of a hormone may be determined and, together with the mean plasma concentration (PC), allows calculation of the production rate (PR) by the formula $PR = MCR \times PC$. In either case, the measurement of hormone production rates remains primarily a research procedure.

DYNAMIC TESTS OF ENDOCRINE FUNCTION

Unfortunately, the range of hormone values obtained from static measurements of one or more plasma samples from normal subjects can overlap substantially with values obtained from patients with abnormal endocrine function. A more stringent test for endocrine abnormalities is to utilize the factors known to regulate production of those hormones in dynamic testing. In general, if one suspects that hormone production is low, one tries to stimulate its production; conversely, if one suspects that hormone production is excessive, one tries to suppress it. By obtaining normative data for these studies performed on normal controls and on patients known to have disease, investigators have developed criteria that distinguish subjects with and without disease more reliably than do static hormone measurements.

Stimulation Tests

A typical stimulation test involves administering of a standard dose of a trophic hormone and measuring the increase in hormone production from the target gland.

The trophic hormone can be a hypothalamic releasing factor such as thyrotropin-releasing hormone (TRH) or a pituitary hormone equivalent (cosyntropin for ACTH or hCG for LH). Alternatively, a stimulatory test may employ a physiological stimulus that evokes an increase in the secretion of an endogenous trophic hormone, which in turn increases production of hormone from the target gland. For instance, hypoglycemia induced by an intravenous insulin bolus evokes a counterregulatory response from higher brain centers. Corticotropin (and subsequently cortisol), GH, and prolactin all rise during hypoglycemia, as do glucagon and epinephrine (see Chapter 14). The specific test chosen depends on which levels of the endocrine axis require assessment and what clinical and practical circumstances prevail. Cosyntropin testing is safe and simple but directly evaluates the only the adrenal gland with a supraphysiological challenge. Insulin-induced hypoglycemia evaluates the hypothalamus, pituitary, and adrenal glands simultaneously with a more physiological stimulus but is cumbersome and can be dangerous for older or sick patients who will not tolerate hypoglycemia. A poor rise in plasma hormone concentrations in response to a stimulus is very good evidence of hormone insufficiency. Abnormal or paradoxically excessive responses to provocative challenges can also be used to diagnose tumors, such as a GH rise in response to TRH in acromegaly or an exaggerated calcitonin rise in response to pentagastrin administration in the early stages of medullary thyroid carcinoma (C-cell hyperplasia).

The ultimate functional test of endocrine function is to demonstrate a normal physiological response in target tissues to stimuli that evoke endogenous hormone production. For example, if a patient's urine is maximally concentrated in response to water deprivation, one can infer that the osmolality-sensing mechanisms in the hypothalamus, the secretion of vasopressin, the V_2 receptor for vasopressin, and postreceptor events in vasopressin action in the kidney are all normal (see Chapter 7). If the urine fails to concentrate, plasma vasopressin measurements and urine osmolality changes in response to a vasopressin injection can determine if vasopressin production or renal responsiveness is abnormal. However, such *in vivo* tests of tissue effects have not been developed for most endocrine systems and do not always identify the locus of the defect. Stimulation testing can sometimes be used not only to evaluate hormone production but also to assess responsiveness of target tissues to hormones, which is abnormal in hormone resistance syndromes. The increase in urinary cyclic adenosine monophosphate (AMP) and phosphate that normally follows PTH administration is blunted or absent in patients with PTH resistance (pseudohypoparathyroidism) but is normal in patients with hypoparathyroidism due to PTH deficiency.

Suppression Tests

If the negative feedback control mechanisms are intact, administration of a supraphysiological dose of a hormone or a synthetic derivative will suppress endogenous hormone secretion. For example, the glucocorticoid dexamethasone is given to persons with suspected hypercortisolism to assess its capacity to inhibit ACTH secretion and thus cortisol production by the adrenals. In a suppression test, failure to suppress indicates autonomous secretion either of the hormone of the target endocrine gland (cortisol) or of the trophic hormone (ACTH). Other suppression tests use physiological challenges that suppress hormone production, such as oral glucose administration in suspected GH excess and salt loading in the assessment of excess aldosterone secretion.

Problems in Interpreting Dynamic Tests

To correctly interpret responses to provocative tests, it is imperative that normative data from affected patients and from appropriate control subjects have been obtained under identical conditions using similar hormone assays. Medications may interfere with dynamic tests by directly suppressing pituitary function (glucocorticoids and TSH), stimulating pituitary function (antipsychotic drugs like risperidol prolactin), or altering metabolism of test agents (anticonvulsant drugs like phenytoin and dexamethasone). Intercurrent medical or psychiatric illnesses, pregnancy, and other conditions may alter the response to provocative tests. Furthermore, criteria for dynamic tests based on pharmacological challenges are empirical and thus not completely reliable. Prior treatment with hormones often alters test results, and patients with prolonged hormone deficiencies may respond differently to an initial challenge than to repetitive stimulations. For example, men with long-standing hypothalamic disease may show a subnormal LH response to an initial bolus of luteinizing hormone-releasing hormone (LHRH), but following a week of pulsatile LHRH administration, their LH response may be normal. Such a comparison may help to distinguish between hypothalamic and pituitary hypogonadism (Fig. 5-5). Similarly, older children often respond abnormally to provocative stimuli for GH secretion unless first primed with sex steroids; furthermore, hypothyroidism, hyperthyroidism, and hypercortisolism all may impair GH responsiveness.

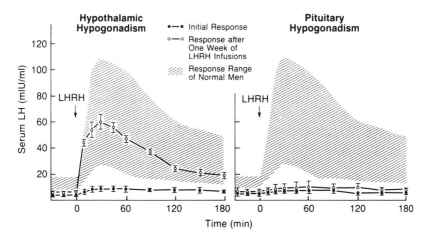

Fig. 5-5 Mean serum luteinizing hormone (LH) responses of 10 men with hypogonadotropic hypogonadism to a 250 mg intravenous bolus dose of luteinizing hormone-releasing hormone (LHRH) before and after daily infusions (500 mg over 4 hours) of LHRH for 1 week. Five men had presumed hypothalamic disease and five had presumed pituitary disease. (From Snyder PJ et al: Repetitive infusion of gonadotropin-releasing hormone distinguishes hypothalamic from pituitary hypogonadism. J Clin Endocrinol Metab 48:864–868, 1979; © 1979, The Endocrine Society.)

MEASUREMENT OF HORMONE RECEPTORS

The major forms of endocrine pathology in which receptor measurements are useful are hormone resistance syndromes, and these assays are normally functional studies such as hormone-binding assays. In general, the characteristic of such states is the lack or incompleteness of the expected hormone's effects in the presence of normal or increased circulating concentrations of the hormone. The types of tissues used for hormone receptor measurements vary with the hormone and receptor of interest and include lymphocytes, red blood cells, tissue biopsy samples, and cultured skin fibroblasts. Alternatively, genetic testing may identify mutations in the gene for the hormone receptor, and the mutant protein may be expressed in cultured cells for convenient functional studies. Intracellular androgen receptors from genital skin fibroblasts of patients with androgen insensitivity often fail to bind testosterone or bind testosterone but fail to activate expression of target genes. Cell surface LH receptors can be nonfunctional in Leydig cell hypoplasia or constitutively active in familial male precocious puberty (testotoxicosis), yielding under- or overproduction of testosterone, respectively.

Disorders may also result from postreceptor proteins that help to transduce the hormone signal within target cells. Guanosine triphosphate (GTP)-binding proteins, a component of cell surface receptor signal pathways, can be constitutively active in the McCune-Albright syndrome, leading to hyperfunction of several endocrine glands. Conversely, inactive GTP-binding proteins can cause resistance to one or more hormones, such as PTH resistance in pseudohypoparathyroidism type I.

Hormone receptor measurements help to guide therapy and add prognostic information in at least one form of hormone-responsive malignancy, cancer of the breast. Quantitating the content of estrogen receptor and of progesterone receptor, the latter made in breast tissue in response to estrogen acting through its receptor, has proven useful in predicting the response of such tumors to hormonal manipulation.

SUGGESTED READING

Gorden P and Weintraub BD: Radioreceptor and other functional hormone assays. In: *Williams Textbook of Endocrinology*, 8th ed., JD Wilson and DW Foster, eds., Saunders, Philadelphia, pp. 1647–1661, 1992.

Griffin JE: Dynamic tests of endocrine function. In: *Williams Textbook of Endocrinology*, 8th ed., JD Wilson and DW Foster, eds., Saunders, Philadelphia, pp. 1663–1670, 1992.

Klee G: Laboratory techniques for recognition of endocrine disorders. In: *Williams Textbook of Endocrinology*, 10th ed., PR Larson, HM Kronenberg, S Melmed, and KS Polonsky, eds., Saunders, Philadelphia, pp. 65–79, 2003.

Lefkowitz RJ: Clinical implications of basic research. N Engl J Med 332:186–187, 1995.

Pardridge WM: Transport of protein-bound hormones into tissues in vivo. Endocr Rev 2:103–123, 1981.

Pardridge WM: Serum bioavailability of sex steroid hormones. J Clin Endocrinol Metab 15:259–278, 1986.

Price CP and Newman DJ, eds: *Principles and Practice of Immunoassay*, 2nd ed., Stockton, New York, 1997.

Segre GV and Brown EN: Measurement of hormones. In: *Williams Textbook of Endocrinology*, 9th ed., JD Wilson, DW Foster, HM Kronenberg, and PR Larsen, eds., Saunders, Philadelphia, pp. 43–54, 1998.

Sevier ED, David GS, Martinis J, Desmond WJ, Bartholomew RM, and Wang R: Monoclonal antibodies in clinical immunology. Clin Chem 27:1797–1806, 1981.

Spencer CA, LoPresti JS, Patel A, Guttler RB, Eigen A, Shen D, Gray D, and Nicoloff JT: Applications of a new chemiluminometric thyrotropin assay to subnormal measurement. J Clin Endocrinol Metab 70:453–460, 1990.

Spencer CA, Takeuchi M, and Kazarosyan M: Current status and performance goals for serum thyrotropin (TSH) assays. Clin Chem 42:140–145, 1996.

Spiegel AM, Weinstein LS, and Shenker A: Abnormalities in G-protein-coupled signal transduction pathways in human disease. J Clin Invest 92:1119–1125, 1993.

Verhoeven GFM and Wilson JD: The syndromes of primary hormone resistance. Metabolism 28:253–289, 1979.

Ward G, McKinnon L, Badrick T, and Hickman PE: Heterophilic antibodies remain a problem for the immunoassay laboratory. Am J Clin Pathol 108:417–421, 1997.

6

The Anterior Pituitary and Hypothalamus

SERGIO R. OJEDA

The core of the neuroendocrine system is represented by the hypothalamic–pituitary complex. The hypothalamus is composed of a diversity of neurosecretory cells arranged in groups, which secrete their products either into the portal blood system that connects the hypothalamus to the adenohypophysis (see below) or directly into the general circulation after storage in the neurohypophysis (see Chapter 7). Because of the nature of their actions, the hypothalamic hormones are classified as releasing or inhibiting hormones (Table 6-1).

The hypothalamic hormones delivered to the portal blood system are transported to the adenohypophysis, where they stimulate or inhibit the synthesis and secretion of different trophic hormones. In turn, these hormones regulate gonadal, thyroid, and adrenal function, in addition to lactation, bodily growth, and somatic development.

No attempt will be made in this chapter to cover the actions of the different pituitary trophic hormones on their target glands, as they are discussed in detail in other chapters. An exception to this is growth hormone (GH). Although Chapter 12 considers several aspects of the control and actions of GH, a broader discussion of its physiological actions will be presented here because GH is the only anterior pituitary hormone that does not have a clear-cut target gland.

ANATOMY

The Pituitary Gland

The pituitary gland (Fig. 6-1) has two parts: the neurohypophysis, of neural origin (see Chapter 7), and the adenohypophysis, of ectodermal origin. In embryonic development, an evagination from the roof of the pharynx pushes dorsally to reach a ventrally directed evagination from the base of the diencephalon. The dorsally projecting evagination, known as *Rathke's pouch,* forms the adenohypophysis, whereas the ventrally directed evagination of neural tissue forms the neurohypophysis. The

Table 6-1 Hypothalamic Releasing and Inhibiting Hormones

Hypothalamic hormone	Purified	Synthesized	Stimulates	Inhibits	Cell bodies in
Vasopressin	Yes	Nonapeptide	ACTH	0	SO, PVN
Corticotropin-releasing hormone (CRH)	Yes	41AA peptide	ACTH	0	PVN
Urocortin I-III	Yes	38-40AA peptides	ACTH	0	PVN, ARC, brain stem
Luteinizing hormone-releasing hormone (LHRH)	Yes	Decapeptide	LH, FSH	0	POA, MBH
Follicle-stimulating hormone (FSH)-releasing factor	Yes	No	FSH	0	PVN/POA?
Thyrotropin-releasing hormone (TRH)	Yes	Tripeptide	TSH, PRL	0	PVN
Growth hormone-releasing hormone (GHRH)	Yes	44AA peptide	GH	0	ARC
Ghrelin	Yes	28AA peptide	GH	0	ARC, stomach(s)
Growth hormone-inhibiting hormone (GHIH) (somatostatin)	Yes	Tetradecapeptide		0	GH, PRL, TSH, APR, gastrin, glucagon, insulin
Prolactin (PRL)-	Yes	Yes	0	PRL	ARC
inhibiting factors (PIFs), dopamine, peptidergic PIF	No	No	0	PRL	?
PRL-releasing factors (PRFs)					
Prolactin-releasing peptide	Yes	20–31AA	PRL	0	DMH, SN
Oxytocin	Yes	Nonapeptide	PRL	0	SO, PVN
TRH, VIP, PHI, AII neurotensin substance P	Yes	—	PRl	0	PVN, SO
Melanocyte-stimulating hormone (MSH)-releasing factor (MRF)	Yes	No	MSH	0	
MSH-inhibiting factor (MIF)	Yes	No	0	MSH	
Pituitary adenylate cyclase-activating peptide (PACAP)	Yes	27 and 38AA	ACTH, GH	0	SO, PVN

AA, amino acid; ACTH, adenocorticotropic hormone; AII, angiotensin II; APR, anterior periventricular region; ARC, arcuate nucleus; DMH, dorsomedial nucleus; MBH, medial basasl hypothalamus; PHI, peptide histidine-isoleucine; POA, preoptic area; PVN, paraventricular nucleus; SN, solitary nucleus; SO, supraoptic nucleus; TSH, thyroid-stimulating hormone; VIP, vasoactive intestinal polypeptide.

neurohypophysis has three parts: the median eminence, the infundibular stem, and the neural lobe itself. The median eminence represents the intrahypothalamic portion and lies just ventral to the floor of the third ventricle protruding slightly in the midline. The main part of the neurohypophysis, the neural lobe, is connected to the median eminence by the infundibular stem. The adenohypophysis can also be divided into three parts: the pars distalis, which is the ventral portion; the pars intermedia, which is that portion adjacent to the neural lobe and separated from the pars distalis by the residual lumen of Rathke's pouch; and the pars tuberalis, which

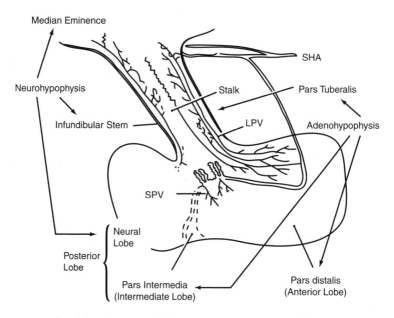

Fig. 6-1 Details of the anatomy of the pituitary gland showing the three components of the neurohypophysis (median eminence, infundibular stem, and neural lobe) and the three components of the adenohypophysis (pars tuberalis, pars distalis, and pars intermedia). The pituitary vasculature represented by the superior hypophyseal arteries (SHA), the long portal vessels (LPV), and the short portal vessels (SPV) is also shown.

spreads dorsally to surround the infundibular stem. The infundibular stem and surrounding pars tuberalis constitute the pituitary stalk. The pars distalis is frequently termed the *anterior lobe* because of its anterior position in most animals. The pars intermedia (which is rudimentary in humans) and the neural lobe constitute the posterior lobe (Fig. 6-1).

There is no significant functional innervation of the adenohypophysis by way of the hypothalamus or neural lobe. Instead, a humoral pathway is provided by means of the hypophyseal portal system of veins (Fig. 6-1). These veins originate from capillary loops in the median eminence and drain blood into parallel veins down the stalk known as *long portal vessels*. In the anterior lobe, the portal vessels break up into sinusoids that provide most of the blood supply to the lobe. Venous blood drains from the gland into the cavernous sinus. In addition to the long portal vessels, there are short portal venous vascular connections that arise in the neural lobe and pass across the pars intermedia to the anterior lobe. These are known as the *short portal vessels*.

Uptake of hormones into and delivery of substances from the vascular system are favored by the presence of fenestrated capillaries within the gland. Because the vascular supply is primarily portal in nature, capillary pressure in the gland is very low and the permeability of these capillaries is high. This arrangement may be analogous to that in hepatic sinusoids with high permeability not only to pituitary protein hormones but also to plasma proteins. Thus, a balance between hydrostatic pres-

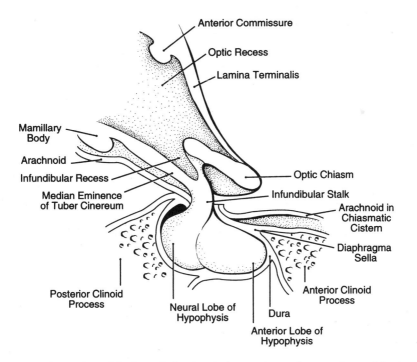

Fig. 6-2 Relationship of the hypothalamic–pituitary unit to other structures of the base of the brain. (Redrawn from Reichlin S: In: *Williams Textbook of Endocrinology,* 7th ed., JD Wilson and DW Foster, eds., Saunders, Philadelphia, p. 495, 1985.)

sure tending to produce ultrafiltration and colloid osmotic pressure tending to cause uptake of extracellular fluid is achieved at a very low sinusoidal pressure.

The Hypothalamus

The hypothalamus is located at the base of the brain, ventral to the thalamus, from which it is separated by the hypothalamic sulcus. Its anterior boundaries are provided by the optic chiasm; laterally, it is separated from the temporal lobes by the hypothalamic sulci. Its posterior limits are defined by the mammillary bodies. The base of the hypothalamus is the tuber cinereum, the central part of which is the median eminence. The anatomical relationships of the hypothalamic–pituitary unit to other structures of the base of the brain are shown in Figure 6-2.

ANTERIOR PITUITARY HORMONES AND THEIR HYPOTHALAMIC CONTROL

As indicated before, the secretion of adenohypophyseal hormones is controlled by releasing and inhibiting hormones that, produced in the hypothalamus, reach the pituitary gland via the portal vessels. Most of these hypothalamic hormones have been identified and their biochemical and genomic structures characterized (Table 6-1).

Hypothalamic Releasing and Inhibiting Hormones

Thyrotropin-Releasing Hormone

This hormone acts on the anterior pituitary gland to release thyroid-stimulating hormone (TSH) as well as prolactin (PRL); it is a tripeptide (pyro-Glu-His-Pro amine) derived from a large precursor that has a molecular weight of about 29,000. The thyrotropin-releasing hormone (TRH) precursor contains five copies of the sequence Gln-His-Pro-Gly, which presumably originates the mature TRH molecule following glutamine cyclization and formation of the terminal amide. Within the hypothalamus, TRH is mainly synthesized in neurons of the parvocellular division of the paraventricular nucleus (Fig. 6-3 and Table 6-1) and also in some cells of the preoptic region. Axons project caudally from these regions and then project ventrally into the median eminence, where the bulk of TRH is stored. In addition, TRH is found outside the hypothalamus, even in the spinal cord, suggesting its involvement in other central nervous system functions.

Prolactin-Releasing Hormone

Although it has been known for years that hypothalamic extracts are capable of stimulating PRL release from the anterior pituitary, the identity of the factors that might contribute to this activity was only partially known. Several neuropeptides, including TRH, oxytocin, and vasoactive intestinal polypeptide (VIP), can elicit PRL release, but their physiological relevance as specific PRL-releasing factors is questionable. More recently, a novel hypothalamic PRL-releasing peptide (PRP) and its cognate pituitary receptor were identified by molecular cloning. The PRP prepro-

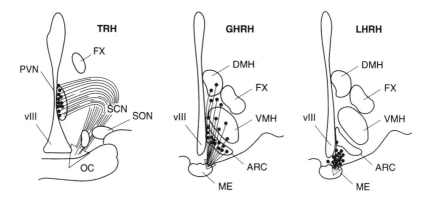

Fig. 6-3 Hypothalamic localization of the neurons that secrete thyrotropin-releasing hormone (TRH), growth hormone–releasing hormone (GHRH), and luteinizing hormone–releasing hormone (LHRH) based on human and animal studies. The neurons (solid dots) are shown in a coronal section through the plane of the densest cell bodies. The projection pathway of axons toward the median eminence is depicted by the solid lines forming an arrow. ARC, arcuate nucleus; DMH, dorsomedial hypothalamic nucleus; FX, fornix; ME, median eminence; OC, optic chiasm; PVN, paraventricular nucleus; SCN, suprachiasmatic nucleus; SON, supraoptic nucleus; vIII, third ventricle; VMH, ventromedial hypothalamic nucleus. (From Riskind PN and Martin JB: In: *Endocrinology*, 2nd ed., Vol. 1, LJ De Groot, ed., Saunders, Philadelphia, p. 101, 1989.)

protein generates two bioactive peptides by proteolytic cleavage, one of 31 amino acids and a shorter form of 20 amino acids. Both peptides release PRL in a specific fashion without affecting other pituitary hormones. They are recognized by a seven-transmembrane domain receptor (see below) previously considered to be an orphan receptor (i.e., a receptor for which there is no known ligand). Although these findings strongly suggest that PRP is a true PRL-releasing hormone (PRH), immuno-histochemical studies have failed to show PRP immunoreactive fibers in the external region of the medial eminence, thus making less likely the possibility that PRP, like other hypophysiotropic hormones, reaches the anterior pituitary via the portal vasculature.

Luteinizing Hormone-Releasing Hormone

This hormone, more commonly known as *gonadotropin hormone–releasing hormone* (GnRH) because it stimulates the release of both luteinizing hormone (LH) and follicle-stimulating hormone (FSH), belongs to a family of decapeptides highly conserved throughout vertebrate evolution. Thus far, 15 different variants have been described in nonmammalian species. Characteristically, the LHRH peptide sequence is followed by that of an associated peptide of variable length. Until recently, it was thought that mammalian LHRH was encoded by a single LHRH gene. Evidence now exists for the existence of a second gene. The first LHRH gene (LHRH-I) encodes a 92 amino acid precursor protein, which upon proteolytic cleavage originates the LHRH decapeptide and a 56-amino acid–associated peptide. The second LHRH gene (LHRH-II) encodes a highly conserved decapeptide that differs from LHRH-I by three amino acids and that has been found to be expressed in a variety of vertebrate species in addition to mammals. The genomic structure of this gene is similar to that of LHRH-I, but the gene is located on a different chromosome (chromosome 20 instead of 8). The LHRH-II gene encodes an associated peptide that is 50% longer than the associated peptide encoded by LHRH-I (84 vs. 56 amino acids). The function of LHRH-II is currently unknown. Although it is expressed in the brain, its abundance is much greater in peripheral tissues such as the kidney, bone marrow, and prostate.

In most mammals examined to date, LHRH-I is contained in neurons scattered throughout the anterior and medial part of the hypothalamus and the preoptic-septal areas. However, in primates—including humans—a substantial fraction of LHRH neurons is also localized to the medial basal hypothalamus and arcuate nucleus (Fig. 6-3 and Table 6-1). The LHRH nerve terminals projecting to the portal vasculature are predominantly localized to the lateral portion of the median eminence, although in humans a medial distribution is also observed. Neurons containing LHRH-II are also found in the hypothalamus, but in different regions from those producing LHRH-I.

Corticotropin-Releasing Hormone

This hormone is a 41-amino acid peptide that stimulates the secretion of adrenocorticotropin (ACTH) and β-endorphin from the adenohypophysis. Corticotropin-releasing hormone is a member of a family of polypeptides that includes at least three other members termed *urocortin I* (40 amino acids), *urocortin II* (38 amino acids), and *urocortin III* (also 30 amino acids). Corticotropin-releasing hormone derives from a 196-amino acid precursor highly conserved among mammalian species. The corticotropin-releasing hormone (CRH) gene contains only two exons separated by a rather short intervening sequence; the mature peptide sequence is entirely encoded by the second exon. Corticotropin-releasing hormone synergizes with vasopressin to stimulate ACTH release. The hypothalamic neurons that produce CRH are mostly found in the medial parvocellular portion of the paraventricular nucleus, where they frequently colocalize with other peptides, particularly vasopressin (Table 6-1). Like TRH, CRH and the urocortins are expressed in both hypothalamic neurons and in several extrahypothalamic areas, suggesting their involvement in nonendocrine functions (see below). Urocortin I is also found in other organs, particularly the heart. Urocortin II is mostly expressed in the nervous system, whereas urocortin III is found, in addition to the brain, in peripheral tissues such as the small intestine and skin.

Somatostatin or Growth Hormone-Inhibiting Hormone

This 14 amino acid peptide (Table 6-1) acts on the pituitary gland to inhibit GH secretion. It can also inhibit TSH release. It has a cyclic structure that results from the formation of two intramolecular disulfide bonds between its two cysteine residues. It is now clear that the original 14-amino acid somatostatin molecule belongs to a family of related peptides, which includes a 28-amino acid peptide, a 12-amino acid fragment derived from the amino terminus of somatostatin 28, and even larger forms having molecular weights of up to 16,000. The somatostatin gene contains two exons separated by a short intervening sequence; both somatostatin 14 and 28 are encoded by sequences present in the second exon. Because there appears to be only one somatostatin gene in mammals, the different somatostatin peptides are likely to derive from alternative processing of the primary mRNA and/or posttranslational modifications of the propeptide.

Somatostatin is widely distributed in the organism, including several regions of the brain, the gastrointestinal tract, and pancreas. Within the hypothalamus, the principal source of somatostatin fibers projecting to the median eminence is neurons of the anterior periventricular area (Table 6-1).

Growth Hormone-Releasing Hormone

This is a 44-amino acid peptide derived from a 108-amino acid precursor protein encoded by a single gene. The growth hormone-releasing hormone (GHRH) gene contains five exons that together with the corresponding intervening sequences span 10 kb of the human genome. Judging from the structure of the GHRH precursor protein, proteolytic processing may yield two peptides of unknown function in addition to GHRH. The GHRH stimulates GH secretion from the pituitary gland. Its location is the most restrictive of all releasing factors. The majority of the GHRH-producing neurons in the hypothalamus are found in and around the arcuate nucleus, close to the median eminence (Fig. 6-3 and Table 6-1).

Growth Hormone Secretagogues

Almost 20 years ago, a synthetic hexapeptide was shown to stimulate growth hormone release from the anterior pituitary. Subsequent studies indicated that this peptide, as well as others of the same class, acted independently of GHRH and somatostatin-mediated pathways, thereby suggesting the existence of both an endogenous factor with GH-releasing activity and a specific receptor for such a peptide. The predicted receptor, termed *growth hormone secretagogue receptor* (GHS-R), is now known to be a seven-transmembrane domain G protein–coupled receptor linked to cyclic adenosine monophosphate (AMP) formation and calcium mobilization. Recently, a novel peptide was isolated from the stomach and shown to potently activate GHS-R and induce GH secretion. This peptide, termed *ghrelin*, consists of 28 amino acids and has an N terminus that is fatty acid acylated. It is produced mainly in the stomach and small intestine, but some of it is also synthesized by hypothalamic neurons.

Anterior Pituitary Hormones

All adenohypophyseal hormones are protein or polypeptide in nature. Their names, number of amino acids, and molecular weights are presented in Table 6-2.

Growth Hormone

As discussed in Chapter 12, there are several forms of GH, but it appears that the predominant species secreted under physiological conditions is a 191 amino acid form with a molecular weight of 22,650. There are at least five GH-related genes

Table 6-2 Human Anterior Pituitary Hormones

	Amino acids	Carbohydrate (CHO)	Molecular weight
I. Corticotropin-related peptide hormones: single small peptides derived from a common precursor.			
1. α-Melanocyte-stimulating hormone (α-MSH) (α-melanotropin)	13AA		1,823
2. Corticotropin (ACTH)	39AA		4,507
3. β-Lipotropin (β-LPH)	91AA		9,500
4. β-Endorphin (β-LPH) (61–91)	31AA		3,100
II. Glycoprotein hormones: composed of two dissimilar peptides. The α-chain is similar in structure or identical. The β-chain differs with each hormone and confers specificity.			
1. Follicle-stimulating hormone (FSH) (follitropin)	α 89AA	18% CHO	32,000
	β 115AA	5% Sialic acid	
2. Luteinizing hormone (LH) (lutropin)	α 89AA	16% CHO	32,000
	β 115AA	1% Sialic acid	
3. Thyrotropin (TSH)	α 89AA	16% CHO	32,000
	β 112AA	1% Sialic acid	
III. Somatomammotropin hormones: single peptide chains with two or three SS[a] bonds; no carbohydrate.			
1. Prolactin (PRL)	198AA		23,510
2. Growth hormone (GH) or somatotropin	191AA		22,650

[a]SS = disulfide.

and pseudogenes in the human genome. All of them have five exons separated by four introns; alternative splicing of exon B leads to the synthesis of a 20 kDa GH variant instead of the predominant 22 kDa form. Growth hormone is stored in secretory granules of cells known as *somatotrophs*. The somatotrophs are the most abundant cell type in the pituitary gland; they store GH in amounts representing 4%–8% of the gland by dry weight.

Growth hormone secretion is regulated by at least two releasing and one inhibiting hormone, namely, GHRH, ghrelin, and somatostatin. Under normal circumstances, the rate of GH release depends on a balance between the stimulatory effect of GHRH/ghrelin and the inhibitory effect of somatostatin. Growth hormone-releasing hormone exerts its biological actions by binding to a membrane-anchored protein shown to be a guanine nucleotide-binding regulatory protein (G protein)–coupled receptor. As such, the GHRH receptor contains seven transmembrane domains. Its activation by GHRH results in cyclic AMP formation. The GHRH receptor gene appears to be expressed only in the anterior pituitary gland, in which two mRNA transcripts of 2.5 and 4 kb can be detected.

The ghrelin receptor (GHS-R) also belongs to the superfamily of seven-transmembrane domain, G protein–coupled receptors. It is a 366-amino acid protein with a molecular weight of about 40,000. A shorter form of 286 amino acids also exists, but both forms appear to be derived from a single gene by alternative splicing of the primary RNA transcript. In addition to being present in the pituitary gland, GHS-R is expressed in the arcuate-ventromedial nuclei of the hypothalamus and the infundibular region of the median eminence. Patients with GHRH deficiency also fail to respond to GHSs, indicating the existence of defects of both GHRH and GHS-R function.

The somatostatin receptor is another seven-transmembrane domain, G protein–coupled receptor. Thus far, five different somatostatin receptors have been described, with an overall sequence homology of 40% to 60%. Despite these large divergences in amino acid sequence, the somatostatin receptors recognize both somatostatin 14 and 28 with high affinity; all of them are negatively coupled to adenylate cyclase. Interestingly, their tissue distribution is also divergent; some have greater expression in the brain than in peripheral tissues and vice versa.

Prolactin

Prolactin (PRL) (Table 6-2) is a 23,000 Da protein hormone that bears considerable structural resemblance to GH. In fact, both hormones appear to have evolved from gene duplication of a common ancestral gene. Despite this, the PRL and GH genes are located on different chromosomes. While in humans there appears to exist a single PRL gene, in rodents there is evidence for at least three related genes, all of which are expressed in the placenta. As in the case of GH, there are several forms of PRL. The predominant form of 199 amino acids has a molecular weight of 23,000. The main function of PRL is to induce mammary gland growth and milk secretion in the properly prepared breast following delivery of the infant (see Chapter 9). In laboratory rodents, PRL affects gonadal function and helps maintain the structure and function of accessory sex organs. Whether PRL acts similarly in humans is not known. The fact that PRL receptors have been found in the ovary of nonhuman primates, however, suggests a physiological role for the hormone in higher species.

An important function of PRL is to up-regulate immune function in animals and humans. It does so by stimulating lymphocyte proliferation and by providing, together with GH, the initial signals that prepare these cells for proliferation and differentiation.

The human pituitary contains five times less PRL than GH. Prolactin is produced by cells known as *lactotrophs,* which can constitute up to 25% of the normal population of anterior hypophyseal cells. Both the number and the size of the lactotrophs are increased by estrogen, and this becomes particularly noticeable during pregnancy. Serum PRL levels are higher in nonpregnant women than in men, reflecting the difference in estrogen production between the two sexes. However, not all changes in PRL secretion are related to sex steroids, as shown by the increase in circulating PRL levels that occurs during sleep in both males and females.

Prolactin secretion is controlled by PRL-releasing and PRL-inhibiting factors. Among the former there are several neuropeptides shown to stimulate PRL release, including TRH, oxytocin, VIP, the VIP-related peptide, peptide histidine isoleucine (PHI), angiotensin II, substance P, neurotensin, and PRP. None of them stimulate PRL secretion in a specific fashion with the exception of PRP. The PRP receptor, known as hGR3, GPR10, or UHR-1, binds PRP with high affinity. Its encoding cDNA contains an open reading frame predicting a polypeptide of 370 amino acids that bears significant structural similarities with other members of the G protein–coupled receptor superfamily. A conclusive demonstration that PRP is a physiologically meaningful PRL-releasing factor will require evidence showing that PRP is released into the portal circulation and that inhibition of its expression results in PRL deficiency.

Dopamine is a major PRL-inhibiting factor. Dopamine inhibits PRL secretion by binding to a dopamine receptor of the D_2 subtype expressed in lactotrophs. This receptor contains seven transmembrane domains and inhibits adenylate cyclase via coupling to a G protein of the G_i type. Dopamine, produced by tuberoinfundibular dopaminergic neurons, is released into the portal system for delivery to the pituitary gland (Table 6-1). It is estimated that the concentration of dopamine in portal blood may be sufficient to hold PRL secretion in check, except when stimulated by stress or by the suckling stimulus. The elevation in PRL that occurs under these conditions is probably related not only to withdrawal of dopaminergic inhibition but also to secretion of PRL-releasing factors.

Adrenocorticotropin

Adrenocorticotropin, as its name implies, is the adenohypophyseal hormone that controls the function of the adrenal cortex. It is a relatively small molecular weight polypeptide hormone consisting of a single chain of 39 amino acids (Fig. 6-4, Table 6-2).

Adrenocorticotropin is part of a POMC prohormone molecule (Fig. 6-4). This large peptide is produced in certain specific loci of the brain and in the anterior and intermediate lobes of the pituitary gland. Processing of the prohormone varies depending on its cellular site. In the anterior lobe, it is processed to ACTH and β-endorphin, an endogenous opioid peptide of 31 amino acids. In the intermediate lobe of rodents, pro-opiomelanocortin (POMC) processing results in the production of α-melanocyte-stimulating hormone (α-MSH) (ACTH 1–13) and CLIP (ACTH 18–39). In the brain, it appears that the major products are ACTH, β-endorphin, and α-MSH.

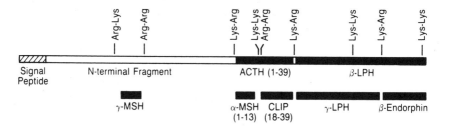

Fig. 6-4 Diagram of the structure of the pro-opiomelanocortin (POMC) molecule and the hormones derived from it by proteolysis. The precursor POMC protein contains a leader sequence (signal peptide) followed by a fragment that contains the sequence of γ-melanocyte-stimulating hormone (γ-MSH) (amino acids 51–62), the adrenocorticotropic hormone (ACTH) molecule (1–39) that contains the sequences for α-MSH (ACTH 1–13) and the corticotropin-like intermediate lobe peptide CLIP (ACTH 18–39), and the β-lipotropin (1–91) molecule that contains the sequences of γ-lipotropin (γ-LPH) (1–58) and β-endorphin (61–91). The last also includes the sequence for met-enkephalin (first five amino acids of β-endorphin). Potential sites for proteolytic cleavage are indicated by the presence of the basic amino acids arginine-lysine (Arg-Lys). (From Reichlin S: In: *Williams Textbook of Endocrinology,* 7th ed., JD Wilson and DW Foster, eds., Saunders, Philadelphia, p. 502, 1985.)

The secretion of ACTH is augmented by noxious stimuli of various sorts termed *stressors*, and this will be discussed in Chapter 14. In addition, ACTH secretion is inhibited by glucocorticoids, an example of classic negative feedback regulation. As indicated above, the hypothalamus controls ACTH secretion via a CRH. The biological actions of CRH are initiated by the binding of the neuropeptide to a membrane protein structurally related to the calcitonin–VIP–GHRH family of G protein–coupled receptors. The CRH receptor (now known as CRH1) is a 415-amino acid protein displaying seven putative transmembrane domains. It is encoded by a 2.7 kb mRNA and is positively coupled to adenylate cyclase. Two types of CRH receptors have been described. CRH1 is expressed mainly in the intermediate and anterior lobes of the pituitary gland, in addition to various sites in the brain, including the cerebral cortex, sensory relay nuclei, and cerebellum. CRH2 expression in brain is more restricted and includes regions of the olfactory bulb, ventromedial hypothalamic nucleus, amygdala, and hippocampus. In addition, CRH2 is expressed in peripheral tissues, including the heart and skeletal muscle. CRH1 mainly recognizes CRH and urocortin I, whereas CRH2 is selectively activated by urocortin II and III.

Vasopressin has a physiological role in the control of ACTH release, as there is a deficiency in ACTH release in animals with hereditary diabetes insipidus; such animals lack endogenous vasopressin. Vasopressin stimulates ACTH release in a dose-related fashion from the pituitary incubated *in vitro* and is present in high concentrations in portal blood at a range capable of stimulating ACTH release. It is now apparent that vasopressin and CRH cooperate in the control of ACTH release, as vasopressin potentiates the action of CRH.

Melanocyte-Stimulating Hormone

Melanocyte-stimulating hormone was isolated from amphibian pituitaries based on its ability to cause skin darkening. As indicated before, MSH is part of a larger pro-hormone, POMC. In reptiles and amphibia, MSH is formed in and secreted by the intermediate lobe of the pituitary gland. In humans, α-MSH cells are more frequently present in the anterior lobe than in the pars intermedia, which is rudimentary. In both, α-MSH colocalizes with ACTH. There are two forms of MSH in nearly all species. The first is known as α-MSH and contains 13 amino acids (Fig. 6-4, Table 6-2). These 13 are identical to the first 13 amino acids of ACTH. The β-MSH consists of 22 amino acids. Amino acids 11–17 of β-MSH and ACTH are identical. In view of the overlap in structure between the MSHs and ACTH, it is not surprising that ACTH has MSH-like activity. The converse, however, is not true, as MSH has no ACTH-like activity. Five receptors, numbered MC1–MC5 R, have been cloned for the melanocortin peptides. These receptors have differing distributions in the body and differing affinities for the melanocortin peptides. All of them bind α-MSH with high affinity with the exception of MC2 R, which only binds ACTH with high affinity. All the melanocortin receptors couple through G_s to increase the activity of adenylyl cyclase and elevate intracellular cyclic AMP.

In broad terms, MC1 R is involved in the paracrine control of skin coloration; MC2 R mediates the actions of ACTH on adrenal function; MC3 R is expressed in the brain, where it appears to function as an autoreceptor limiting the activation of melanocortin neurons; MC4 R mediates the effects of melanocortins to inhibit food intake and increase energy expenditure; and MC5 R controls the secretion of exocrine glands. Central MC3 and MC4 receptor activity is modulated by an endogenous receptor antagonist known as *agouti-related peptide* (AgRP). This peptide acts centrally to exert an effect similar to that of the paracrine factor agouti, which antagonizes MC1 R activity in peripheral tissues.

Although the secretion of MSH has been postulated to be controlled by both MSH-releasing and MSH-inhibiting factors, both the identity and the physiological significance of these factors remain to be determined.

Pituitary Glycoprotein Hormones

The pituitary hormones discussed above are relatively simple proteins. The adenohypophysis secretes other, more complex hormones that have a carbohydrate moiety attached to the protein component, which in turn is composed of two interconnected amino acid chains. These hormones are called *glycoproteins* because of their carbohydrate moiety. They are secreted by basophilic cells, that is, cells showing an affinity for basic dyes. There are three pituitary glycoprotein hormones—TSH, FSH, and LH—each with a molecular weight of about 30,000. They consist of two subunits, an α-subunit that is identical in the three hormones and three different β-subunits that confer biological specificity to each hormone (Table 6-2). The α- and β-chains are synthesized separately, and they are combined before joining the carbohydrate moieties. At the time of secretion, an excess of α-chains is secreted, so one can detect α-chain in the plasma. When the secretion rate is elevated, a small amount of free β-chain may also appear.

Thyroid-Stimulating Hormone

As discussed in Chapter 13, this hormone stimulates secretion of the hormones thyroxine and triiodothyronine by the thyroid gland. There is a high degree of conservation in the amino acid sequence of the TSH-β subunit among different mammalian species. In all cases, the subunit appears to be encoded by a single gene, the expression of which is subjected to regulatory control by thyroid hormones. Like other glycoprotein hormones in the pituitary, TSH is secreted by cells termed *thyrotrophs;* these cells are characterized by the presence of abundant, relatively small secretory granules. The thyrotrophs make up to 15% of the cells of the adenohypophysis. The secretion of TSH is under negative feedback control by thyroid hormones (see Chapter 13) and is stimulated by the hypothalamic peptide TRH. Thyrotropin-releasing hormone initiates its biological actions by binding to a membrane-anchored receptor that, like the GHRH, somatostatin, and CRH receptors, belongs to a family of G protein–coupled receptors containing seven highly conserved transmembrane domains. The TRH receptor is a protein of 393–412 amino acids and appears to be the product of a single gene. Binding of TRH to the receptor results in phospholipase C activation, calcium mobilization, and cAMP formation (see below).

Gonadotropins

In females, follicle-stimulating hormone (FSH) stimulates the growth of ovarian follicles. In the male, FSH acts to promote spermatogenesis. Further details of these actions are given in Chapters 9 and 10. Follicle-stimulating hormone is produced by cells called *gonadotrophs.* Some of these secrete only FSH, but others secrete both FSH and LH. Follicle-stimulating hormone is produced in cells that have very small secretory granules relative to those of other pituitary cells. The synthesis and secretion of FSH are controlled by LHRH (see below).

Pituitary control of gonadal function requires still another glycoprotein hormone, LH, also known as *interstitial cell-stimulating hormone* (ICSH) because it stimulates the interstitial cells of both ovaries and testes. The function of this hormone is to induce ovulation and the formation of the corpus luteum in the female, and to stimulate steroid secretion in both the ovaries and the testes (see Chapters 9 and 10). The hormone is structurally similar to FSH and again possesses the common α-chain. Its β-chain is different from that of FSH and TSH and confers specific biological activity to the molecule. As in the case of FSH, some gonadotrophs secrete only LH, but others secrete both FSH and LH. The secretion of LH is stimulated by LHRH. The LHRH receptor (LHRH-R) is a 327-amino acid protein with a molecular weight of 37,000. Like the GHRH, somatostatin, CRH, and TRH receptors, LHRH-R contains seven transmembrane domains characteristic of G protein–coupled receptors. Surprisingly, LHRH-R lacks the cytoplasmic C-terminal region, which appears to be important for the biological activity of other G protein–coupled receptors. Very recently, an LHRH receptor that selectively recognizes LHRH-II was identified in the human genome and was molecularly cloned from the rhesus monkey pituitary gland. This receptor is also a G protein coupled, seven transmembrane domain receptor, but unlike LHRH-R, the LHRH receptor II (LHRH-RII) has a C-terminal cytoplasmic tail. The LHRH-RII gene contains three exons and is located in chromosome 1. Surprisingly, LHRH-RII mRNA is ubiquitously expressed throughout the body, including tissues as diverse as the brain, liver, and skeletal muscle. The specific functions that LHRH-RII and its ligand may have in these tissues remain to be determined.

With the elucidation of the structures of these releasing and inhibiting hormones, it has been possible to prepare analogs of each of these peptides. In the case of LHRH, the initial aim was to obtain inhibitory analogs that might suppress fertility. However, it was accidentally found that analogs more active than the natural compound could easily be prepared if unnatural amino acids were substituted at positions likely to be subject to proteolysis. Because prolonged administration of these agonist analogs down-regulates LHRH receptors, the agonist analogs have proven to be clinically important in the treatment of gonadotropin hypersecretion, such as that seen in sexual precocity of central origin.

Mechanism of Action of Releasing Hormones

Cyclic Adenosine Monophosphate

The best-known mechanism used by hypothalamic releasing hormones to alter pituitary hormone release involves activation of adenylate cyclase with the generation of cyclic AMP. It appears that activation of protein kinases by cyclic AMP results in phosphorylation of certain membrane constituents that promote exocytosis, the mechanism for secretion. The secretory granules migrate to the cell surface and fuse with the cell membrane, and the granular core containing the hormone is extruded into the extracellular space, particularly at the vascular pole of the cell. The release of GH, PRL, ACTH, and TSH by their respective hypothalamic releasing hormones is mediated by such cyclic AMP–dependent mechanisms. However, in gonadotrophs the cyclic AMP system plays a minor role, possibly only in enhancing synthesis of LH.

Calcium

Extracellular calcium is required for optimal release of all pituitary hormones. It may also be mobilized from intracellular stores in the case of some of the hormones as well. For those releasing factors that operate via the cyclic AMP mechanism, a cyclic AMP–dependent protein kinase may be involved in opening calcium channels, allowing entrance of the ion and possibly mobilizing it from intracellular stores.

Arachidonic Acid Metabolites

The products of arachidonic acid metabolism can promote exocytosis, and—as in the case of cyclic AMP—their relative importance varies with the pituitary cell type. Prostaglandins appear to be important in the release of GH and ACTH, and they can activate the production of cyclic AMP. In other cells such as the gonadotrophs, it appears that metabolites of arachidonic acid different from prostaglandins, such as the leukotrienes and epoxides, may also be involved in the exocytosis process.

Arachidonic acid release from the cell membrane may result from a receptor-mediated activation of phospholipase C, a membrane-bound enzyme that catalyzes the hydrolysis of polyphosphoinositides into inositol triphosphate and diacylglycerol. The latter not only contains arachidonate, which is then made available to phospholipase A for subsequent metabolism, but also interacts with protein kinase C, a calcium-dependent, phospholipid-activated enzyme. Protein kinase C phosphorylates several proteins that then participate in the process of hormone release. Inositol triphosphate, the other product of phospholipase C activity, mobilizes intracellular calcium from the endoplasmic reticulum.

The releasing hormones act on the cell very rapidly (within less than a minute) to promote release of particular pituitary hormones. In addition, they stimulate hormone biosynthesis by increasing mRNA levels. This effect appears to be exerted via both an increase in gene transcription and mRNA stability. In the case of LH and FSH, it has been shown that the pattern of pulsatile LHRH secretion is critical for the induction of changes in gonadotropin subunit mRNA expression. Thus, a rapid frequency of LHRH pulses increases subunit α, LH-β, and FSH-β gene expression, whereas slow-frequency pulses increase only FSH-β mRNA levels.

Releasing hormones such as TRH and LHRH utilize the same intracellular signal transduction pathways to exert their stimulatory effects on TSH-PRL and LH-FSH release. The mechanism underlying the ability of each of these releasing hormones to differentially release TSH versus PRL or LH versus FSH is unknown. The TRH receptors in thyrotrophs and lactotrophs are coupled to the same G proteins and activate a phosphoinositide-protein kinase C–mediated pathway. Activation by TRH results in the stimulation of phospholipase C, enhanced phosphoinositide turnover, calcium mobilization, cyclic AMP formation, and arachidonic acid release. The same is true for LHRH receptors in LH- and FSH-secreting cells. Perhaps the differential release of TSH versus PRL or LH versus FSH is provided by binding to additional G proteins and/or differential activation of a family of serine/threonine protein kinases known as *mitogen-activated protein kinases* (MAPKs) or extracellular *signal-related kinases* (ERKs). These kinases, which are rapidly activated by both growth factors and releasing hormones, appear to play an essential role in a number of signaling cascades leading to nonproliferative changes in cell activity.

Mechanism of Action of Inhibiting Hypothalamic Hormones

The inhibiting hormones, somatostatin and dopamine, also use cyclic AMP and calcium-dependent pathways to decrease pituitary hormone secretion. They act in part by inhibition of adenylate cyclase and in part by other mechanisms, such as decreasing the availability of calcium to the cell.

Effect of Hormones Secreted by Target Glands on the Responsiveness of the Adenohypophysis to Releasing and Inhibiting Hormones

In general, all hormones produced by target glands, such as the thyroid gland, adrenals, and gonads, feed back on the adenohypophysis to inhibit hormone secretion (Fig. 6-5) and thus modulate the stimulatory effect of hypothalamic releasing hormones. This inhibitory effect is also exerted on the hypothalamus, where they inhibit the secretion of releasing hormones.

Part of the mechanism by which these inhibitory effects are exerted include transcriptional repression of gene expression and down-regulation of releasing hormone receptors in the pituitary. In the case of the LHRH-gonadotropin releasing system, there is an added level of complexity, as the ovarian hormone estradiol shows a biphasic effect on gonadotrophin secretion, first inhibition (negative feed-

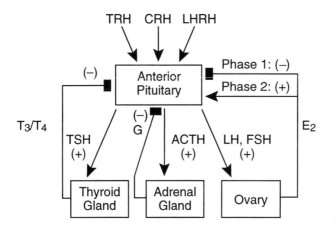

Fig. 6-5 Modulation of anterior pituitary responsiveness to hypothalamic releasing hormones. (−) inhibits the response to the releasing hormone; (+) facilitates the response. ACTH, adrenocorticotropic hormone; CRH, corticotropin-releasing hormone; E_2, estradiol; FSH, follicle-stimulating hormone; G, glucocorticoids; LH, luteinizing hormone; LHRH, luteinizing hormone-releasing hormone; TRH, thyrotropin-releasing hormone; TSH, thyroid-stimulating hormone; T_3, triiodothyronine; T_4, thyroxine; Phase 1, early phase; Phase 2, later phase, only in females.

back) and then stimulation (positive feedback) (see Fig. 6-5). This latter effect is critically important because it is responsible for the preovulatory surge of gonadotropins that occurs in every menstrual cycle (see Chapter 9).

Putative Synaptic Transmitters Involved in Controlling the Release of Releasing Hormones

The neurons that produce releasing factors are in synaptic contact with a host of putative neurotransmitters. The most abundant neurotransmitters present in the hypothalamus are the excitatory amino acid glutamate and the inhibitory amino acid gamma-aminobutyric acid (GABA). Both are present in more than 98% of the synaptic contacts found in this region of the brain. Other neurotransmitters include the catecholamines dopamine and epinephrine, in addition to serotonin and acetylcholine. Hypothalamic neurons also utilize peptides for transsynaptic communication. The most important peptides regulating the secretion of hypothalamic releasing and inhibiting hormones are neuropeptide Y (NPY) and opioids (β-endorphin, dynorphin, and enkephalins).

Each of the aforementioned neurotransmitters and neuropeptides has been shown to affect the hypothalamic release of both releasing and inhibiting hormones. The most extensive studies have been carried out on the transsynaptic regulation of LHRH secretion, and the picture that has emerged is one in which the dominant neurotransmitter systems controlling LHRH secretion are those that use glutamate and GABA for synaptic transmission. The activity of LHRH neurons is directly increased by glutamate and indirectly (via other neurons) inhibited by GABA. Catecholamines and peptides, such as NPY, appear to stimulate LHRH release only in the presence of gonadal steroids, that is, in animals with intact gonads. While less is known in the case of other releasing/inhibitory hormones, it appears clear that catecholamines stimulate the release of CRH and GHRH, whereas dopamine itself acts as an inhibitory hormone to suppress PRL release.

Of great interest to the field of neuroendocrinology is the potential role played by peptides originally thought to be localized in other organs and that have now been found in the brain. Among these are angiotensin II, which was first thought to be formed only in the circulation after release of renin from the juxtaglomerular apparatus of the kidney. There are angiotensin II–producing neurons within the hypothalamus, and they may play a stimulatory role in controlling ACTH and PRL secretion. Others are the atrial natriuretic peptides, which were originally discovered in the atria of the heart and have now been found within neurons in the hypothalamus. They may suppress ACTH as well as vasopressin secretion (see Chapter 7). The almost ubiquitous peptide pituitary adenylate cyclase activating peptide (PACAP; Table 6-1) is apparently released into the portal vessels, and acts in the pituitary to induce cyclic AMP formation and regulate POMC gene transcription. Examples of gastrointestinal peptides found in brain neuronal systems, which may control pituitary hormone secretion via both hypothalamic and pituitary actions are VIP and cholecystokinin, which may control neurosecretion via activation of the cyclic AMP system.

Short Loop Feedback of Pituitary Hormones to Alter Their Own Release

A variety of pituitary hormones exert short loop negative feedback actions to suppress their own release. They exert this effect without reaching the general circulation (Fig. 6-6). This is in contrast to the so-called long loop feedback of pituitary target gland hormones described earlier. Pituitary hormones may reach the hypothalamus via reverse flow of the portal circulation and/or from sites of production within the brain itself. For instance, ACTH may be secreted by POMC neurons of the arcuate nucleus of the medial basal hypothalamus, and PRL and LH may be secreted by neurons of the hypothalamus found to express the genes encoding these hormones. Regardless of the means used by pituitary hormones to reach the hypothalamus, the ability of these hormones to exert short loop negative feedback ef-

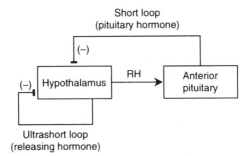

Fig. 6-6   Short and ultrashort loop feedback systems in the hypothalamic–pituitary unit. RH, releasing hormone.

fects on releasing hormone secretion has been clearly established for LH, FSH, ACTH, PRL, and GH. In the last case, the feedback may be mediated not only by GH itself but also by insulin-like growth factor I (see below), either delivered via the peripheral circulation or made directly in the brain.

Ultrashort Loop Feedback of Releasing and Inhibiting Hormones to Modify Their Own Release

Ultrashort loop feedback is an alteration in the release of hypothalamic peptide induced by the peptide itself acting within the brain. It may occur as direct recurrent inhibition or via interaction with an interneuron that in turn alters the discharge rate of the peptidergic neuron (Fig. 6-6). Experimental evidence for ultrashort loop negative feedback has been provided in the case of somatostatin, GHRH, and LHRH.

Extrapituitary Actions of Releasing Hormones

The distribution of releasing hormones in brain regions outside the hypothalamus (e.g., brain stem, cortex) suggests that they exert extrapituitary actions. As indicated earlier, TRH is found in other brain regions and even in the spinal cord; somatostatin is distributed widely throughout the nervous system and also has been found in the delta cells of the pancreatic islets of Langerhans. Because somatostatin can inhibit the release of both insulin and glucagon, it probably acts locally to control the release of these hormones from the islets.

A behavioral effect of releasing hormones is the induction of mating behavior by LHRH in animals. The physiological importance of this effect remains to be determined.

Perhaps the best example of extrapituitary actions of releasing hormones is provided by the CRH family of peptides. Corticotropin-releasing hormone not only stimulates ACTH release but also has a variety of other effects on the central nervous system that mimic the response to stress. Thus, CRH induces anxiogenic effects, increases cardiovascular activity, induces anorexia, and inhibits LHRH secretion. All of these effects are independent of its stimulatory effects on glucocorticoid secretion. Urocortin I influences feeding, anxiety, and auditory processing. Mutant mice lacking urocortin I show hearing impairment and increased anxiety-like behavior. Urocortin I is a more potent suppressor of appetite/feeding behavior than CRH. It also has more potent effects on the cardiovascular system than CRH, suggesting that urocortin may play a critical role in the cardiovascular response to stress. Urocortin II, on the other hand, decreases feeding behavior and appears to play a role in delaying gastric emptying.

PITUITARY GROWTH HORMONE, ITS ACTION AND ITS CONTROL

Now that the overall hypothalamic control of anterior pituitary hormone secretion has been considered, the actions of GH and control of its secretion will be discussed in more detail.

Actions of Growth Hormone

Growth hormone has powerful effects on growth and metabolism. Its absence is associated with dwarfism. Its excessive secretion leads to giantism or acromegaly (see below).

Metabolic Effects of Growth Hormone

Growth hormone affects metabolism by:

1. Decreasing blood amino acid concentrations.
2. Decreasing blood urea nitrogen.
3. Increasing the positive nitrogen balance, defined as the difference between daily nitrogen intake in food and excretion in urine and feces as nitrogenous wastes.
4. Increasing DNA, RNA, and protein synthesis, that is, producing a protein anabolic effect.
5. Elevating blood glucose levels via decreased utilization of carbohydrates and decreased sensitivity to the plasma glucose–lowering action of insulin.
6. Increasing oxidation of fat, leading to a decrease in the respiratory quotient ($RQ = CO_2$ output divided by O_2 intake). The RQ for the metabolism of carbohydrates to CO_2 and water is 1.0, whereas that for the metabolism of fats is 0.7. Protein metabolism leads to an RQ of about 0.8. The increased utilization of fats is often accompanied by an elevation of the free fatty acids in blood because of lipid mobilization from fat stores and by an increase in ketone body formation (β-hydroxybutyric acid, acetoacetic acid, acetone) associated with the increased fatty acid oxidation (see Chapter 16).

Growth Effects of Growth Hormone

Growth hormone stimulates growth by increasing protein synthesis and promoting the utilization of fat as a source of energy so as to spare amino acids for protein synthesis. In addition to increasing protein synthesis via direct genomic effects, GH stimulates the uptake of amino acids by muscle and liver cells.

Growth hormone is a powerful stimulus for cartilage and bone metabolism. Long bones grow by proliferation of cartilage cells in the epiphyseal plate, which is followed by growth due to ossification occurring in diaphyseal and epiphyseal ossification centers. In the absence of GH in hypophysectomized animals, the epiphyseal ossification center atrophies and there is a very thin epiphyseal plate of cartilage. Administration of GH causes a thickening of this cartilage plate, and this has served as a bioassay for the hormone.

As will be discussed in Chapter 12, these actions of GH on cartilage and bone growth are mediated by somatomedic C, most commonly known as *insulin-like growth factor I* (IGF-I). This is produced by the liver and other tissues under the stimulatory control of GH.

Mechanism of Action of Growth Hormone

Growth hormone initiates its actions by binding to a single transmembrane domain, membrane-anchored receptor that is a member of the cytokinine/hematopoietin receptor superfamily. Other members of this family include receptors for ciliary neurotrophic factor, erythropoietin, and interleukin-2, among others. The GH receptor is encoded by a 4.7 kb mRNA that appears to be the product of a single gene. The nucleotide sequence predicts a mature protein of 620 amino acids with a molecular weight of 70,000. The difference between this estimation and the actual molecular weight (130,000) determined by gel analysis appears to be due to the heavy glycosylation of the receptor's extracellular domain. The GH receptor is covalently linked to ubiquitin, a proteolytic molecule that appears to be responsible for the short half-life of the receptor. Binding of GH to its receptor results in the activation of JAK2 (Janus kinase 2), a tyrosine kinase. This initial step is followed by the phosphorylation of several members of the signal transducers and activators of transcription (STAT) family, which regulate the transcription of a variety of genes including several transcription factors, IGF-I and metabolic enzymes involved in glucose transport, protein synthesis, and lipogenesis. Another signaling pathway involved in GH action is the Ras-MAP (mitogen-activated protein) kinase pathway, which is also activated by JAK2.

Control of Growth Hormone Secretion

Episodic Growth Hormone Secretion

Growth hormone is secreted in a pulsatile fashion throughout life. The pattern of secretion has an ultradian rhythm, with a frequency of about one pulse every 2 to 3 hours, and appears to be caused by changes in the secretory activity of those hypothalamic neuroendocrine cells involved in regulating the secretion of GH from the pituitary gland (i.e., GHRH and somatostatin neurons). The bursts of secretion are caused by an increase in GHRH output, the troughs by an enhanced production of somatostatin. Studies in sheep, however, have shown that such a relationship is not always apparent.

Episodic GH secretion is influenced by sex, age, and sleep. Women secrete more GH than do men; they show a higher GH baseline, larger bursts of secretion, and an overall higher 24-hour total secretory output of the hormone. In both sexes, however, the rate of secretion is elevated during the first few days after birth, decreasing thereafter, possibly as a consequence of an enhanced IGF-I negative feedback. At puberty, GH secretion increases again in both sexes, paralleling the changes in height velocity associated with the attainment of sexual maturity. After completion of linear growth and attainment of adulthood, the rate of GH secretion returns to prepubertal levels. It remains stable throughout at least the fifth decade of life, decreasing again during aging. In all these instances, the most prominent episodes of GH release occur at night. The release of the hormone increases during the onset of deep sleep (stages III and IV) and decreases during the phase of rapid eye movement (REM) sleep, which is associated with dreaming. It is not clear, however, that sleep is absolutely required for nocturnal GH secretion to increase, as nocturnal episodes of GH release may occur in the absence of slow-wave sleep. It would appear that sleep and circadian activation of GH release are independent but coincidental events (Fig. 6-7).

Central Mechanism Controlling Growth Hormone Secretion

As indicated above, GH secretion is controlled by a regulatory mechanism that involves two hypothalamic peptides—GHRH and somatostatin—and a peripherally

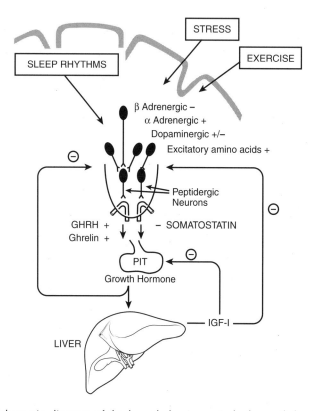

Fig. 6-7 Schematic diagram of the hypothalamic control of growth hormone secretion. For details see text. GHRH, growth hormone-releasing hormone; IGF-I, insulin-like growth factor-I; PIT, anterior pituitary gland. (Modified from Reichlin S: In: *Williams Textbook of Endocrinology,* 7th ed., JD Wilson and DW Foster, eds., Saunders, Philadelphia, p. 529, 1985.)

originated peptide, ghrelin, that is produced mainly in the stomach. Although neurons of the arcuate nucleus of the hypothalamus have been shown to contain ghrelin, it appears that the main source of ghrelin stimulating GH release is the stomach. Ghrelin secretion is stimulated by fasting, probably through a decrease in blood glucose concentration.

As indicated earlier, the neuroendocrine neurons producing GHRH are mostly located in the arcuate, ventromedial, and dorsomedial nuclei of the basal hypothalamus. Lesions of this area, particularly in the ventromedial nucleus, impair GH secretion. Conversely, stimulation of this region results in GH release. Thus, these changes mainly reflect alterations in GHRH output and are not compromised by potential changes in somatostatin release, which may occur because somatostatin-producing neurons are also present in the arcuate and ventromedial nuclei. Indeed, most of the somatostatin neurons projecting to the median eminence are located elsewhere, in the anterior periventricular area of the hypothalamus.

Several neurotransmitter systems are involved in the control of GH secretion. They do so mainly via regulation of GHRH and somatostatin release from the hypothalamus. Thus, catecholamines acting via α_2-adrenergic receptors, dopamine acting via D_1 or D_2 receptors, and excitatory amino acids acting via both N-methyl-D-aspartate (NMDA) and non-NMDA receptors stimulate GH secretion by activating GHRH and inhibiting somatostatin release. Dopamine, however, may also have inhibitory effects, possibly mediated by stimulation of somatostatin release. In contrast to the stimulatory effect of α-adrenoreceptor–mediated neurotransmission, activation of β-adrenergic receptors suppresses GH release, presumably by facilitating somatostatin output.

An additional central mechanism involved in the control of GH secretion is an ultrashort loop feedback effect exerted by both somatostatin and GHRH on their own secretion.

Metabolic Signals Regulating Growth Hormone Secretion

Glucose, amino acids and nonesterified fatty acids play an important role in the regulation of GH secretion. Administration of insulin to produce hypoglycemia results in a prompt increase in GH release caused by the hypoglycemia. Because of this effect, insulin-induced hypoglycemia is used as a provocative test to stimulate GH secretion in individuals with suspected GH deficiency. Part of the effect of hypoglycemia on GH secretion may be mediated by ghrelin (see above). Certain amino acids, particularly arginine given orally or intravenously, are extremely potent in inducing GH secretion, an effect that appears to be mediated by a concomitant increase in GHRH output and a decreased secretion of somatostatin. Some of these effects may be mediated by the conversion of arginine to nitric oxide, a gaseous neurotransmitter recently found to be involved in the hypothalamic control of anterior pituitary function. Nonesterified fatty acids reduce GH secretion, but the mechanisms underlying this effect are not well understood.

Other Hormones Influencing Growth Hormone Secretion

Glucocorticoids exert a dual effect on GH secretion: first they stimulate and then they inhibit it. Thyroid hormones are required for normal GH output, and the gonadal steroids, estrogen and androgens, facilitate the secretion of the hormone throughout the life of the individual. The lipostatic hormone leptin also stimulates GH secretion, likely via inhibition of NPY neurosecretion. A leptin-induced increase in GH secretion appears important for the activation of metabolic processes aimed at regulating changes in body weight and preventing obesity.

Other Factors Controlling Growth Hormone Secretion

Exercise and stress are two *nonspecific* but potent stimulants of GH secretion. It is likely that they release GH as part of a preparatory *fight-or-flight* response that shifts metabolism from carbohydrates to fat.

CLINICAL ASSESSMENT OF ANTERIOR PITUITARY FUNCTION

Clinical assessment of anterior pituitary function includes a history of the condition, a physical examination, and usually some form of laboratory testing. Because physiological regulation of anterior pituitary hormone secretion needs to be considered in assessing pituitary function, the evaluation for a possible deficiency or excess of each of the clinically relevant anterior pituitary hormones is briefly discussed in this section (but also see Chapter 5).

Growth Hormone

A random serum GH measurement is not useful for assessing the adequacy of secretion, as GH levels may be low in normal individuals. Provocative tests are necessary. Screening tests include the measurement of GH following exercise or 90 minutes after the onset of sleep. If the results of screening tests are abnormal, more definitive tests are required. The two most commonly used definitive tests are the measurement of GH following insulin-induced hypoglycemia and the administration of l-dopa.

As with possible GH deficiency, a random serum GH measurement may not be reliable in assessing GH excess. Because GH is secreted episodically, if the random sample is drawn at the height of a secretory episode, seemingly elevated levels may be found in normal individuals. Growth hormone levels are normally suppressed by the rise in glucose that occurs 30 to 90 minutes following an oral glucose load. Patients with GH excess do not suppress and often have a paradoxical increase in GH after glucose administration. In addition, IGF-I levels are measured to assess the possibility of GH excess (see Chapter 12).

Prolactin

Although PRL secretion can be stimulated by a number of agents (including commercially available TRH) and inhibited by l-dopa, it is not necessary to perform such maneuvers for routine clinical assessment. A single basal serum PRL determination is usually sufficient to determine the presence of PRL excess, and PRL deficiency is not usually a clinical concern. Because PRL is the only anterior pituitary hormone with predominant negative control by the hypothalamus, it is often elevated by lesions that interfere with hypothalamic–pituitary portal blood flow. Such elevation is less pronounced than that seen with primary overproduction of PRL by adenomas of the pituitary (see below).

Thyroid-Stimulating Hormone

Deficiency of TSH may be assessed by a single serum measurement. As with all anterior pituitary hormones that have target endocrine glands, however, the interpretation of the adequacy of TSH secretion requires measurement of the other member of the hormone pair, thyroxine. Deficiency of TSH secretion is not usually manifested by a lower than normal serum TSH value; instead, the TSH is inappropriately normal in the presence of low serum thyroxine (see also Chapter 5).

Likewise, TSH excess may be assessed by a single serum measurement. Uncommonly, thyroid hormone excess is associated with inappropriately normal or increased levels of TSH. This is in contrast to the usual form of thyroid hormone overproduction, in which the TSH level is below normal or undetectable (see Chapter

13). Thus, TSH levels must be interpreted in light of the other member of the hormone pair, thyroxine, because excess TSH may only be manifested as an inappropriately normal level.

Gonadotropins (Luteinizing Hormone, Follicle-Stimulating Hormone)

In a woman, the presence of normal spontaneous cyclic menses indicates that gonadotropin secretion is normal (see Chapter 9). In women who do not have evidence of normal ovarian estrogen secretion, a single serum sample for measuring LH and FSH is sufficient to determine whether primary ovarian failure is present (elevated gonadotropins) or whether hypothalamic–pituitary abnormalities exist (low or normal gonadotropins). Similarly, in a man, gonadotropins must be interpreted in light of testicular function (see Chapter 10). Because LH is secreted in pulses, with resultant pulses of testosterone secretion, aliquots from three serum samples obtained at 20-minute intervals should be pooled for a more accurate estimate of basal levels of LH and testosterone. Again, elevated levels of gonadotropins with low testosterone indicate primary testicular failure, whereas low or normal gonadotropin levels signal hypothalamic or pituitary disease. Thus, LHRH testing may help distinguish hypothalamic from pituitary causes of low circulating gonadotropin levels (see Chapter 10).

Gonadotropin excess unrelated to gonadal failure may occur in women or men as a result of a pituitary adenoma and may be assessed by basal plasma levels. The α-subunit common to all the glycoprotein hormones is often secreted in excess by such gonadotroph cell adenomas.

Adrenocorticotropic Hormone

The clinical assessment of ACTH secretion usually involves the measurement of a product of the target gland (e.g., cortisol). Thus, ACTH deficiency is assessed by screening for sufficiency of the pituitary–adrenal axis. This is done with the short ACTH stimulation test by measuring the serum cortisol 1 hour after ACTH injection. Basal cortisol levels alone are not sufficient for diagnostic screening. If the response to the short ACTH stimulation test is abnormal, either hypothalamic–pituitary or adrenal abnormalities may be present. Prolonged ACTH administration may then be used to identify an adrenal problem, or ACTH and glucocorticoid secretion may be stimulated by insulin-induced hypoglycemia or the drug metyrapone to identify a pituitary problem (see Chapter 14).

Excess ACTH as a possible cause of excess cortisol secretion is determined by suppression tests, as basal cortisol levels are not reliable indicators of glucocorticoid excess and plasma ACTH may not be elevated in patients with pituitary-dependent cortisol excess. Dexamethasone, a synthetic potent glucocorticoid, is given at 11:00 P.M., and the serum cortisol is measured at 8:00 A.M. the next day. If the individual is normal, ACTH and consequently cortisol will be low the morning after dexamethasone is given. Failure of the cortisol level to decrease below 5 μg/dl indicates the need for definitive testing with a prolonged suppression test to determine the cause of the adrenal hyperfunction (see Chapter 14).

DERANGED HYPOTHALAMIC–PITUITARY FUNCTION

Hypothalamic Disease

A variety of hypothalamic disorders including tumors, trauma, infections, congenital malformations, genetic defects, and vascular alterations can affect the secretion of different releasing hormones either selectively or collectively, depending on the location and extent of the lesion. In general, lesions of the median eminence–tuber cinereum region decrease pituitary function. An exception to this is the secretion of PRL, which increases after such lesions develop because of the loss of its inhibitory hypothalamic tone.

A deficit of individual hypothalamic hormones results in isolated pituitary hormone deficiency. Prominent examples of this condition are the syndromes of hypothalamic hypothyroidism caused by TRH deficiency, olfactory-genital dysplasia (Kallmann's syndrome or isolated gonadotropin deficiency) characterized by a deficit in LHRH secretion associated with hyposmia, and idiopathic dwarfism caused by GHRH deficiency. Kallmann's syndrome is particularly interesting because the deficit in LHRH secretion is related to the failure of embryonic LHRH neurons to migrate from their site of origin (the olfactory placode) to their final destination in the hypothalamus, possibly due to a defect in a neuroadhesion molecule.

Hypopituitarism

If hypopituitarism develops in a child, the defect in GH secretion leads to the development of a pituitary dwarf. In this condition there is a proportional reduction in body size, in contrast to the conspicuous shortening of the long bones in the so-called achondroplastic dwarf. If the deficiency extends to other anterior pituitary hormones, other symptoms and signs will be present. These can include weakness, fatigue, and headaches, but they are of little diagnostic significance. The development of hypopituitarism in adulthood may also produce weakness, fatigue, and headaches, plus signs and symptoms associated with decreased secretion of gonadotropins such as loss of axillary and pubic hair and breast atrophy. The reduction in GH is probably at least in part responsible for the pallor and fine wrinkling of the facial skin seen in adult hypopituitarism. In women, the menstrual cycle ceases and there is genital atrophy. In men, secondary testicular failure can cause loss of libido and potency, muscle strength, beard growth, and testicular size, the decrease in testis size because of the diminished gonadotropin secretion, the decreased libido, strength and beard because of the loss of testosterone. Hypopituitarism may be caused by hypothalamic disease or by disorders that directly affect the pituitary gland, such as inactivating mutations of releasing hormone receptors, tumors, infarct, and damage by radiation therapy (see also Chapter 12).

Acromegaly and Gigantism

An excess of GH release leads to the development of gigantism if the hypersecretion has been present during early life (a rare condition) and to acromegaly if hypersecretion occurs after body growth has stopped. In the case of gigantism, a rather symmetrical enlargement of the body results in a true giant with overgrowth of long bones, connective tissue, and visceral organs. In the case of acromegaly, the epiphyseal and diaphyseal centers of the long bones (femur, tibia, etc.) fuse, and elongation of these bones is no longer possible. In this condition there is an overgrowth of cancellous bones, resulting in a protruding jaw, termed *prognathism*, thickening of the phalanges, overgrowth of soft tissue that thickens the skin, and overgrowth of the visceral organs. Acromegaly and gigantism are caused by eosinophilic adenomas consisting of somatotrophs, leading to the excessive secretion of GH.

Hyperprolactinemia

This is the most common example of pituitary hyperfunction and is brought about by microadenomas of the lactotrophs. Hyperprolactinemia can also result from treatment with the dopamine receptor blockers that are commonly prescribed for psychiatric illness. In women, hyperprolactinemia frequently leads to amenorrhea and galactorrhea. The amenorrhea is caused by the disturbance in gonadotropin secretion arising from prolactin excess. Galactorrhea is caused by the direct effect of PRL on the breast. In men, galactorrhea is not common; however, hyperprolactinemia can cause loss of libido, impotence, and decreased sperm density, usually associated with a decrease in the plasma levels of LH and testosterone. The diagnosis can be made by measuring plasma PRL and then examining for the presence of microor macroadenomas of the pituitary by computed tomographic scanning or magnetic resonance imaging. Hyperprolactinemia can be treated with a dopamine agonist, such as bromocriptine, or by surgical removal of the adenoma.

SUGGESTED READING

Gershengorn MC and Osman R: Molecular and cellular biology of thyrotropin-releasing hormone receptors. Physiol Rev 76:175–191, 1996.

Herrington J and Carter-Su C: Signaling pathways activated by the growth hormone receptor. TEM 12:252–257, 2001.

Hinuma S, Habata Y, Fujii R, Kawamata Y, Hosoya M, Fukusumi S, Kitada C, Masuo Y, Asano T, Matsumoto H, Sekiguchi M, Kurokawa T, Nishimura O, Onda H, and Fujino M: A prolactin-releasing peptide in the brain. Nature 393:272–276, 1998.

Kojima M, Hosoda H, Date Y, Nakazato M, Matsuo H, and Kangawa K: Ghrelin is a growth-hormone-releasing acylated peptide from stomach. Nature 402:656–660, 1999.

Kourides IA, Gurr JA, and Wolf O: The regulation and organization of thyroid-stimulating hormone genes. Recent Prog Horm Res 40:79–120, 1984.

Krieger DT, Liotta AS, and Brownstein MJ: ACTH, β-lipotropin and related peptides in brain, pituitary and blood. Recent Prog Horm Res 36:272–344, 1980.

Marshall JC: Regulation of gonadotropin synthesis and secretion. In: *Endocrinology*, 4th ed., Vol. 3. LJ DeGroot and JL Jameson, eds., Saunders, New York, 2001, pp. 1916–1925.

Müller EE, Locatelli V, and Cocchi D: Neuroendocrine control of growth hormone secretion. Physiol Rev 79:511–607, 1999.

Neill JD, Duck LW, Sellers JC, and Musgrove LC: A gonadotropin-releasing hormone (GnRH) receptor specific for GnRH in primates. Biochem Biophys Res Commun 282: 1012–1018, 2001.

Reichlin S: Neuroendocrinology. In: *Williams Textbook of Endocrinology,* 8th ed., JD Wilson and DW Foster, eds., Saunders, Philadelphia, pp. 135–219, 1992.

Reisine T and Bell GI: Molecular biology of somatostatin receptors. Endocr Rev 16:427–442, 1995.

Riskind PN and Martin JB: Functional anatomy of the hypothalamic-anterior pituitary complex. In: *Endocrinology,* 2nd ed., Vol. 1, LJ DeGroot, ed., Saunders, Philadelphia, pp. 97–107, 1989.

Sealfon SC, Weinstein H, and Millar RP: Molecular mechanisms of ligand interaction with the gonadotropin-releasing hormone receptor. Endocrinol Rev 18:180–205, 1997.

Venihaki M and Majzoub JA: Animal models of CRH deficiency. Front Neuroendocrinol 20:122–145, 1999.

7

The Posterior Pituitary and Water Metabolism

WILLIS K. SAMSON

STRUCTURE OF THE POSTERIOR PITUITARY GLAND

The neurohypophysis, also called the *posterior pituitary* or *neural lobe,* is the ventral extension of hypothalamic tissue derived from a developmental downgrowth of the neuroectoderm forming the floor of the third cerebroventricle. It weighs approximately 0.10–0.15 g in humans and is well developed at birth, having been present since the fifth month of intrauterine life. In addition to containing glial elements called *pituicytes,* the posterior pituitary is composed of unmyelinated nerve fibers and axon terminals of neurons whose cell bodies reside primarily in the supraoptic and paraventricular hypothalamic nuclei (Fig. 7-1). These hypothalamo–neurohypophyseal fibers deliver the two primary posterior pituitary hormones, oxytocin (OT) and arginine vasopressin (AVP), to the neural lobe in association with specific proteins, the neurophysins, once thought to be carrier proteins but now known to be portions of the OT and AVP precursor molecules.

The neurons produce either OT or AVP, never both, and recent studies indicate that in addition to one of these two hormones, other neuropeptides, such as corticotropin-releasing hormone (CRH), and neurotransmitters are also produced in OT- or AVP-containing cells. The phenomenon of colocalization of neuromodulatory agents has aroused a great deal of clinical interest in the role of neuropeptides such as OT and AVP in brain function. Both OT- and AVP-containing nerve fibers originating in the supraoptic and paraventricular nuclei also project to a variety of other brain structures that are thought to be the sites of their observed central nervous system actions, and to the vicinity of the hypophyseal portal vessels in the median eminence. Release from these fibers of both OT and AVP explains the high levels of these hormones in portal blood and provides the framework for the actions of OT and AVP as modulators of anterior pituitary function.

The arterial blood supply of the posterior pituitary is via the inferior (and to some degree the superior) hypophyseal arteries, which originate from the cavernous and postclinoid portions of the internal carotid artery. The venous drainage is composed of efferent vessels joining the intercavernous sinuses and eventually the internal jugular vein.

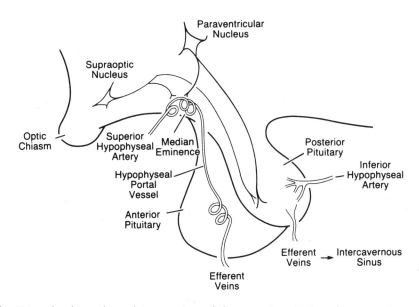

Fig. 7-1 Blood supply and innervation of the posterior pituitary by oxytocin- and vasopressin-containing neurons.

POSTERIOR PITUITARY HORMONES

Both OT and AVP (also called *antidiuretic hormone,* ADH) are nonapeptides containing internal disulfide bonds linking cystine residues at positions 1 and 6, giving them a ring structure that is necessary for some of the peptides' biological activity (Fig. 7-2). Both are assembled on the ribosomes as parts of large precursor molecules that consist of the respective hormone and its associated carrier protein (α-neurophysin, approximately 10,000 molecular weight). The AVP-associated neurophysin, nicotine-stimulated neurophysin, is a polypeptide with a C-terminal extension that contains the 39-amino acid, AVP-associated C-terminal glycoprotein. Estrogen-stimulated neurophysin, associated with OT, is a polypeptide that lacks the C-terminal glycoprotein extension. After ribosomal assembly, the precursor molecules are transferred to the Golgi complex and packaged into neurosecretory granules that move along the axon at a flow rate of 8 mm/hr (faster than normal axoplasmic flow). The precursor and the associated neurophysins have not been demonstrated conclusively to possess biological activity; however, during axoplasmic transport the neurophysin carrier is proteolytically cleaved from the associated neurohormone, and both the neurophysin and neurohormones (OT or AVP) are released into the capillary spaces in the posterior pituitary. These hypothalamo–neurohypophyseal cells are neurons that can generate and propagate action potentials that, on arrival at the nerve terminals, cause depolarization and exocytosis of the secretory granule contents (stimulus–secretion coupling). Both OT and AVP circulate in the blood unbound to other proteins and are rapidly removed (mainly by the kidney but also by the liver and brain) from the circulation. The older literature reflects a plasma half-life ($t_{1/2}$) for both hormones of about 5 minutes; however,

ARGININE VASOPRESSIN

```
      ┌─────S──────S──┐
Cys-Tyr-Phe-Gln-Asn-Cys-Pro-Arg-Gly-NH₂
```

m.w. 1084

OXYTOCIN

```
      ┌─────S──────S──┐
Cys-Tyr-Ile-Gln-Asn-Cys-Pro-Leu-Gly-NH₂
```

m.w. 1007

ATRIAL NATRIURETIC FACTOR (ANP 99-126)

```
Ser-Leu-Arg-Arg-Ser-Ser-Cys-Phe-Gly-Gly-Arg-Met-
                        └S──S──┐
Asp-Arg-Ile-Gly-Ala-Gln-Ser-Gly-Leu-Gly-Cys-Asn-Ser-Phe-Arg-Tyr-NH₂
```

m.w. 3081

Fig. 7-2 Structures of arginine vasopressin, oxytocin, and atrial natriuretic factor.

studies employing sensitive radioimmunoassays for each peptide and calculations based on more physiological circumstances reveal a two-component disappearance curve with a much faster $t_{1/2}$ (less than 1 minute) and a second component of approximately 2–3 minutes.

VASOPRESSIN

Primary Action: Antidiuresis

Vasopressin, which circulates at basal levels of around 1 pg/ml plasma (10^{-12} M), binds to a specific membrane receptor (Table 7-1), the V_2 receptor, on the peritubular (serosal) surface of cells of the distal convoluted tubules and medullary collecting ducts inducing adenylyl cyclase activity. The cyclic adenosine monophosphate (cAMP) formed is responsible for activation of a protein kinase, which initiates a phosphorylation cascade resulting in the insertion of the protein, aquaporin, in the luminal membrane and thereby enhances the permeability of the cell to water. This AVP-dependent increase in membrane permeability to water permits back diffusion of solute-free water remaining in the urine after proximal tubule handling down the osmotic gradient from hypotonic urine to the hypertonic interstitium of the renal medulla, resulting in an increase in urine osmolality (relative

Table 7-1 Vasopressin Receptors

Receptor subtype	Location	Function
V_1	Blood vessels	Vasoconstriction
V_2	Renal collecting duct epithelium	Increased water permeability
V_3	Anterior pituitary gland	Stimulation of adrenocorticotropin release

to glomerular filtrate or plasma). The net result is an increase in urine osmolality and a decrease in urine flow.

Control of Secretion

Plasma Osmolality

Water deprivation results in increased plasma osmolality, which is thought to be sensed by specialized brain cells, called *osmoreceptors*, located in two highly vascularized regions (where the blood–brain barrier is absent) of the central nervous system (CNS): the vascular organ of the lamina terminalis and the subfornical organ. The increased osmolality of plasma results in loss of intracellular water from the osmoreceptors and stimulation of AVP release. The osmoreceptor cells themselves do not release AVP; instead, as revealed in animal studies, they are thought to communicate with the AVP neurons using acetylcholine as their neurotransmitter. The sensitivity of the osmoreceptor to changes in plasma osmolality is increased by angiotensin II, which potentiates AVP release in response to osmotic stimuli. As can be seen in Figure 7-3, the AVP response to changes in plasma osmolality is extremely sensitive; indeed, increases as small as 1% result in enhanced AVP secretion.

Nonosmotic Factors

A fall in blood volume of greater than 8% (hemorrhage), quiet standing (orthostatic hypotension), and positive pressure breathing, all of which reduce cardiac output and therefore central blood volume, are potent stimuli for AVP release (Fig. 7-3), whereas maneuvers that increase total blood volume (isotonic saline or blood infusion, cold water immersion) suppress AVP release. Low (left atrial) and high (carotid and aortic) pressure baroreceptors sense small alterations in blood volume and communicate with CNS structures via medullary afferents of the 9th and 10th cranial nerves. These pressure receptors normally exert a tonic inhibition on AVP release via medullary efferents to the hypothalamus; thus, decreases in blood volume unload the baroreceptors (decrease afferent flow), resulting in less inhibition (α-adrenergic) of AVP release and increased circulating AVP. Hypovolemia also results in renin release from the juxtaglomerular apparatus of the kidney (see Chapter 14) and the formation of angiotensin II, both of which sensitize the osmoreceptor cells of the hypothalamus, leading to enhanced AVP release. Therefore, altering blood volume can *reset* the central osmotic threshold and possibly the sensitivity for AVP release (Fig. 7-3) such that the AVP response to any given increase in plasma osmolality is more accentuated as the level of volume depletion increases. A variety of other stimuli can affect AVP release. Increased partial pressure of carbon dioxide ($PaCO_2$) or reduced partial pressure of oxygen (PaO_2), pain, stress, increased temperature, β-adrenergic agents, estrogens, progesterone, opiates, barbiturates, nicotine, and prostaglandins have been demonstrated to stimulate AVP release. A decrease in temperature, α-adrenergic agents, ethanol, and cardiac hormones can exert inhibitory actions on AVP release.

Secondary Actions

It has been demonstrated that AVP acts within the CNS to lower body temperature and to facilitate memory consolidation and retrieval. Indeed, studies in aged humans

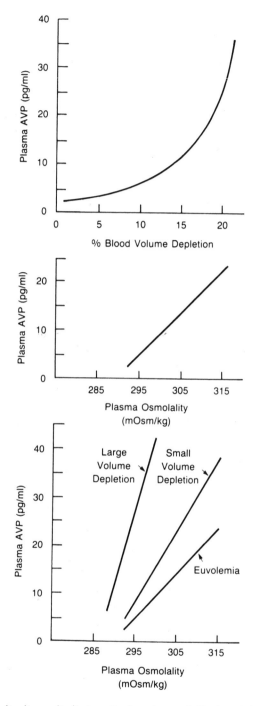

Fig. 7-3 Effects of volume depletion (*top*) and osmolality (*center*) on arginine vaso-pressin (AVP) release. Interaction of the two variables (*bottom*) is also illustrated. (Idealized for humans from rat data reported by Dunn FL et al: J Clin Invest 52:3212–3219, 1973.)

revealed the improvement of short-term memory after AVP administration. Vasopressin-containing fibers that project to the hypophyseal portal plexus in the median eminence deliver AVP to the portal blood and anterior pituitary, where AVP acts via a subtype of AVP receptor, which differs from that in the kidney and vasculature, to potentiate the release of adrenocorticotropin (ACTH) in response to CRH. This action of AVP seems coordinated to potentiate the adrenocorticotropin response to stress.

In addition to its effects in the kidney, via V_2 receptors, AVP exerts potent vascular actions. Interaction of AVP with specific (V_1) receptors on vascular smooth muscle results in profound contraction, shunting of blood away from the periphery, and elevated central venous pressures. Total peripheral resistance increases in a linear fashion, with increases in circulating AVP. However, the rise in total peripheral resistance seen in response to AVP is buffered by baroreceptor-mediated falls in cardiac output and general sympathetic tone, so that except for having a prolonged effect on regional distribution of blood flow, the overall increase in arterial pressure is minimal.

Disorders of Arginine Vasopressin Secretion

Deficient Secretion

Usually caused by destruction or dysfunction of the hypothalamo–neurohypophyseal complex, diabetes insipidus is characterized by the inability to produce a concentrated urine, frequent urination (with low specific gravity and osmolality), and often excessive thirst. Treatment of this disorder involves use of a vasopressin analog, desmopressin, which fails at therapeutic doses to react with vascular (V_1) AVP receptors (and therefore is a nonpressor), yet is recognized by renal tubular (V_2) receptors; it has the additional advantage of a prolonged duration due to a longer ($t_{1/2}$) in plasma and enhanced antidiuretic potency.

Patients with diabetes insipidus cannot reduce urine flow during standard water deprivation testing because of their inability to concentrate their urine. Diabetes insipidus can result from CNS lesions (failure to secrete AVP) or from a renal disorder (failure to respond to AVP). The differential diagnosis can be made by AVP administration. Patients with diabetes insipidus of central origin respond, whereas those with nephrogenic diabetes insipidus do not. The renal form of diabetes insipidus is primarily a local lesion characterized by unresponsiveness of the tubule to appropriate levels of AVP and is not associated with lesions of the hypothalamus or posterior pituitary gland. Failure of the renal tubule to respond to AVP can be attributed to at least two causes: genetic and acquired hyporesponsiveness. Congenital nephrogenic diabetes insipidus is usually deteted in the first week of life and can be caused by a mutation in the V_2 receptor itself or in the aquaporin water channel protein. Acquired hyporesponsiveness can be caused by multiple factors, most of which result in structural damage to the kidney, and also by drug interactions (e.g., lithium).

Inappropriate Production

Release of AVP exceeding that predicted by plasma volume or tonicity can result from CNS disease or trauma, drug interactions, or ectopic production by tumors resulting in water retention and concentration of urine in excess of plasma. Paradoxically, sodium excretion into the urine increases despite the low serum sodium level (probably due to elevated levels of atrial natriuretic factors caused by the expanded plasma volume; see below). Symptoms include altered mental status, headache, drowsiness, nausea, and often coma. Fluid restriction is appropriate treatment; however, acute administration of hypertonic saline is often considered to raise plasma osmolality. In the longer term, treatment with naloxone (to decrease central AVP release) or demeclocycline (to block AVP action on the kidney) is often employed. This so-called syndrome of inappropriate antidiuretic hormone (SIADH) secretion is characterized by normal renal and adrenal function, yet by

1. Hyponatremia (serum sodium concentrations of 100–115 mEq/liter)
2. Continued renal sodium excretion
3. Absence of clinical evidence of volume depletion or edema
4. Inappropriately high urine osmolality

OXYTOCIN

Primary Action

Oxytocin stimulates milk ejection by contracting the myoepithelial cells surrounding the alveoli and ducts in the mammary gland. Additionally, it stimulates rhythmic myometrial contractions in the uterus, aiding in expulsion of the fetus. Although not necessary for its initiation, labor proceeds more slowly in the absence of OT. Therapeutically, OT (also called *pitocin*) is employed postpartum to sustain contractions and to decrease bleeding.

Control of Release

Oxytocin is normally present at barely detectable levels (1–10 pg/ml in plasma) but is present in readily detectable quantities during ovulation, parturition, and lactation, as well as in males and females during certain mild stresses. Vaginal stimulation during intercourse or delivery and stimulation of touch receptors in the nipples result in afferent neural input (via the spinothalamic tract and a variety of brain stem relays) to OT-producing cells in the paraventricular and supraoptic nuclei. The stimulatory neurotransmitter involved is thought to be acetylcholine or dopamine. Extremely severe pain, increased temperature, and loud noise can inhibit OT release (probably via an opioid mechanism), whereas hemorrhage and psychogenic stress (restraint, novel environment, mild apprehension, and fear) stimulate OT secretion. The OT release seen during the immediate preovulatory period is possibly due to rising estrogen levels present at that time (remember, the OT-associated carrier is also known as the *estrogen-stimulated neurophysin*). Indeed, administration of exogenous estrogens can stimulate OT release.

Secondary Actions

In addition to possessing some renal and vascular actions mimicking those of AVP, probably due at least in part to an interaction with the AV receptor, OT can potentiate CRH-induced adrenocorticotropin release, again by interacting with the AVP receptor. Central nervous system actions of OT include amnestic effects and stimulation of maternal behavior. Recently, OT has been shown to act within the CNS to curb the appetite for salt. Increases in OT levels in plasma often parallel those of prolactin (during mild stress, ovulation, and lactation), and recent evidence indicates that OT can act directly at the lactotroph to stimulate prolactin release, suggesting a physiological role for OT as a prolactin-releasing factor.

Disorders of Oxytocin Secretion

Oxytocin excess has not been clearly demonstrated. Deficient OT secretion normally results in difficulty in nursing due to inadequate milk ejection.

CARDIOVASCULAR HORMONES AND THE INTEGRATED CONTROL OF FLUID AND ELECTROLYTE HOMEOSTASIS

It has been recognized for some time that hypothalamic peptides (AVP and OT) interact with hormones from the adrenal gland (glucocorticoids and mineralocorticoids) and angiotensin II to coordinate the mechanisms regulating fluid and electrolyte homeostasis. Only recently has it become clear that several additional families of peptides, derived primarily from vascular tissues but produced also in the adrenal gland, kidney and brain, play important roles and, indeed, contribute to the physiology and pathophysiology of sodium and water balance. These discoveries have led to the definition of a new discipline, cardiovascular endocrinology, which focuses on the interactions of hormonal and cardiorenal mechanisms protecting vascular status (tissue perfusion) and plasma osmolarity (electrolyte balance). Cardiovascular hormones can be functionally divided into procontractile/promitogenic factors and vasodilatory/antimitogenic factors, a categorization that identifies two important characteristics of their biological actions.

Procontractile Cardiovascular Peptides

Heading the list in this category is angiotensin II (A II). Produced in the circulation and in some tissues (i.e., brain and vascular cells) through conversion of the precursor angiotensin I by angiotensin converting enzyme (ACE), this octapeptide has potent vasoconstrictive and promitogenic effects. As detailed in Chapter 14, angiotensin I is cleaved from the plasma protein angiotensinogen by renin released from the juxtaglomerular apparatus of the kidney in response to decreased renal perfusion pressure or decreased renal tubular sodium delivery to the macula densa. The hallmark actions of A II are many, most closely related to a physiological compensation for loss of fluid and electrolytes (Table 7-2).

There are two major subclasses of angiotensin receptors, AT1 and AT2, with the first class further subdivided on the basis of gene cloning into the AT1A and AT1B receptors. All are seven transmembrane domain receptors and members of the G protein–coupled receptor family. In kidney, adrenal cortex, and vascular smooth muscle cells, the action of A II is transduced via the AT1 receptor coupled

Table 7-2 Physiologic Actions of Angiotensin II

Vascular

Vasoconstriction (increased total peripheral resistance by direct actions on the contractile elements and indirectly via enhancement of norepinephrine release from nerve terminals innervating the blood vessels, increased sympathetic discharge, and increased medullary epinephrine release)

Remodeling (enhanced migration, proliferation and hypertrophy of vascular smooth muscle cells, cardiomyocytes and fibroblasts; increased matrix formation; indirect stimulation of cardiomyocyte proliferation and hypertrophy by the increased cardiac afterload due to volume expansion secondary to sodium retention)

Renal/Adrenal

Antinatriuresis (direct proximal tubule effect to stimulate sodium reabsorption and indirect effect via stimulation of aldosterone release and subsequent sodium reabsorption in distal tubule)
Hemodynamic (renal vasoconstriction; increased renal sympathetic tone)

Brain

Sympathostimulation and attenuation of the baroreceptor reflex
Dipsogenesis
Stimulation of salt appetite
Stimulation of arginine vasopressin and oxytocin secretion

Pituitary Gland

Synergism with corticotropin-releasing hormone to stimulate adrenocorticotropin secretion

to a pertussis-toxin–insensitive class of G proteins (G_q of G11) and subsequent activation of phospholipase C. There and in other tissues such as the pituitary gland, A II also activates AT1 receptors coupled via G proteins (G_s or G_i) to adenylyl cyclase. Coupling of the AT1 receptor to phospholipase A2 and phospholipase D has also been reported. The mitogenic actions of A II are expressed via activation of mitogen-activated protein kinases (MAP kinases) and tyrosine kinases. The function of the AT2 receptors is less clear; however, it is known that they are present in fetal tissues and adult brain, suggesting developmental and neurotropic effects. The activation of AT2 receptors initiates G protein–linked signaling as well as non–G protein–linked signaling via tyrosine phosphatase and MAP kinase inactivation. This perhaps explains the observed functional antagonism of the AT1 and AT2 receptors, with AT1 receptor activation leading to a hyperplastic response and AT2 receptor activation leading to cell inactivation and death (i.e., apoptosis).

The second major procontractile vascular hormone is a family of peptides know as the *endothelins* (ETs). Three unique and ancestrally related gene products, ET-1, ET-2, and ET-3, comprise this family. All are 21-amino acid peptides containing two intramolecular disulfide bonds necessary for biological activity. These peptides are produced in endothelial cells lining the blood vessels; fortunately, because of their potent vasoconstrictive effects, under normal conditions they are secreted abluminally—that is, away from the vessel lumen. Thus, in most cases these peptides act as local paracrine or autocrine factors. One of the peptides, ET-3, appears to be

Table 7-3 Biological Actions of the Endothelins

Tissue	Receptor subtype	Signaling mechanism	Actions
Lung	ET-A	Phospholipases D and A2	Prostanoid production
Vascular smooth muscle	ET-A	Phospholipase C Activation of K^+ channels Activation of adenylyl cyclase	Contraction, mitogenesis
Myocardium	ET-A	G protein–mediated closing of Cl^- and L-type Ca^{2+} channels, with opening of K^+ channels leading to decreased electrical activity	Tissue damage in myocardial infarction
Endothelium	ET-B	Nitric oxide synthase activation, PLC activation, and Ca^{2+} mobilization, CNP release Opens Na^+-H^+ antiporter Inhibits adenylyl cyclase	Transient vasodilation
Astrocytes	ET-B	PKC activation of MAP kinase	Mitogenesis

CNP, C-type natriuretic peptide; MAP, mitogen-activated protein; NOS, nitric oxide synthase; PKC, protein kinase C; PLC, phospholipase C.

preferentially produced in brain, where it exerts potent mitogenic actions on astrocytes. Two distinct ET receptors have been identified, both seven transmembrane spanning domain proteins. The ET-A receptor displays a rank order of binding affinity preferring ET-1 (ET-1 $\geq$ ET-2 >> ET-3). This is the primary ET receptor on vascular smooth muscle cells and cardiomyocytes. The ET-B receptor binds all three isoforms with equal affinity. The actions of the ETs are diverse in nature and are mediated via multiple signaling mechanisms (Table 7-3).

Because of their powerful vasconstrictive effects, the ETs were hypothesized to play a role in the pathogenesis of hypertension. However, mice lacking the ET-1 gene are not hypotensive; rather, they are paradoxically hypertensive, and thus a definitive role for the ETs in blood pressure regulation remains unestablished. Good evidence does exist for a role for endogenous ET in reperfusion injury. Blockade of the action of locally released ET with antibodies or antagonists significantly reduced tissue damage distal to transient coronary artery ligation and in a model of myocardial infarction. Thus, ET antagonists may have clinical utility in the prevention of reperfusion injury.

Some of the best evidence for a therapeutic value of the ET antagonists comes from the improvement of renal function in genetic models of hypertension and the prevention, by these antagonists, of ischemia-induced renal failure. Finally, cyclosporine-induced nephrotoxicity must be due, at least in part, to the local release of endogenous ET (and the subsequent constriction of the afferent arteriole), as the renal toxicity of immunosuppressant therapy was blocked by ET antagonist administration. The potential pathological roles for the ETs in disease states are listed in Table 7-4.

Table 7-4 Endothelins in Human Disease

Proven pathological roles	Proposed pathological roles
Myocardial damage from vascular insult	Acute vascular insult (vasospasm in brain)
Cyclosporine-induced nephrotoxicity	Patent ductus arteriosus
Postischemic renal failure	Pulmonary hypertension and fibrosis
Vasospasm secondary to subarachnoid hemorrhage	Gastric ulceration
Hirschsprung's disease	Heart failure manifestations
	Hepatorenal syndrome (cirrhosis)
	Unstable angina
	Raynaud's phenomenon
	Shock
	Glomerulonephritis
	Inflammatory bowel disease
	Dysmenorrhea
	Asthma
	Pre-eclampsia

While A II can be viewed as a physiologically relevant circulating hormone that regulates cardiovascular and renal function by affecting not only volume status (and therefore pressure) but also sodium homeostasis, the effects of the ETs are more closely related to abnormal alterations in blood pressure and regional flow, as well as renal perfusion. Thus, only under pathological conditions may the ETs be important regulators of fluid and electrolyte balance.

Vasodilatory Cardiovascular Peptides

Two families of peptides, the natriuretic peptides and peptides derived from the adrenomedullin gene product, not only express vasodilatory and antimitogenic actions opposed to those of A II and the ETs, but also exert potent actions related to the control of fluid and electrolyte homeostasis. Biological activities shared between the two families of peptides are exerted at numerous tissue sites, all seemingly coordinated to regulate sodium intake and excretion and, at the same time, volume status.

The Natriuretic Peptides

It has been recognized for some time that atrial distention results in profound diuresis (increased urine flow). The proposed mechanisms for this effect include not only neuronal reflex activation of CNS structures (vagal afferents) but also the possible release of a volume regulatory substance from the heart. Infusion of extracts of mammalian cardiac atrial tissue were found to stimulate significant increases in urine volume and urinary sodium excretion (natriuresis). Additionally, these extracts were shown to relax precontracted vascular and gastrointestinal smooth muscle strips *in vitro* (a spasmolytic action). The peptide responsible for the diuretic, natriuretic, and spasmolytic actions was identified to be 28 amino acids in length and to be produced primarily in atrial myocytes under normal physiological conditions. Because of the original localization and the spectrum of biological activity, this peptide was named *atrial natriuretic peptide* (ANP). Expression of ANP increases under volume overload conditions, as does the production of a second member of the family, the 32 amino acid B-type natriuretic peptide (BNP). The third member of the family, C-type natriuretic peptide (CNP, 22 amino acids), was later isolated and found to be produced in endothelial cells and brain, but not normally in cardiac myocytes. Atrial natriuretic peptide is the major circulating member of the family, and normal plasma levels range from 50 to 150 pg/ml. Highest levels are present in the aorta (vena cava to aorta concentration gradient 76–177 pg/ml, identifying the heart as the major site of release), and the plasma half-life is about 1–3 minutes. In addition to being filtered into the urine, major degradation sites include kidney, liver, lung, and brain.

Stimuli for Release. Cardiac myocytes are located in a position to detect pressure changes accompanying increases in venous return or afterload. Indeed, stretch associated with increases in venous return is the major stimulus for ANP release, as interventions (head down tilt, passive leg elevation, cold water immersion, saline or blood loading) that result in increases in right atrial pressure and an increase in right atrial dimension result in concomitant increases in ANP release and diuresis. Therefore, the heart responds to an increase in venous return (Fig. 7-4) by releasing hormones that act at the kidney (and other sites; see below), resulting in a lowering of fluid volume (via diuresis) and a decrease in venous return. Recent evidence indicates that an increase in plasma osmolality also releases ANP, perhaps reflecting the natriuretic action as well. Increasing the sodium intake in normal volunteers from 10 to 200 mmol/day resulted in a twofold elevation in plasma ANP. Furthermore, these subjects released even more ANP in response to subsequent interventions that elevated venous return.

Natriuretic Peptide Receptors. Three subtypes of natriuretic peptide receptors have been cloned and sequenced. Two have extracellular binding domains linked via a transmembrane spanning segment with an intracellular particulate guanylyl cyclase. The third lacks the intracellular extension, and although it has been designated the nonbiological clearance receptor (originally thought to function only as a biological sponge that removed the natriuretic peptides from the circulation), it is now apparent that this subtype transduces important antimitogenic signals of the natriuretic peptides and is linked to activation of inositol phosphate hydrolysis and inhibition of adenylyl cyclase. Table 7-5 summarizes the three receptor subtypes.

Renal Actions. The hallmark renal actions of ANP are natriuresis and diuresis. Infusion of ANP into healthy volunteers results in increases in urine volume, creatinine clearance, free water clearance, and the excretion rates of sodium and chloride. These effects are at least partially due to ANP's ability to increase the glomerular filtration rate, a reflection of its action to stimulate postglomerular vasoconstriction. Additionally, ANP exerts a direct tubular effect to inhibit sodium transport in the distal nephron and antagonizes the effect of AVP in the tubule and duct. A final renal action of ANP is exerted directly at the level of the juxtaglomerular apparatus to inhibit renin secretion, thus reducing A II formation.

Adrenal Actions. In addition to preventing A II formation by inhibiting renin release, ANP blocks the action of A II in the adrenal. Indeed, both basal and stimu-

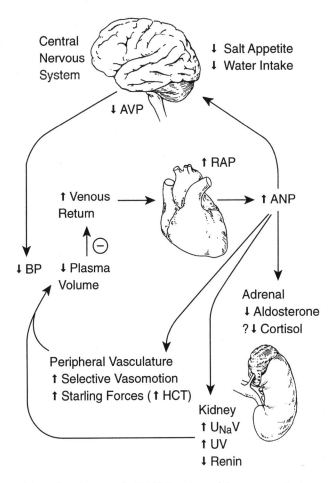

Fig. 7-4 Atrial natriuretic peptide (ANP) is released in response to increased venous return and the associated increase in right atrial pressure (RAP). It acts in the brain, adrenal, kidney, and peripheral vasculature to produce a drop in blood pressure (BP) and venous return, thus eliminating the signal for its release. AVP, arginine vasopressin; HCT, hematocrit; $U_{Na}V$, urine sodium excretion; UV, urine volume.

Table 7-5 The Natriuretic Peptide Receptor (NPR) Family

Receptor subtype	Ligand preference	Signalling mechanism
NPR$_A$ receptor (guanylyl cyclase A, GC-A)	ANP > BNP >> CNP	Particular guanylyl cyclase
NPR$_B$ receptor (guanylyl cyclase B, GC-B)	CNP > ANP > BNP	Particular guanylyl cyclase
NPR$_C$ receptor (clearance receptor)	ANP = BNP = CNP	Inositol phosphase turnover, adenylyl cyclase

ANP, atrial natriuretic peptide; BNP, B-type natriuretic peptide; CNP, C-type natriuretic peptide.

lated (A II and ACTH) aldosterone secretion are inhibited by cardiac hormones. Although the renal effect of ANP (natriuresis) is too rapid to be explained by alterations in aldosterone levels, in chronic volume expansion ANP may play a part in the suppression of aldosterone levels.

Vascular Actions. Intravenous infusion of ANP in humans results in decreased mean arterial blood pressure and decreased cardiac output. The decrease in mean arterial pressure could be due solely to an *in vivo* vasodilatory effect of ANP that matches its *in vitro* spasmolytic action. Increases in forearm blood flow have been observed; however, in certain vascular regions, vasoconstrictive effects are seen (efferent renal artery). Alternatively, the drop in mean arterial pressure could be secondary to the observed decrease in cardiac output caused by decreased venous return. Strong evidence in favor of this exists. Detailed experiments have revealed that ANP reduces circulatory capacitance as a result of decreased blood volume (and vascular recoil) and active vasoconstriction, thereby decreasing venous return. In addition to urinary fluid loss, the observed increase in hematocrit during ANP infusion may be due to transcapillary fluid shifts initiated by increases in postcapillary resistance. No direct chronotropic or inotropic effects have been observed *in vitro* in isolated heart preparations.

The abundant production of CNP in vascular endothelial cells reflects a paracrine action of the peptide to control vascular tone in concert with several other vasorelaxant and vasoconstrictive factors produced locally. Circulating ET-3 or locally produced ET-1, members of a powerful family of vasoconstrictor peptides, stimulate the release from the endothelial cells of both CNP and nitric oxide (NO). These factors are released abluminally, away from the vascular lumen toward the surrounding smooth muscle, and induce vasodilation by unique but potentially convergent mechanisms. While CNP activates particulate guanylyl cyclase via the natriuretic peptide receptor B subtype (NPR_B) receptor, NO diffuses into the vascular smooth muscle cell and activates soluble guanylyl cyclase, both resulting in elevated cytosolic cyclic guanosine monophosphate (cGMP). Thus, there exists at the endothelial interface with the vascular smooth muscle a balance of redundant vasodilatory substances including CNP and NO, and additional endothelial-derived factors such as prostacyclins and adrenomedullin (see below), with local vasconstrictors such as ET-1. An interplay of these agents, together with local neural influences, determines vascular tone and therefore blood pressure. The ability of CNP to potently dilate coronary vessels suggests a possible therapeutic use for CNP or selective NPRB agonists in the treatment of myocardial ischemia.

Central Nervous System Actions. In addition to its renal, adrenal, and vascular actions, ANP exerts a profound influence on CNS-mediated events related to fluid and electrolyte homeostasis. Natriuretic peptide receptors have been localized to discrete brain regions, and the production of ANP and, to a greater extent, CNP in neuronal elements is well established. Natriuretic peptide–containing neurons terminate in regions known to be important in the neuroendocrine and neuronal control of renal and cardiovascular function. Indeed, ANP exerts a profound inhibitory action on AVP release (Fig. 7-4) and significantly impairs fluid consumption by inhibiting water intake and salt appetite. These central actions match well the peripheral effects of the hormone, such that in addition to exerting an opposite action (diuresis) in the kidney, ANP inhibits the release of AVP (the antidiuretic hormone). Also, the renal diuretic and natriuretic actions are suitably paired with ANP's CNS actions to inhibit water and salt intake.

Pathophysiology of the Natriuretic Peptide. Whereas derangements in ANP and BNP secretion have been observed (i.e., elevation during congestive heart failure [CHF], supraventricular tachycardia, chronic renal failure, and primary hyperaldosteronism), these conditions with elevated plasma peptide levels usually reflect an exaggerated drive for release of the hormone. In fact, it is in volume overload states such as CHF, that expression of BNP, particularly in ventricular myocytes, increases. The elevated circulating levels of BNP in CHF are considered by many to be diagnostic of the early stages of the disease. The extreme elevations in circulating ANP and BNP in the face of continued water reabsorption during CHF suggests not a derangement of hormone levels per se, but instead a combination of possibly altered natriuretic peptide receptor mechanisms (i.e., down-regulation), reduced renal perfusion, or simultaneous activation of the renin–angiotensin system. Just the same, exaggerated ANP release might be an important factor in SIADH (see above) and aldosterone escape (see Chapter 14).

Plasma levels of CNP are remarkably elevated in septic shock, but not in CHF or hypertension. A variety of circulating cytokines and growth factors (including interleukin-1a and -1b, tumor necrosis factor-α [TNF-α], and transforming growth factor-β), as well as ANP and BNP, can stimulate CNP release from endothelial cells. As a result, the endothelial cells can, via CNP secretion, both transduce the antimitogenic effects of circulating ANP and BNP and buffer the proliferative effects of circulating cytokines and growth factors.

How Physiologically Relevant Are These Effects? Transgenic overexpression models reveal that ANP must play some role in the maintenance of normal blood pressure, as animals with the ANP transgene display lower mean arterial blood pressure than do nontransgenic littermates under basal conditions. However, under basal conditions, renal function is not altered. It is only when challenged, in this case by volume expansion, that the renal excretory function of the animals with excessive ANP production exceeds that of normal, nontransgenic littermates. Another way to address the issue of physiological relevance is to create animals lacking ANP, so-called gene knockouts (i.e., null mutations). Homozygous mice lacking the ANP gene are more likely to develop hypertension when maintained on a high-salt diet than normal, ANP gene–intact animals. These findings tell us that ANP is not necessary for normal embryological and postnatal development (i.e., knockouts survive and thrive under unstressed conditions) but that endogenous ANP must protect against the development of hypertension.

The Adrenomedullins

Recently, a second family of vascular hormones has been identified with even more potent vasodilatory and diuretic actions than the natriuretic peptides. Discovered originally in extracts of a pheochromocytoma (tumor of the adrenal medulla), the first member of the family was named *adrenomedullin* (AM). This 52-amino acid peptide was later found to be produced in endothelial cells and in neurons and to exert many actions similar to those of ANP. Once the structure of the AM gene product was identified, it became clear that a second peptide was also encoded, this being 20 amino acids in length, residing in the N terminus of the prohormone. That peptide, called *proadrenomedullin N-terminal 20 peptide* (PAMP), is also a potent vasodilatory agent, albeit via a different mechanism than that of AM. Adrenomedullin circulates in plasma like other vasoactive peptides at very low levels (10–100 pg/ml) and has a plasma half-life of approximately 20 minutes.

Physiological Actions. Both AM and PAMP appear to play important roles in the regulation of vascular tone, hormone secretion from the anterior pituitary gland, and adrenal function. Profound renal actions have been demonstrated as well. In general, these peptides, like the natriuretic peptides, seem to function to maintain appropriate vascular volume and therefore ensure adequate tissue perfusion. This is accomplished by multiple tissue sites of action related to both fluid and electrolyte homeostasis.

Vascular Actions. Adrenomedullin is a potent hypotensive agent. This action is blocked by pretreatment with false substrates for the enzyme nitric oxide synthase (NOS); thus, the majority of the actions of AM in the vascular tree are mediated via NO. The effects of endogenous AM on vascular tone are probably not due to changes in circulating hormone levels, but instead to a paracrine action of the peptide, since it was necessary in human trials to elevate plasma levels of AM past those observed in pathological states to cause hypotension. Does this mean that this vascular effect is solely pharmacological in nature? Indeed, it does not. It is clear that proinflammatory cytokines such as interleukin-1 and TNF-α are potent stimulators of AM gene transcription and peptide release both from cultured vascular smooth muscle and endothelial cells *in vitro* and from the blood vessels *in vivo*. Thus, the hypotensive crisis of septic shock has been directly correlated with AM release in this condition, and it is thought that the elevated AM levels of septic shock are responsible not only for the profound drops in mean arterial pressure but, more importantly, for the maintenance of renal perfusion during this life-threatening event (AM increases renal blood flow). Hence, the release of AM in inflammatory states is in fact a positive compensatory event. The other peptide encoded by the AM gene product, PAMP, also exerts vasodilatory actions; however, these effects are not due to a direct action on the vascular smooth muscle or endothelial cells. Instead, PAMP, released in the adrenal medulla, actually decreases the amount of epinephrine released (i.e., local autocrine negative feedback, since both epinephrine and PAMP are released from the chromaffin cells) and additionally acts in the vasculature to inhibit norepinephrine release from sympathetic fibers innervating the vessels.

Renal Actions. Although in humans the threshold for vascular actions may be lower than that for renal actions, it is clear that AM, but not PAMP, is a renotropic agent. The diuretic and natriuretic effects of AM are due to inceases in renal blood flow and direct tubular actions. The tubular actions occur at lower doses than do the blood flow changes, suggesting that AM produced in the kidney, particularly in the glomerulus, cortical, and medullary collecting ducts (but not in the medullary thick ascending limb), acts in a paracrine fashion to control sodium excretion and free water clearance. Osmotic permeability of the inner medullary collecting duct is increased by AM, and a complementary action of the peptide is expressed in the brain, where it inhibits AVP release, and in the adrenal gland, where it inhibits aldosterone secretion.

Increases in renal blood flow stimulated by AM are due to a prostaglandin-mediated and inhibitory effect on renal vascular resistance and to an inhibition of mesangial cell proliferation. Also, AM directly stimulates renin secretion, an effect that joins other actions in brain and heart to provide a measure of cardioprotection during septic shock.

Adrenal Actions. Both AM and PAMP are potent inhibitors of A II and potassium-induced release of aldosterone. These actions complement both the natriuretic actions of AM in the renal tubule and the actions of both peptides to inhibit ACTH secretion from the anterior pituitary gland. Thus, in several tissues, the actions of these peptides seem coordinated to ensure the appropriate excretion of sodium into the urine and therefore the normalization of plasma volume and electrolyte content.

Cardiac Actions. Plasma AM levels are elevated in human disease states characterized by volume or pressure overload, including pulmonary hypertension, heart failure, essential hypertension, renal failure, liver disease with ascites, and thyrotoxicosis. This suggested that, like ANP, AM may be produced in cardiac myocytes and, indeed, this is the case. Direct cardiac actions have also been described. Adrenomedullin blocks A II–induced protein synthesis in cultured cardiomyocytes and coronary smooth muscle cell migration, and thus may play an important role in the prevention of cardiac muscle growth and coronary vessel remodeling. Also, AM may prevent pathological vascular remodeling in the general circulation, as it inhibits vascular smooth muscle cell migration and proliferation. In endothelial cells, AM acts as a survival factor, suppressing apoptosis.

Just as in kidney, where the effect of AM on renal perfusion may protect against failure in septic shock, positive cardioprotective effects have been demonstrated. Adrenomedullin exerts direct effects in heart to increase the heart rate, cardiac output, and force of contractility. These effects, together with the peptide's ability to act in brain to activate the sympathetic nervous system, provide a measure of protection against circulatory collapse in sepsis or heart failure. This portfolio of biological actions makes AM an excellent candidate for the potential treatment of volume-expanded and pressure overload states such as CHF (Table 7-6).

How Physiologically Relevant Are These Effects? Although the only pharmacological action of AM yet to be demonstrated to have physiological relevance is its ability to inhibit salt appetite and therefore regulate the ingested sodium load, many clinical conditions exist in which plasma levels of AM are markedly elevated. Do these elevations reflect compensatory roles for AM gene products or merely tissue damage? Recent experiments strongly suggest a potential role for AM and PAMP in the body's response to pathological conditions and the possible therapeutic benefit of selective AM or PAMP agonists.

Plasma AM levels are elevated in a variety of human hypertensive conditions. In stroke-prone, spontaneously hypertensive animal models, plasma AM levels are very low, perhaps reflecting the loss of the protective vasodilatory effect of the

Table 7-6 Actions of the Adrenomedullins (Adrenomedullin and/or Proadrenomedullin N-Terminal 20 Peptide)

Tissue	Effect
Vasculature	Hypotension (vasodilation)
	Decreased total peripheral resistance
	Increased renal blood flow
	Antimitogenesis
Heart	Positive chronotropism and inotropism
	Inhibition of myocyte hypertrophy and vascular hyperplasia
Lung	Pulmonary vasodilation
Adrenal gland	Inhibition of cholinergic stimulation of catecholamine release
	Inhibition of stimulated aldosterone secretion
Kidney	Diuresis
	Natriuresis
Pituitary gland	Inhibition of ACTH release
Brain	Inhibition of water drinking and salt appetite
	Stimulation of sympathetic nervous system activity
	Inhibition of AVP release

ACTH, adrenocorticotropin; AVP, arginine vasopressin.

peptide. In another genetic model of spontaneous hypertension, AM gene delivery significantly lowered blood pressure to levels observed in normal littermates. This suggests that the elevated AM plasma levels in hypertensive humans reflect a compensatory mechanism counteracting the elevation in pressure.

Patients in heart failure also display elevated plasma AM levels. When heart failure is induced in laboratory animals, AM gene transcription in heart increases in parallel with the observed cardiac hypertrophy. Additionally, infusion of AM into these animals at doses too low to cause hypotension initiates ameliorative responses in kidney (i.e., diuresis and natriuresis). It had long been hoped that ANP infusion would be a clinical tool for lowering plasma volume and therefore cardiac afterload in heart failure; however, the natriuretic peptide receptors in kidney appear to be down-regulated in response to continued elevation of plasma ANP and BNP levels in this condition, thereby limiting the efficacy of this approach. It is now possible that AM infusion will provide the therapeutic benefit originally hypothesized for ANP.

The antimitogenic actions of AM demonstrated *in vitro* may have a physiological correlate. The peptide is produced in cardiomyocytes, endothelial cells, and mesangial cells and has been demonstrated to express its antimitogenic actions in these cell types. It was recently shown that antiserum against AM accentuated A II–induced protein and platelet-derived growth factor–stimulated DNA synthesis in cultured myocytes and endothelial and mesangial cells, respectively. Thus, endogenously produced AM may act in an autocrine fashion to prevent cell proliferation and uncontrolled growth.

The best evidence for a physiological role for AM comes from studies of sepsis, in which plasma AM levels parallel the inflammatory and hypotensive course of the disease. It is now recognized that proinflammatory cytokines stimulate AM gene transcription and peptide secretion. Additionally, a positive correlation exists between circulating hormone levels and survival rate. It appears that the increased plasma AM levels, in addition to causing vasodilation, spare the kidney by concomitantly elevating, even in the face of exaggerated drops in mean arterial pressure, renal plasma flow and therefore preventing renal failure.

INTEGRATED CONTROL OF WATER AND SODIUM HOMEOSTASIS

The integrated control of body fluid homeostasis requires a balance of renal, adrenal, vascular, cardiac, brain, and endocrine influences (Fig. 7-5). Most importantly, all of these converge on the kidney as the final site of regulation. It is not surprising, therefore, that multiple endocrine peptides with profound effects on fluid and electrolyte homeostasis have as a major site of action the kidney. Thus, A II itself is antinatriuretic, as is aldosterone. Both of these hormonal actions contribute to sodium retention, and, as a result, to both water retention and the restoration of plasma volume and perfusion pressure. The counterregulatory hormones ANP and AM act in the opposite fashion, stimulating urinary sodium and water excretion and thereby contributing to volume regulation by unloading the vascular tree. These two hormones also act to inhibit the antidiuretic actions of AVP, the major determinant of free water reabsorption from the urine, again ensuring the reduction in plasma volume in electrolyte and/or volume overload states.

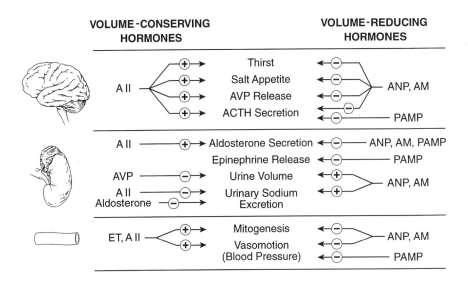

Fig. 7-5 The endocrine regulation of fluid and electrolyte homeostasis. The volume-conserving hormones angiotensin II (A II), aldosterone, arginine vasopressin (AVP), and endothelin (ET) act to restore plasma volume and maintain tissue perfusion. The volume-reducing hormones atrial natriuretic peptide (ANP), adrenomedullin (AM), and proadrenomedullin N-terminal 20 peptide (PAMP) act directly or indirectly to lower plasma volume and to decrease tissue perfusion, with the exception of renal blood flow, which is stimulated by AM.

The level of integration of the actions of these potent volume regulatory hormones is even more complex than those renal actions would suggest. In fact, in numerous tissues, these opposing hormones *push and pull* the physiological mechanisms by which fluid and electrolyte homeostasis is maintained (Fig. 7-5). The natriuretic and diuretic actions of AM and ANP expressed in kidney are complemented in brain by effects of the peptides to inhibit water drinking (thirst) and salt appetite. These actions in brain are antagonistic to those of A II, which oppositely stimulates both thirst and salt appetite. In the adrenal gland as well, the stimulatory effect of A II on aldosterone secretion is blocked by both ANP and AM and by the other AM gene product, PAMP. In the anterior pituitary gland, the ability of A II to stimulate ACTH secretion is opposed by ANP, AM, and PAMP. The release of AVP from nerve terminals in the posterior pituitary gland is stimulated by A II and inhibited by ANP and AM.

The opposing actions of the volume-conserving versus the volume-depleting hormones extend into the vasculature as well (Fig. 7-5). Whereas A II and ET are vasoconstrictors, ANP, AM, and PAMP exert vasodilatory effects, actions well suited to their roles in other tissues to regulate plasma volume and tissue perfusion pressures. The antimitogenic actions of ANP and AM also are opposed by the promitogenic effects of A II and ET, and thus a common thread is revealed. In most cases, the overall physiological effects of the procontractile/promitogenic/volume-conserving peptides are opposed by those of the vasorelaxant/antimitogenic/volume-reducing hormones, and only the integration of these multiple signals can explain the normal maintenance of fluid and electrolyte homeostasis. Clearly, any alteration in the production, release, or bioactivity (including the response to) of any one of these hormones can result in imbalances in volume status and plasma osmolar state. In addition, over- or underproduction of these hormones leads to hypertensive states that threaten life if left untreated. Thus, the peptides themselves may be diagnostic of underlying cardiovascular disease and may prove useful as therapeutic agents in a variety of disease states.

SUGGESTED READING

Birnbaumer M: Vasopressin receptors. Trends Endocrinol Metab 11:406–410, 2000.

D'Orleans-Juste P, Labonte J, Bkaily G, Choufani S, Plante M, and Honore JC: Function of the endothelin(B) receptor in cardiovascular physiology and pathophysiology. Pharmacol Ther 95:221–238, 2002.

Poulain D, Oliet S, and Theodosis D: *Vasopressin and Oxytocin: From Genes to Clinical Applications*, Elsevier, Amsterdam, 2001.

Robinson AG and Verbalis JG: Posterior pituitary gland. In: *Williams Textbook of Endocrinology*, 10th ed., PR Larsen, HM Kronenberg, S Melmed, and KS Polonsky, eds., Saunders, Philadelphia, pp. 281–329, 2003.

Samson WK and Levin ER: *Natriuretic Peptides in Health and Disease*, Humana Press, Totowa, NJ, 1997.

Taylor MM, Shimosawa T, and Samson WK: Endocrine and metabolic actions of adrenomedullin. The Endocrinologist 11:171–177, 2001.

Varagic J and Frohlich ED: Local cardiac renin–angiotensin system: hypertension and cardiac failure. *J Mol Cell Cardiol* 34:1435–1442, 2002.

8

Sexual Differentiation

KEITH L. PARKER

Sexual differentiation is a sequential process that begins at fertilization with the establishment of chromosomal sex, continues with the determination of gonadal sex, and culminates in the development of secondary sexual characteristics that comprise the male and female phenotypes. This basic paradigm (Fig. 8-1) was formulated by Alfred Jost to explain the results of castration experiments in fetal rabbits. If the gonads (ovaries or testes) were removed before sexual differentiation, female sexual differentiation inevitably ensued. The male pathway could be partly restored by testosterone implants, suggesting that hormones produced by the testes mediate male sexual development. Thus, the concept arose that the testes induce a male pattern of differentiation on an embryo that otherwise would follow the female pathway. Cytogenetic studies shortly thereafter showed that the critical genetic determinant of sex is the presence or absence of the Y chromosome, leading to the proposal that the Y chromosome directs the gonad to differentiate into a testis, which then produces hormone(s) that cause male sexual differentiation.

The chromosomal sex of the embryo generally corresponds to its phenotypic sex. Occasionally, however, the process of sexual differentiation goes awry, resulting in individuals with abnormal sexual differentiation. Clinically recognized disorders of sexual development occur at many levels, ranging from relatively common disorders in the terminal steps of male differentiation (e.g., testicular descent, growth of the penis) to more fundamental abnormalities that lead to varying degrees of ambiguity of phenotypic sex. Although most of these abnormalities impair reproduction, they usually are not life-threatening. Thus, humans and experimental animals with naturally occurring defects in sexual differentiation survive to reach the attention of physicians and scientists. This chapter reviews the sequence of events in normal sexual development and describes disorders of this process—many of which result from single-gene mutations—that have provided valuable insights into the mechanisms of sexual differentiation.

DEVELOPMENT OF CHROMOSOMAL SEX

Normally, human somatic cells have 22 pairs of autosomes and 1 pair of sex chromosomes. The critical genetic determinant of sex is the presence or absence of the

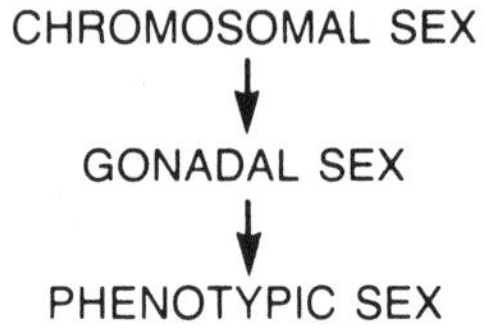

CHROMOSOMAL SEX

↓

GONADAL SEX

↓

PHENOTYPIC SEX

Fig. 8-1   The Jost paradigm for sexual differentiation.

Y chromosome; thus, the normal female genotype is 46,XX, while the normal male genotype is 46,XY. Meiosis in the germ cells reduces their chromosomal complement to the haploid state, so that oocytes are 23,X and spermatocytes are either 23,X or 23,Y. Fertilization restores the diploid state and—depending on the presence or absence of the Y chromosome—specifies the genetic sex as either 46,XX (female) or 46,XY (male).

The most striking function of the Y chromosome is in sex determination. Analyses of human subjects whose phenotypic sex did not correlate with genetic sex (i.e., the presence or absence of a Y chromosome) led to the isolation of a gene called *SRY* (Sex-determining Region, Y chromosome) that is both necessary and sufficient for male sex determination. The *SRY* gene encodes a putative transcriptional regulator proposed to trigger a cascade of events that result in development of the testes. The term *sex determination* is used to describe the initiation of the male pathway by *SRY*, and the subsequent events in the production and action of testicular hormones are referred to as *male sexual differentiation.*

Although it is one of the smallest human chromosomes, the Y chromosome contains more than 30 genes that contribute to functions such as spermatogenesis, skeletal growth, and tooth development. The Y chromosome also contains a putative locus near the centromere—designated GBY for Gonadoblastoma, Y chromosome—that predisposes to the development of germ cell tumors in subjects with disorders of gonadal sex.

The Y chromosome presumably arose from an ancestral homolog of the X chromosome and retains regions of homology at its ends—termed the *pseudoautosomal regions*—that permit it to pair with the X chromosome during meiosis. Between these pseudoautosomal regions lie discontinuous stretches of X-Y homology mixed with regions that are unique to the Y chromosome. *SRY*, the critical mediator of male sex determination, is located on the short arm of the Y chromosome just inside the pseudoautosomal region. Because of its position directly adjacent to the pseudoautosomal region, in which X-Y recombination normally occurs, *SRY* occasionally is transferred from the Y to the X chromosome, leading to either 46,XX males or 46,XY females (see below under Disorders of Gonadal Sex).

DEVELOPMENT OF GONADAL SEX

An overview of the events in the development of the male and female phenotypes is presented in Figure 8-2.

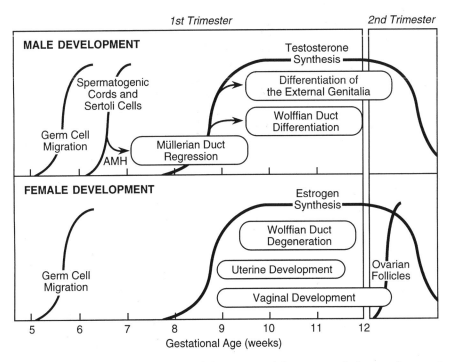

Fig. 8-2 Gonadal differentiation and the timing of the events of phenotypic sexual differentiation. AMH, antimüllerian hormone.

Indifferent Phase

Both male and female gonads develop from the urogenital ridges—structures containing cell lineages that ultimately contribute to the kidneys, the gonads, and the adrenal cortex. The gonads initially are identical in both sexes and therefore are termed *indifferent gonads*. These indifferent gonads differentiate into distinct cell types that have functional counterparts in testes and ovaries: supporting cells (Sertoli or granulosa cells), stromal cells (Leydig or theca cells), and primordial germ cells (spermatogonia or oocytes). The supporting cells derive from the coelomic epithelium of the gonadal ridge (although cells derived from the mesonephros also may contribute in some species), stromal cells derive from the mesenchyme of the gonadal ridge, and primordial germ cells originate in the proximal epiblast and migrate into the gonadal ridge by the fifth week of gestation. The differentiation of these cell lineages to form the indifferent gonad requires the action of several transcription factors, which presumably regulate the expression of target genes needed for gonadogenesis.

Before ~7–8 weeks of gestation, during the indifferent phase, the sex of the embryo cannot be recognized. At this time, all embryos acquire dual ductal systems that are precursors to the male and female internal genitalia (Fig. 8-3, top). The first ducts to form are the wolffian (or mesonephric) ducts, which serve as excretory ducts for the mesonephric (embryonic) kidney and are attached directly to the in-

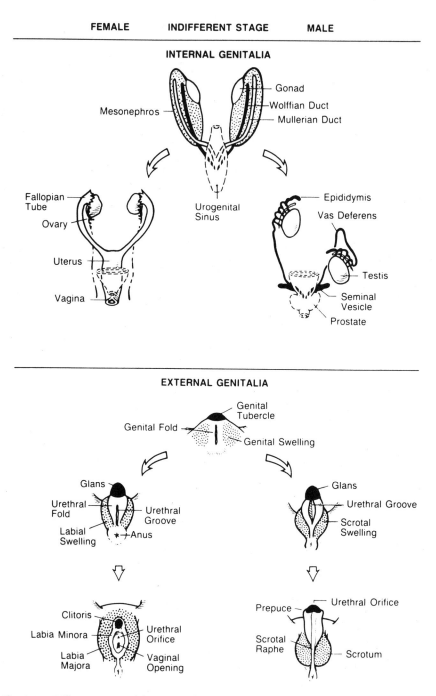

Fig. 8-3 Differentiation of the internal and external genitalia of the human fetus.

different gonad. Caudally, as the wolffian ducts join the primitive urogenital sinus, an outgrowth of their dorsomedial wall—the ureteric bud—gives rise to the excretory ducts and collecting tubules of the metanephric (permanent) kidney. The internal male accessory organs of reproduction—the seminal vesicles, vas deferens, and epididymis—develop from these wolffian ducts.

The paramesonephric (müllerian) ducts begin to form at 6 weeks of gestation as an evagination of the coelomic epithelium into the mesonephros just lateral to the wolffian ducts. These müllerian ducts in females ultimately give rise to the internal reproductive tract (fallopian tubes, uterus, and upper vagina), whereas they regress in males. The external genitalia of both sexes, which arise from the genital tubercle, the urethral folds and groove, and the labioscrotal swellings, again are indistinguishable before sexual differentiation. Thus, the male and female internal genitalia develop from different embryonic anlagen, whereas the external genitalia arise from a common anlage (Fig. 8-3, bottom).

Male Development

The initial event in the virilization of the male urogenital tract is regression of the müllerian ducts shortly after the organization of the testes into spermatogenic cords at approximately 8 weeks of gestation. Soon thereafter, the male genital tract begins to develop from the wolffian ducts (Fig. 8-2). Those mesonephric tubules adjacent to the testis lose their primitive glomeruli and establish contact with the developing rete and spermatogenic tubules of the testis to form the efferent ductules. The portion of the wolffian duct immediately caudal to the efferent ductules becomes elongated and convoluted to form the epididymis, and the middle portion of the duct develops thick muscular walls to become the vas deferens (Fig. 8-3, top). At about the thirteenth week of gestation, the lower portions of the wolffian ducts near the urogenital sinus begin to form the seminal vesicles. The terminal portions of the ducts between the seminal vesicles and the urethra become the ejaculatory ducts and ampullae of the vas deferens.

The prostatic and membranous segments of the male urethra develop from the pelvic portion of the urogenital sinus. At approximately 10 weeks of gestation, the prostatic buds begin to form in the mesenchyme surrounding the pelvic urethra. This budding is most extensive in the area surrounding the entry of the wolffian ducts (the ejaculatory ducts) into the male urethra. Although initial differentiation of the prostate occurs early in embryogenesis, growth and development of the gland continue after birth.

Beginning in the ninth week of gestation and continuing through the twelfth week, the external genitalia of the male and female become sexually differentiated (Fig. 8-3, bottom). The genital swellings in the male enlarge and migrate posteriorly to form the scrotum, and the genital folds fuse over the urethral groove to form the penile urethra. The line of closure remains marked by the penile raphe. Incomplete fusion of the genital folds over the urethral groove results in a condition known as *hypospadias*. When the formation of the penile urethra is almost complete, the prepuce begins to develop, completely covering the glans penis by 15 weeks of gestation.

Although the formation of the male genital tract is largely accomplished between 7 and 13 weeks of gestation, two additional aspects of male development occur later in gestation—growth of the external genitalia and testicular descent.

At approximately 11 weeks of gestation, when formation of the male urethra is largely complete, the male and female phalluses are comparable in size. During the last two trimesters of pregnancy, the male external genitalia, prostate, and structures derived from the wolffian ducts grow progressively. As a consequence, the male external genitalia at birth are considerably larger than those of the female.

The complex events of testicular descent remain incompletely understood, although this descent is essential to reproductive function because spermatogenesis requires the lower temperature present in the scrotum. A failure of the process—termed *cryptorchidism*—occurs in at least one testis in approximately 3% of full-term male infants, making it one of the most common congenital abnormalities. Testicular descent involves two stages: the *transabdominal* phase, which occurs between 10 and 15 weeks of gestation, and the *inguinoscrotal* phase, which usually occurs between 26 and 35 weeks of gestation. During the transabdominal phase, the cranial suspensory ligaments regress, and outgrowth of a posterior fold of peritoneum called the *gubernaculum* causes the testes to migrate from the dorsal abdominal wall to the internal inguinal ring. During the third month of gestation, prompted at least partly by increased intra-abdominal pressure, the processus vaginalis develops as a herniation in the coelomic cavity along the course of the gubernaculum. In the inguinoscrotal phase, the portion of the gubernaculum that contacts the testes regresses, and the testes pass through the inguinal canal into the scrotum. This event normally occurs at about the seventh month of gestation, although it does not take place in some infants until the first year of life.

At least two hormones contribute to testicular descent. The increased incidence of cryptorchidism in human subjects with impaired testosterone biosynthesis or action implicates androgens in this process, predominantly in the inguinoscrotal phase. In addition, studies in knockout mice demonstrate that the Leydig insulin-like hormone INSL3, a secreted member of the insulin-like hormone superfamily, is essential for development of the gubernaculum and the transabdominal phase of testicular descent.

Female Development

In females, the internal reproductive tract forms from the müllerian ducts, and the wolffian ducts largely degenerate. The cephalic ends of the müllerian ducts—which are derived from coelemic epithelium—are the anlagen of the fallopian tubes, while the caudal portion fuses to form the uterus (Fig. 8-3, top). The uterine cervix is recognizable by 9 weeks of gestation, and the formation of the myometrium from mesenchyme surrounding the müllerian ducts is completed by 17 weeks of development.

Vaginal development begins at approximately 9 weeks of gestation with the formation of a solid mass of cells—the uterovaginal plate—between the caudal buds of the müllerian ducts and the dorsal wall of the urogenital sinus. The cells of the uterovaginal plate subsequently degenerate, thus increasing the distance between the uterus and the urogenital sinus. The upper one-third of the vagina derives from the müllerian ducts, and the remainder derives from the urogenital sinus.

After 10 weeks of gestation, the genital tubercle begins to bend caudally, the lateral portions of the genital swellings enlarge to form the labia majora, and the posterior portions fuse to form the posterior fourchette. The urethral folds flanking the urogenital orifice do not fuse but persist as the labia minora (Fig. 8-3, bottom). Thus, most of the urogenital sinus of the female remains exposed on the surface as a cleft into which the vagina and urethra open.

Breast Development

At 5 weeks of development, paired lines of epidermal thickening extend on the ventral surface of the embryo from the forelimb to the hindlimb. Between 6 and 8 weeks of development, these *mammary lines* largely disappear, except for a small portion on either side of the thoracic region that condenses and penetrates the underlying mesenchyme. This single pair of mammary buds undergoes little change until the fifth month of embryonic development, when secondary epithelial buds appear and the nipples begin to form. Although some species exhibit sexual dimorphism in embryonic breast development, such dimorphism has never been demonstrated in humans, and breast development is identical in males and females before the onset of puberty.

ENDOCRINE CONTROL OF PHENOTYPIC DIFFERENTIATION

The fetal castration experiments of Jost demonstrated definitively that the fetal testes are necessary for male phenotypic development. Two products of the fetal testis are essential for male development: the glycoprotein hormone *anti-müllerian hormone* (AMH; also called *müllerian-inhibiting substance*, or MIS)—which causes regression of the müllerian ducts—and testosterone—which virilizes the wolffian ducts, urogenital sinus, and genital tubercle. In contrast, female differentiation apparently does not require hormone production by the fetal ovaries, as female phenotypic development occurs in the absence of gonads.

Onset of Endocrine Function of Testes and Ovaries

Fetal ovaries and testes first become distinct histologically at approximately 7 weeks of gestation, when the testes form primitive spermatogenic tubules that contain fetal Sertoli cells and primordial germ cells. The fetal Sertoli cells produce AMH, which causes the first discernible event in male phenotypic differentiation: regression of the müllerian ducts. Shortly thereafter, at ~8–9 weeks of gestation, mesenchymal cells in the interstitium differentiate into Leydig cells and initiate testosterone synthesis (Fig. 8-2). Although the role of pituitary or placental gonadotropins in the earliest stages of androgen production is debated, virilization in the latter two-thirds of gestation—such as penile growth—probably requires gonadotropins (see Chapter 11). No effects on female sexual differentiation have been attributed to ovarian hormones, and the fetal ovaries do not actually form primordial follicles until the fifth month of development, but they nonetheless initiate estrogen biosynthesis at approximately 9 weeks of gestation (Fig. 8-2).

Role of Testicular Hormones in Male Development

Müllerian Duct Regression

Müllerian duct regression in male fetuses begins at 8–9 weeks of gestation, and is mediated by AMH, a member of the transforming-growth factor β (TGF-β) family of signaling molecules that is secreted by fetal Sertoli cells. By interacting with its type 2 receptor on mesenchymal cells surrounding the müllerian ducts, this 140 kDa glycoprotein activates an apoptotic pathway that ultimately causes müllerian duct regression. As discussed below, mutations in either the *AMH* gene or its receptor cause the persistent müllerian duct syndrome. In the female, it is essential that AMH is not expressed during fetal development of the urogenital tract, as the female internal genitalia otherwise would not develop. Perhaps to maintain this extremely tight regulation, the *AMH* gene is regulated by a number of transcription factors involved in gonadal development, including steroidogenic factor 1 (SF-1), Wilms' tumor–related 1 (WT1), and SOX9 (see below).

Virilization

Virilization of the male fetus results from the action of androgens on the wolffian ducts, urogenital sinus, and external genitalia. Although testosterone is the principal androgen secreted by the fetal and adult testes, many of the differentiating, growth-promoting, and functional actions of androgens are mediated by its 5α-reduced metabolite, dihydrotestosterone (Fig. 8-4).

Androgens act via a specific receptor found in androgen-responsive cells (Fig. 8-4). The androgen receptor is a member of the nuclear hormone receptor superfamily, structurally related, zinc finger transcription factors that mediate the action of a large group of hydrophobic ligands, including steroid hormones, thyroid hormone, retinoids, vitamin D, bile acids, and oxysterols. Following secretion by the testes, testosterone enters target cells by passive diffusion. In certain target tissues, the type 2 isozyme of 5α-reductase converts testosterone to dihydrotestosterone. After binding testosterone or dihydrotestosterone, the androgen receptor regulates the expression of target genes by binding to recognition sequences in their promoter regions.

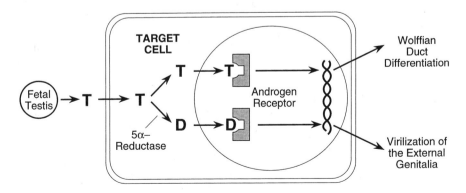

Fig. 8-4 Mechanisms of androgen action in target tissues. D, dihydrotestosterone; T, testosterone.

Genetic studies (see below) clearly demonstrate that a single androgen receptor mediates the action of both testosterone and dihydrotestosterone. Nonetheless, there is a dichotomy of androgen action in different androgen-responsive tissues. Testosterone itself regulates gonadotropin release and virilizes the wolffian ducts during male sexual differentiation, whereas conversion to dihydrotestosterone is required for virilization of the external genitalia during embryonic development and for the development at puberty of most male secondary sex characteristics. Definitive support for the differential roles of the two androgenic hormones comes from the study of patients with inherited deficiency of dihydrotestosterone due to the absence of 5α-reductase activity; such patients have normally differentiated structures derived from the wolffian ducts but exhibit failure of external virilization.

DISORDERS OF CHROMOSOMAL SEX

Two disorders of chromosomal sex resulting from nondisjunction of the sex chromosomes during meiosis—Klinefelter syndrome (47,XXY) and Turner syndrome (most commonly 45,X)—illustrate the roles of the sex chromosomes in controlling gonadal development.

Klinefelter Syndrome

Individuals with Klinefelter syndrome, which affects 1 in 500 newborn males, typically have a 47,XXY karyotype and a predominantly male phenotype. Before puberty, patients have small testes and decreased numbers of spermatogonia but otherwise have a normal male phenotype. After the time of normal puberty, patients often exhibit incomplete virilization and breast enlargement (gynecomastia). After puberty, consistent clinical features include male phenotype, bilaterally small testes (always <3 cm and generally <1.5 cm in length), and absence of sperm in the ejaculate (azospermia).

Endocrine findings include low to normal plasma testosterone levels and elevated circulating levels of estradiol; the relative imbalance of androgen to estrogen causes varying degrees of impaired virilization and enhanced feminization. Circulating gonadotropins—particularly follicle-stimulating hormone (FSH)—are elevated owing to impaired feedback at hypothalamic/pituitary levels.

Various karyotypes are associated with Klinefelter syndrome, almost all of which include two or more X chromosomes and a Y chromosome (e.g., 47,XXY [classic form]; 46,XY/47,XXY [mosaic form]). Other individuals with the Klinefelter phenotype have a single Y chromosome and more than two X chromosomes, demonstrating that a single Y chromosome is sufficient to induce testicular differentiation and male phenotypic development irrespective of the number of X chromosomes. The classic form of Klinefelter syndrome results most frequently from nondisjunction of the sex chromosomes during the first or second meiotic division; thus, increased maternal age is an important risk factor.

Turner Syndrome

Classically, Turner syndrome is seen in phenotypic females who exhibit short stature, primary amenorrhea, lack of secondary sexual characteristics (sexual infantilism), multiple congenital abnormalities, and bilateral streak gonads (i.e., bands of fibrous tissue that lack histological features of either testicular or ovarian organization). These congenital defects include aortic coarctation, bicuspid aortic valve, horseshoe kidney, webbed neck, and various skeletal abnormalities. Although it was originally ascribed to a 45,X genotype, we now recognize that Turner syndrome is associated with a range of karyotypes—all of which involve complete or partial absence of one sex chromosome or monosomy X. Moreover, Turner syndrome patients frequently carry two or more cell lines with distinct karyotypes (i.e., they are mosaic). A larger percentage of 46,XX cells in these mosaic patients correlates with a milder phenotype.

With the advent of more frequent karyotypic analysis, it now is apparent that spontaneous abortion also is a frequent manifestation of Turner syndrome. Because an estimated 2% of all human conceptuses are 45,X—less than 1% of which survive to term—Turner syndrome collectively accounts for up to 10% of spontaneous abortions.

Although the only universal feature in live-born Turner patients is short stature, apparently secondary to haploinsufficiency of the Short Homeobox-containing gene (SHOX) located in the pseudoautosomal region of the X chromosome, individuals with Turner syndrome frequently present with sexual infantilism, and a large majority have primary ovarian failure. Primordial germ cells migrate normally into the gonads and the number of oogonia is relatively normal until the stage of primary follicle formation at approximately 20 weeks of gestation, but oocytes undergo markedly accelerated atresia after birth, leading to premature ovarian failure. The deficiency of ovarian steroid hormones results in primary amenorrhea and failure to develop female secondary sexual characteristics. Turner syndrome is the most common cause of primary amenorrhea.

DISORDERS OF GONADAL SEX

Disorders of gonadal sex occur when chromosomal sex is normal (i.e., either 46,XX or 46,XY), but differentiation of the gonads is abnormal. Phenotypic sex will vary, depending on when the gonadal defect becomes manifest during embryogenesis.

Pure Gonadal Dysgenesis

Pure gonadal dysgenesis denotes a syndrome in which bilateral streak gonads are associated with an immature female phenotype. In contrast to patients with 45,X gonadal dysgenesis, these patients are of normal height, do not have associated somatic defects, and, most importantly, have a normal 46,XX or 46,XY karyotype. Because gonadal development is arrested before AMH and androgens are produced, the sexual phenotype is female. Little is known about the pathogenesis of 46,XX gonadal dysgenesis. A few of these subjects have homozygous mutations in the FSH receptor, resulting in hypoplastic ovaries that retain some primary follicles. Within the same kindreds, 46,XY males homozygous for the identical mutation exhibit variably impaired spermatogenesis without azospermia.

SRY and 46,XY Complete Gonadal Dysgenesis

The demonstration of point mutations in *SRY* in some subjects with 46,XY complete gonadal dysgenesis established the essential role of *SRY* in testis determination and subsequent male sexual differentiation. More extensive studies have identified SRY mutations in approximately 10%–20% of these subjects; most cases of 46,XY gonadal dysgenesis therefore result from mutations in other genes (see below). Subjects with 46,XY pure gonadal dysgenesis—whether associated with *SRY* mutations or with mutations in other genes described below—have an increased incidence of gonadoblastoma, possibly associated with the *GBY* locus near the centromere of the Y chromosome.

Other Genes Implicated in Complete Gonadal Dysgenesis

Three autosomal genes and one gene on the X chromosome have been implicated in 46,XY complete gonadal dysgenesis (Table 8-1). Intriguingly, these genes all encode transcription factors that are proposed to regulate the expression of target genes essential for gonadal survival. The cascade of gene regulation within the developing gonads apparently is very sensitive, because changing either the relative amounts of these transcription factors or the time when their expression commences can impair normal gonadal development.

Wilms' Tumor–Related 1. The first autosomal gene to be linked specifically to 46,XY complete gonadal dysgenesis was the Wilms' tumor–related gene *WT1*, which maps to chromosome 11p13; it was isolated through analyses of patients with familial Wilms' tumor, an embryonic kidney tumor arising from abnormal proliferation of the metanephric blastema. Although Wilms' tumors generally present sporadically, approximately 1% occur in patients with similarly affected first-degree relatives, suggesting that these families carry mutations in a tumor-suppressor gene.

The *WT1* mutations cause two distinct syndromes of gonadal dysgenesis—Denys-Drash syndrome and Frasier syndrome. Denys-Drash syndrome is an autosomal dominant disorder characterized by gonadal and urogenital abnormalities in conjunction with diffuse mesangial sclerosis. The gonadal abnormalities vary but are relatively severe, with streak gonads and female external and internal genitalia at one extreme and varying degrees of impaired virilization in less severely affected 46,XY males. Denys-Drash syndrome almost always results from point mutations in the zinc finger region of WT1 that abrogate DNA binding; these mutated proteins are predicted to inhibit function of the protein encoded by the wild-type allele. The degree of inhibition of WT1 action generally correlates with the impairment of genitourinary development, with the most severe mutations leading to early gonadal dysgenesis and sex reversal of external and internal genitalia. Genetic mod-

Table 8-1 Genes Associated with 46,XY Gonadal Dysgenesis

Gene	Chromosomal location	Associated disorder	Target genes
WT1	11p13	Denys-Drash syndrome Frasier syndrome	*AMH*
SF-1	9q33	Adrenal insufficiency	*AMH*, steroid hydroxylases, ACTH receptor, StAR
SOX9	17q21	Campomelic dysplasia	*AMH*
DAX-1	Xp21	Adrenal hypoplasia congenita	*StAR* (inhibits)

ACTH, adrenocorticotropin; AMH, anti-müllerian hormone; StAR, steroidogenic acute regulatory protein.

ifiers also affect the severity of the phenotype, as demonstrated by studies of Denys-Drash families in which the fathers were phenotypically normal despite carrying the same *WT1* mutation as the affected offspring.

Patients with Frasier syndrome present with gonadal dysgenesis, impaired virilization, and focal glomerular sclerosis, but they do not develop Wilms' tumors. The *WT1* mutations that cause Frasier syndrome cluster within intron 9 of the *WT1* gene, apparently interfering with the synthesis of specific splice variants of *WT1* that are essential for gonadal development but are not required to suppress the development of Wilms' tumors.

Steroidogenic Factor 1. Development of the indifferent gonads also requires steroidogenic factor 1 (SF-1), officially designated NR5A1. Initially, SF-1 was identified as a transcription factor that regulated the cell-specific expression of the cytochrome P450 steroid hydroxylases that catalyze most steroidogenic conversions. Like the androgen receptor, SF-1 belongs to the nuclear hormone receptor superfamily. Subsequent studies have shown that SF-1 regulates the expression of a diverse array of genes involved in steroidogenesis, including 3β-hydroxysteroid dehydrogenase, the adrenocorticotropin (ACTH) receptor, the steroidogenic acute regulatory protein (StAR), and the high-density lipoprotein receptor SR-B1. In addition to its roles in steroidogenesis, including testosterone production, SF-1 also regulates the production of the two other hormones that mediate male sexual differentiation: AMH and INSL3. SF-1 transcripts also are expressed in pituitary gonadotropes and the ventromedial nucleus of the hypothalamus (VMH), suggesting that it regulates endocrine function at all three levels of the hypothalamic–pituitary–gonadal axis.

Knockout mice lacking SF-1 exhibit adrenal and gonadal agenesis, with female internal and external urogenital tracts, confirming its essential roles in gonadal development and sexual differentiation. The human *SF-1* gene, located on chromosome 9q33, shares extensive homology with its mouse counterpart and is expressed in many of the same sites, suggesting that SF-1 also has important roles in human endocrine development. This model is supported by human subjects with adrenal insufficiency and 46,XY gonadal dysgenesis who carry *SF-1* mutations that impair function.. These studies demonstrate that SF-1 in humans also plays essential roles in embryonic development of the adrenal glands and gonads.

SOX9. Gonadal dysgenesis is seen in most 46,XY patients with campomelic dysplasia, an autosomal dominant syndrome that includes skeletal, renal, and cardiac abnormalities. Campomelic dysplasia results from heterozygous mutations in *SOX9*, a close relative of *SRY* that maps to chromosome 17q21. SOX9 is expressed at high levels in testes—where it is proposed to regulate the transcription of key mediators of male differentiation such as AMH—and at lower levels in ovaries. Presumably, homozygous *SOX9* mutations are incompatible with fetal survival owing to the essential roles of this gene in chondrogenesis.

DAX-1 and Dosage-Sensitive Sex Reversal. 46,XY gonadal dysgenesis also is associated with duplication of the short arm of the X chromosome (Xp21), a phenomenon termed *dosage-sensitive sex reversal.* The critical region of Xp21 for dosage-sensitive sex reversal contains a gene, *DAX-1*, that is mutated in boys with adrenal hypoplasia congenita (AHC). In addition to adrenal insufficiency, AHC patients have a compound hypothalamic/pituitary defect that causes hypogonadotropic hypogonadism at the time of normal puberty, and exhibit impaired spermatogenesis even if treated with gonadotropins. The *DAX-1* gene encodes an atypical member of the nuclear receptor family that retains the conserved ligand-binding domain but lacks the typical zinc finger DNA-binding motif. This finding suggests that DAX-1 may interact directly with other proteins involved in the cascade of gonadal development. Consistent with this model, DAX-1 and SF-1 are coexpressed in many sites, including the gonads, adrenal cortex, pituitary gonadotropes, and VMH. Moreover, several studies indicate that DAX-1 inhibits the expression of SF-1-dependent target genes, providing a potential mechanism by which an excess of DAX-1 in patients with Xp21 duplication could cause impaired sexual differentiation in 46,XY subjects.

The Vanishing Testis Syndrome

A spectrum of phenotypes has been described in 46,XY males with absent or rudimentary testes in whom endocrine function of the testis was present at some time during sexual differentiation. The disorder varies in its manifestations from complete failure of virilization, through varying degrees of incomplete virilization of the external genitalia, to otherwise normal males with anorchia. The most severely affected individuals are 46,XY phenotypic females who lack testes and accessory male reproductive organs and are sexually infantile. The disorder in these individuals differs from the 46,XY form of pure gonadal dysgenesis in that no müllerian duct derivatives are present. Thus, testicular failure in these individuals must have occurred in the interval between the onset of AMH biosynthesis and the secretion of testosterone. In other patients, the clinical features suggest that testicular failure occurred later in gestation, while at the other extreme are phenotypic men with anorchia who lack müllerian derivatives and are completely virilized except for the absence of the epididymis.

DISORDERS OF PHENOTYPIC SEX

Disorders of phenotypic sex are classified as those disorders in which the phenotypic sex is ambiguous or is completely in disagreement with the chromosomal and gonadal sex. Conceptually, as detailed below, such disorders generally result from a failure of synthesis or action of hormones that mediate male sexual differentiation (male pseudohermaphroditism) or from the inappropriate synthesis of androgens (female pseudohermaphroditism).

Female Pseudohermaphroditism

This condition occurs in individuals who have ovaries and müllerian derivatives but exhibit varying degrees of virilization of the external genitalia. This process requires exposure *in utero* to androgens, and the degree of virilization depends on the stage of sexual differentiation at the time of androgen exposure. Following the twelfth week of gestation, when the vagina has formed from the urogenital sinus, androgen exposure causes only clitoromegaly. Because AMH is not produced, the uterus and fallopian tubes are normal.

The most common cause of virilization in newborn females is a condition called *congenital adrenal hyperplasia* (CAH), which results most frequently from mutations in the 21-hydroxylase enzyme (see the pathway of steroid biosynthesis in Fig. 8-5). Less commonly, CAH with female pseudohermaphroditism results from defects in 11β-hydroxylase or 3β-hydroxysteroid dehydrogenase. The common feature in these disorders is an enzymatic defect that impairs cortisol synthesis in the adrenal cortex and disrupts the normal feedback mechanism by which circulating cortisol inhibits corticotropin (ACTH) secretion by the pituitary. Elevated ACTH levels stimulate the flow of cholesterol precursor down the steroidogenic pathway in adrenocortical cells, with consequent buildup of steroids proximal to the enzymatic block (e.g., progesterone and 17-hydroxyprogesterone in 21-hydroxylase deficiency). The steroid intermediates can be converted peripherally to more potent androgens, thus virilizing the females *in utero*.

The genitalia of females with virilizing CAH exhibit a spectrum of masculinization from simple clitoral enlargement to complete labioscrotal fusion and a penile urethra. The internal female structures and ovaries are unaltered, and male wolffian duct derivatives are not present. These facts indicate either that the onset of increased adrenal androgen occurs after the critical period for wolffian duct differentiation or that these ducts are not capable of responding to the adrenal androgens. The labial folds are rugated and resemble an empty scrotum. Thus, the external appearance of affected females is similar to that of males with bilateral cryptorchidism and hypospadias. Occasionally, when virilization is so severe that a complete penile urethra is formed, errors in sex assignment are made at birth.

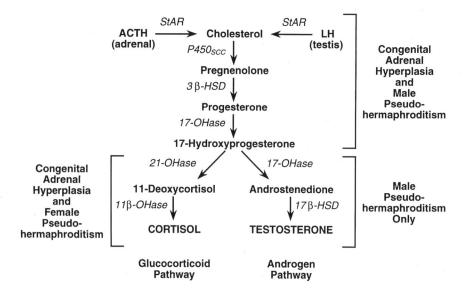

Fig. 8-5 Pathway for synthesis of glucocorticoid and androgenic hormones from cholesterol in adrenal and testis.

Placental aromatase deficiency, a rare autosomal recessive disorder, provides striking evidence for the protective role of the placenta against excess androgen exposure *in utero*. During pregnancy, the placenta receives large amounts of androgen precursors from the fetal and maternal adrenal glands, which it converts into androgens such as androstenedione. Placental aromatase converts the C19 androstenedione into C18 estrogens, thus removing the potential source of excess androgen. In the absence of this protective barrier, androgen exposure in 46,XX subjects results in clitoromegaly, varying degrees of posterior fusion, scrotalization of the labioscrotal folds, and occasionally a single perineal orifice. At puberty, subjects with aromatase deficiency develop hypergonadotropic hypogonadism and polycystic ovaries with progressive virilization.

Male Pseudohermaphroditism

Defective virilization of the 46,XY embryo with testes (male pseudohermaphroditism) can result from defects in androgen synthesis in the testis, defects in androgen action in target cells, or defects in müllerian duct regression.

Disorders of Androgen Biosynthesis

Defects in Testosterone Synthesis. Figure 8-5 summarizes the pathway by which testosterone is synthesized from cholesterol in the testis. As discussed above, many of the same enzymes are involved in corticosteroid production in the adrenal cortex. Thus, defects in the early steps of the pathway—which are required for the biosynthesis of both corticosteroids and androgens—cause both adrenal insufficiency and male pseudohermaphroditism. Steroidogenic enzymes whose mutations can cause this combined clinical presentation include the cholesterol side chain cleavage enzyme (CYP11A) 3β-hydroxysteroid dehydrogenase and 17α-hydroxylase (CYP17). The regulated production of all classes of steroid hormones also requires a mitochondrial phosphoprotein—the steroidogenic acute regulatory protein (StAR)—that is essential for the delivery of cholesterol to the steroidogenic complex inside the mitochondria. Mutations in *StAR* cause the rare autosomal recessive disorder *congenital lipoid adrenal hyperplasia*.

Defects in the glucocorticoid pathway distal to 17-hydroxyprogesterone result in both adrenal insufficiency and virilization of females by adrenal androgens (see Female Pseudohermaphroditism). Finally, isolated male pseudohermaphroditism results from defects in the androgen synthetic pathway distal to the formation of 17-hydroxyprogesterone (e.g., the C17–20 lyase reaction of CYP17 and the conversions catalyzed by the type 3 isozyme of 17β-hydroxysteroid dehydrogenase).

Impaired androgen production also is associated with Leydig cell hypoplasia or agenesis. This condition results from inactivating mutations in the gene encoding the receptor for luteinizing hormone (LH). In 46,XY subjects with the most severe form of this disorder, the external genitalia appear female; milder defects may cause microphallus and hypoplastic external genitalia. Some virilization of structures derived from the wolffian ducts can occur, suggesting some capacity at early stages of gestation for autonomous production of androgens. The absence of Leydig cell hypoplasia/aplasia in patients with deficient secretion of pituitary gonadotropins suggests that fetal testosterone production during the critical period of virilization of the external genitalia may be driven by human chorionic gonadotropin.

Unlike patients with gonadal dysgenesis, in these patients AMH production is normal and müllerian structures regress normally. Presumably, impaired development of Leydig cells due to the absence of LH receptor signaling prevents adequate production of testosterone, with consequent failure of virilization. Thus, 46,XX individuals with homozygous inactivating mutations of the LH receptor have normal development of secondary sexual characteristics at puberty but have elevated LH levels and amenorrhea.

Defects in Androgen Action

Testosterone synthesis is normal in more than 80% of male pseudohermaphrodites; thus, most disorders of male phenotypic development presumably result from impaired androgen action. In these disorders, testosterone synthesis and müllerian duct regression are normal, but male development is incomplete owing to impaired action of androgen in target cells. These subjects can have defects either in the conversion of testosterone to dihydrotestosterone by 5α-reductase or in the androgen receptor.

5α-Reductase Deficiency. Deficiency of 5α-reductase—which converts testosterone to the potent androgen dihydrotestosterone in peripheral tissues—is a rare cause of androgen resistance in humans. This disorder results from mutations in the gene encoding the type 2 isozyme of 5α-reductase, which maps to chromosome 2p23. Subjects with this disorder have a predominantly female phenotype. The urethral opening is commonly at the base of a small phallus, and a blind-ending vaginal pouch usually opens near the urethral orifice in the urogenital sinus. Female internal genitalia are not present, and the male internal genitalia (epididymis, vas deferens, and seminal vesicles) are well developed. The fact that the defect in embryonic virilization in these individuals is limited to the urogenital sinus and the external genitalia proved that testosterone itself can mediate virilization of the wolffian ducts, while dihydrotestosterone is absolutely required for differentiation of the prostate and external genitalia.

Androgen Receptor Defects. The most severe form of androgen resistance—the complete androgen insensitivity syndrome, previously called *testicular feminization*—is caused by mutations that severely impair androgen receptor action. Subjects with this condition generally come to medical attention at puberty when they are evaluated for primary amenorrhea. The karyotype is 46,XY but the external genitalia are those of a normal female, except that the vagina is short and blind-ending. The testes are of normal size and can be located in the abdomen, along the course of the inguinal canal, or in the labia majora. Neither müllerian duct– nor wolffian duct–derived structures are present internally. Although breast development is normal, axillary, pubic, and facial hair is absent or scanty. Biochemically, circulating testosterone levels are elevated, and 5α-reductase activity in peripheral tissues is normal.

Molecular analyses of the androgen receptor—which is encoded on the X chromosome—have defined the molecular basis for complete androgen insensitivity in most patients. These androgen receptor mutations run the full gamut, including deletions, expansion of a CAG triplet repeat, those that interfere with splicing, and nonsense, missense, and frameshift mutations. Most subjects with complete androgen insensitivity have point mutations in the hormone-binding domain of the androgen receptor that impair androgen binding. Less commonly, point mutations in the DNA-binding domain interfere with its activation of target genes despite normal hormone binding.

Less severe mutations in the androgen receptor—the partial androgen insensitivity syndrome—can cause relatively minor degrees of undervirilization and/or infertility. The partial androgen insensitivity syndrome includes hypospadias, cryptorchidism, and oligospermia, although most patients with these conditions have normal androgen receptors. Patients with partial androgen insensitivity often develop gynecomastia at the time of puberty due to increased production of estradiol.

Syndrome of Persistent Müllerian Ducts

The persistence of the müllerian ducts (uterus and fallopian tubes) in a genotypic and otherwise normal phenotypic male is a rare condition. This syndrome generally is diagnosed at the time of surgery, often when it is noted that inguinal hernias contain müllerian derivatives (fallopian tubes and/or uterus). The testes are often cryptorchid, most likely secondary to interference of normal descent by the female structures rather than a direct requirement for AMH in testicular descent. The patients generally are fully virilized, although the intra-abdominal location of the testes often impairs spermatogenesis. Approximately half of the patients with persistent müllerian ducts have mutations in the *AMH* gene on chromosome 19p13 that interfere with its biosynthesis or processing. The remainder have mutations in the type 2 AMH receptor—a serine threonine kinase that bears homology to receptors for other members of the TGF-β family—which presumably interfere with AMH binding or downstream signaling events.

CONCLUSION

Figure 8-6 summarizes our current understanding of the processes of sex determination and differentiation, indicating specific sites where dysfunction can lead to abnormal sexual development. Some genes, such as *SF-1* and *WT1*, are expressed very early in gonadogenesis and are essential for survival of the indifferent gonads; mutations of these genes cause early gonadal degeneration with impaired male sex differentiation. Thereafter, *SRY* in males induces the indifferent gonads to differentiate into testes and synthesize the two key effectors of male sexual development: AMH and androgens. SOX9 has been proposed to support SRY in the induction of testes development, whereas *SF-1* has been proposed to act as a direct upstream regulator of genes involved in both arms of male sexual differentiation. Anti-müllerian hormone—secreted by fetal Sertoli cells—interacts with specific receptors to induce regression of the müllerian ducts. Testosterone—secreted by fetal Leydig cells—interacts with the androgen receptor to virilize the male internal genitalia, while virilization of the external genitalia and prostate further requires the conversion of testosterone to dihydrotestosterone by 5α-reductase. Anything that

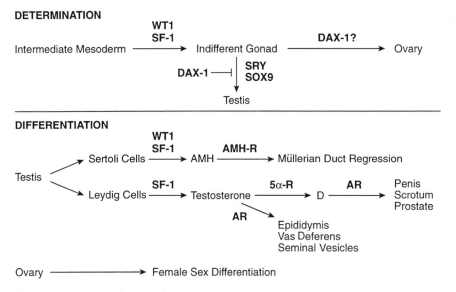

Fig. 8-6 Summary of the molecular events in mammalian sex determination and differentiation. As discussed in this chapter, the positions of genes believed to mediate key events in sex determination and differentiation are indicated. AMH, anti-müllerian hormone; AMH-R, AMH receptor; AR, androgen receptor; D, dihydrotestosterone; 5αR, 5α-reductase.

impairs the synthesis or function of these two testicular hormones causes aberrant or incomplete male sexual development.

Conversely, virilization of females can result from exposure *in utero* to androgens at critical periods of development, as seen most commonly in patients with congenital adrenal hyperplasia due to 21-hydroxylase deficiency. Thus, phenotypic sex differentiation is controlled by the presence (in males) or absence (in females) of specific hormonal signals during embryogenesis.

Although recent studies have defined in considerable detail the hormonal and genetic factors necessary for mammalian sexual differentiation, many fundamental issues in the embryogenesis of the urogenital tract remain poorly understood. Issues such as the nature and timing of chromosomal signals and cellular changes that cause gonadal differentiation, as well as the mechanisms by which the same hormonal signal from androgens is translated into distinct physiological effects in different tissues, must be clarified before we understand fully the developmental program that underlies phenotypic sexual differentiation.

SUGGESTED READING

Donohoue PA, Parker KL, and Migeon CJ: Congenital adrenal hyperplasia. In: *The Metabolic and Molecular Bases of Inherited Disease,* 8th ed., CR Scriver, AL Beaudet, WS Sly, and D Valle, eds., McGraw-Hill, New York, pp. 4077–4116, 2000.
Hughes IA: Minireview: sex differentiation. Endocrinology 142:3281–3287, 2001.

Jost A, Vigier B, Prepin J, and Perchellet J: Studies on sex differentiation in mammals. Recent Prog Horm Res 29:1–41, 1973.

McPhaul MJ: Molecular defects of the androgen receptor. Recent Prog Horm Res 57:181–194, 2002.

Parker KL, Schedl A, and Schimmer BP: Gene interactions in gonadal development. Annu Rev Physiol 61:417–433, 1999.

Swain A and Lovell-Badge R: Mammalian sex determination: a molecular drama. Genes Dev 13:755–767, 1999.

Teixeira J, Maheswaran S, and Donahoe PK: Müllerian inhibiting substance: an instructive developmental hormone with diagnostic and possible therapeutic applications. Endoc Rev 22:657–674, 2002.

Vialain E: Anomalies of human sexual development: clinical aspects and genetic analysis. Novartis Found Symp 244:43–53, 2002.

White PD and Speiser PW: Congenital adrenal hyperplasia due to 21-hydroxylase deficiency. Endocr Rev 21:245–291, 2000.

Wilson JD: The role of 5-alpha-reduction in steroid hormone physiology. Reprod Fertil Dev 13:673–678.

9

Female Reproductive Function

SERGIO R. OJEDA

The production of germ cells is essential for the continuation of a species. In the female this function is accomplished by the ovaries. In addition, the ovaries secrete steroidal and nonsteroidal hormones that not only regulate the secretion of anterior pituitary hormones but also act on various target organs including the ovaries themselves, the uterus, fallopian tubes, vagina, mammary gland, and bone.

STRUCTURAL ORGANIZATION OF THE OVARY

Morphologically, the ovary has three regions: an outer cortex that contains the oocytes and represents most of the mass of the ovary; the inner medulla, formed by stromal cells and cells with steroid-producing characteristics; and the hilum, which, in addition to serving as the point of entry of the nerves and blood vessels, represents the attachment region of the gland to the mesovarium (Fig. 9-1).

The cortex, which is enveloped by the germinal epithelium, contains the follicles, which are the functional units of the ovary. They are present in different states of development or degeneration (atresia), each enclosing an oocyte. In addition to the oocyte, ovarian follicles have two other cellular components: granulosa cells, which surround the oocyte, and thecal cells, which are separated from the granulosa cells by a basal membrane and are arranged in concentric layers around this membrane. The follicles are embedded in the stroma, which is composed of supportive connective cells similar to that of other tissues, interstitial secretory cells, and neurovascular elements.

The medulla has a heterogeneous population of cells, some of which are morphologically similar to the Leydig cells in the testes. These cells predominate in the ovarian hilum; their neoplastic transformation results in excess androgen production.

OVARIAN HORMONES

The ovary produces both steroidal and peptidergic hormones. Whereas the steroids are synthesized in both interstitial and follicular cells, peptidergic hormones are primarily produced in follicular cells and, after ovulation, by cells of the corpus luteum.

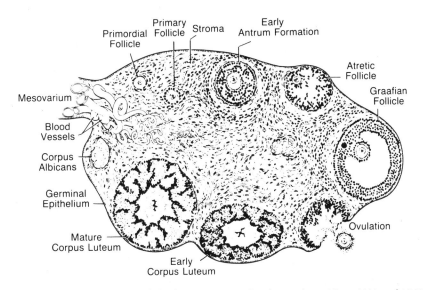

Fig. 9-1 Microscopic view of the human ovary. (Redrawn from Ham AW and Li TS: *Histology,* 4th ed., Lippincott, Philadelphia, p. 802, 1961, with permission.)

Biosynthesis, Transport, and Metabolism of Steroid Hormones

Biosynthesis

The initial precursor for steroid biosynthesis is cholesterol (Fig. 9-2), which derives from animal fats of the diet or from local synthesis. The cholesterol that arrives at the ovary via the bloodstream is mostly transported in association with low-density lipoproteins (LDL), which bind to specific receptors located in the plasma membrane of ovarian cells. Thereafter, the LDL–receptor complexes are internalized and hydrolyzed within lysosomes that release cholesterol for steroid biosynthesis. Excess cholesterol is esterified and stored in lipid droplets for later use. Under normal conditions, most of the cholesterol utilized in steroid biosynthesis comes from the plasma LDL-associated pool and intracellular lipid droplets. A less important source originates from *de novo* local synthesis.

For cholesterol to be used in steroid biosynthesis, it must be transported to the mitochondria. This process is achieved by a protein termed *steroidogenic acute regulatory protein* (StAR), which promotes the transfer of cholesterol from the outer to the inner mitochondrial membrane. On reaching this location, cholesterol becomes available to an enzyme called *cholesterol side-chain cleavage enzyme* for conversion to pregnenolone (see below). The StAR is, therefore, essential for the acute regulation of steroid biosynthesis. The gene encoding StAR spans 8 kb in the human genome; its mRNA product comprises several transcripts ranging from 1.6 to 7.5 kb and generates a 37 kDa precursor protein that is cleaved in the mitochondria to a 30 kDa mature protein. The cytosolic precursor form is thought to be the steroidogenic active protein acutely synthesized in response to hormonal, cyclic adenosine monophosphate (cAMP)–mediated stimulation. Formation of the 30 kDa

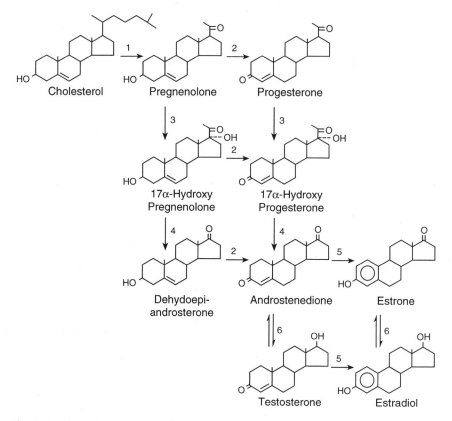

Fig. 9-2 Biosynthesis of steroids in the ovary. 1: Cholesterol side-chain cleavage enzyme complex; 2: 3β-hydroxysteroid dehydrogenase; 3: 17α-hydroxylase; 4: 17,20-lyase; 5: aromatase; 6: 17β-hydroxysteroid dehydrogenase.

mature form in the mitochondria signals the termination of cholesterol transfer, so that new transfer requires additional synthesis of the precursor form.

The main steroids produced by the ovary are progesterone and estradiol (Fig. 9-2). Whereas androgens, particularly androstenedione and testosterone, are also secreted into the bloodstream, a significant portion is converted to estradiol through the action of an aromatase enzyme complex. In addition to these steroids, the ovary secretes estrone, 17α-hydroxyprogesterone, 20α-hydroxyprogesterone, and 5α-reduced androgens such as 5α-dihydrotestosterone and 3α-androstanediol.

The first step in the synthesis of ovarian steroids is the conversion of cholesterol, which has 27 carbons, to the C-21 compound pregnenolone in a reaction catalyzed by cholesterol side-chain cleavage enzyme. The reaction occurs in the mitochondria. Pregnenolone can then be converted into progesterone by the action of a 3β-hydroxysteroid dehydrogenase enzyme, or into 17α-hydroxypregnenolone by a 17α-hydroxylase. Both progesterone and 17α-hydroxypregnenolone can, in turn, be metabolized to 17α-hydroxyprogesterone (Fig. 9-2).

In contrast to cholesterol, progestogen compounds have only 21 carbons. Additional metabolism to androgens and estrogens results in further reduction in the number of carbons to 19 (androgens) and 18 (estrogens).

17α-Hydroxyprogesterone is the substrate for a 17,20-lyase enzyme that, by cleaving the C-20,21 side chain, yields androstenedione. This androgen is either directly metabolized to estrone or, preferentially, converted into testosterone in a reaction catalyzed by the enzyme 17β-hydroxysteroid dehydrogenase. Both androstenedione and testosterone are substrates for estrogen production. Whereas androstenedione is converted into estrone, testosterone metabolism results in estradiol formation. In both cases the reaction is catalyzed by an aromatase enzyme that generates the estrogens through a complex series of reactions involving hydroxylations, oxidations, removal of the C-19 carbon, and aromatization of the A ring of the androgen. All of the reactions involved in the metabolism of progesterone to estradiol, including the initial formation of progesterone from pregnenolone, occur in the endoplasmic reticulum.

With the exception of the 3β- and 17β-hydroxysteroid dehydrogenases, the enzymes involved in ovarian steroid biosynthesis belong to a group called *mixed function oxidases* that utilize different forms of cytochrome P450 and require molecular oxygen and nicotinamide adenine dinucleotide phosphate (NADPH) for their activity. They consist of the cytochrome P450, which binds to the substrate, and an electron transport system. In the case of the cholesterol side-chain cleavage enzyme, the electron transport system consists of an iron-sulfur protein and a flavoprotein, NADPH-adrenodoxin reductase. In the case of the 17α-hydroxylase, 17,20-lyase, and aromatase enzyme systems, the electron transport system is provided by a flavoprotein NADPH–cytochrome P450 reductase.

The synthesis of P450 steroid hydroxylases is regulated by the activation of an orphan nuclear receptor known as *steroidogenic factor-1* (SF-1). Alternative promoter usage and different 39 splicing patterns of the gene encoding SF-1 originates multiple transcripts that appear to serve different functions. In addition to being essential for P450 steroid hydroxylase expression, SF-1 is involved in the regulation of other steroidogenic enzymes such as 3β-hydroxysteroid dehydrogenase and StAR. Unexpectedly, targeted disruption of the SF-1 gene revealed that SF-1 is essential for ovarian and adrenal morphogenesis; in its absence, both glands fail to develop. In addition, SF-1–deficient mice show a reduction in pituitary gonadotropin synthesis and loss of the ventromedial nucleus of the hypothalamus (for additional information see Chapter 8).

The bulk of androgen production occurs in interstitial cells and the cells of the follicular theca (see p. 192 and Fig. 9-3). Estradiol is produced mainly by granulosa cells of antral follicles. Progesterone, in contrast, is secreted by all steroidogenic cells of the ovary, regardless of their localization.

For students interested in the subject, a detailed description of steroid chemistry, pathways, and biosynthetic enzymes can be found in the review by Kellie, and in the book *The Physiology of Reproduction,* by Knobil and Neill, listed at the end of this chapter.

Transport and Metabolism of Steroid Hormones

Both 17β-estradiol and estrone are present in the bloodstream. Whereas estradiol is secreted directly by the ovary, estrone derives largely from peripheral conversion of estradiol or androstenedione. Estrone is further metabolized to estriol, a reaction that occurs predominantly in the liver. Most circulating estrogens ($\sim$70%) are bound to proteins, preferentially albumin, for which they have a low affinity, or to a

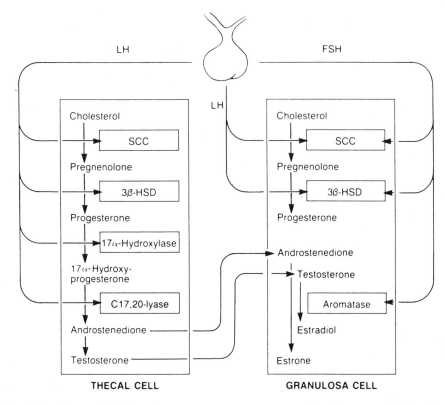

Fig. 9-3 The control of ovarian estrogen, progesterone, and androgen production by luteinizing hormone (LH) and follicle-stimulating hormone (FSH). The LH acts on both thecal and granulosa cells; FSH acts only on granulosa cells. 3β-HSD, 3β-hydroxysteroid dehydrogenase; SCC, cholesterol side chain cleavage enzyme.

steroid-binding protein known as *sex hormone-binding globulin* (SHBG), for which they have a higher affinity. Estrogens have a lower affinity for SHBG than androgens do; this results in a greater availability of estrogens to target tissues because only free steroids can be transported into target cells (see Chapter 5).

Metabolism of estrogens via oxidation or conversion to glucuronide and sulfate conjugates occurs predominantly in the liver. The resulting metabolites are excreted in the bile and reabsorbed into the bloodstream via the enterohepatic circulation. Their final excretion route, however, is the urine.

In women, androgens are produced by both the ovaries and the adrenals. There are three main circulating androgens in women: dehydroepiandrosterone, produced by the adrenal; androstenedione, derived from both the ovary and the adrenal; and testosterone, which in addition to being produced by the ovary and adrenal is formed in peripheral tissues, mainly from androstenedione and to some extent from dehydroepiandrosterone and Δ⁵-androstenediol. Indeed, testosterone is the primary physiologically active androgen in women. It may act on target tissues directly or after its conversion to 5α-dihydrotestosterone. As in men (see Chapter 10), 97%–99% of the total circulating testosterone in women is bound to SHBG. As with estrogens, androgens are excreted mostly in the urine.

Progesterone also circulates bound to a plasma protein, corticosteroid-binding protein (transcortin). Progesterone is converted in the liver to pregnanediol, which, following conjugation to glucuronic acid, is excreted in the urine.

Peptide Hormones of Ovarian Origin

One of the first peptide hormones to be recognized as a product of the ovary was relaxin. It is produced mainly by the corpus luteum during pregnancy but has also been found in decidual tissue and human seminal plasma. The secretion of relaxin from the corpus luteum is stimulated by human chorionic gonadotropin (hCG). In humans, there are two relaxin-related genes. Human relaxin consists of an α- and a β-peptide chain covalently linked by disulfide bonds. Interestingly, both the position of the bonds and the processing of the prohormone to yield mature relaxin are identical to those of insulin, suggesting that both proteins, as well as the insulin-like growth factors (IGFs; see Chapter 12), derive from the duplication of a common ancestral gene. The main effect of relaxin is to induce relaxation of the pelvic bones and ligaments, inhibit myometrial motility, and soften the cervix. In addition, relaxin has been shown to induce uterine growth. It is clear, therefore, that the hormone plays an important role in both maintaining uterine quiescence and favoring the growth and softening of the reproductive tract during pregnancy.

Relaxin Receptors

For many years the identity of relaxin receptors remained elusive. Recently, however, two orphan receptors, LGR7 and LGR8, were found to bind relaxin and mediate its actions via a cAMP-mediated pathway different from that activated by insulin and the IGF family. LGR7 and LGR8 are heterotrimeric guanine nucleotide binding protein (G protein)–coupled receptors. Surprisingly, they appear to be widely expressed throughout the body, including organs such as the brain, kidney, testis, ovary, skin, adrenal gland, bone marrow, and heart. This widespread distribution suggests that relaxin may be involved in a variety of functions different from those related to parturition.

The ovary also produces a peptide hormone that exerts selective inhibitory control over the secretion of follicle-stimulating hormone (FSH). This protein, originally described in testicular extracts and termed *inhibin,* was isolated from follicular fluid and found to be a heterodimeric protein consisting of an α- and a β-polypeptide chain connected by disulfide bonds. Two forms of inhibin (A and B) exist, each with a molecular weight of 32,000. The α-subunits are identical and the β-subunits are different. Combination of the β-subunits of inhibin among themselves via disulfide bond linkage results in the formation of another family of proteins with completely different functions. The first of these functions to be recognized was the selective stimulation of FSH secretion from the adenohypophysis. Because of this activity, this inhibin-associated protein was termed *FSH-releasing protein* (FRP) or *activin.* There are three forms of activin resulting from the differential dimerization of β-subunits, which can form $\beta A/\beta A$, $\beta A/\beta B$, and $\beta B/\beta B$ dimers, respectively.

It now appears that the functions of activin are much more diverse than was originally anticipated. The messenger RNA (mRNA) encoding the βA subunit of activin is expressed in the brain, pituitary gland, germ cells of the testis, and erythropoietic tissue, suggesting a role for activin in cell differentiation. Such a role is supported by studies showing that the differentiation of erythrocytes is promoted by a factor encoded by the same mRNA that encodes the βA-subunit of activin. These nonreproductive functions, though initially surprising, are consistent with the finding that inhibins and activins are members of a large family of peptides that includes transforming growth factor-β (TGF-β), anti-müllerian hormone (AMH; see Chapter 8), and many other peptides involved in the control of growth and differentiation.

In addition to activins and inhibins, follicular cells produce another group of proteins with molecular weights ranging from 32,000 to 43,000, which inhibit FSH secretion. These proteins, termed *follistatins,* bind activins with high affinity and thus are able to neutralize their biological activity.

Still another peptidergic factor, termed *gonadotropin surge-attenuating factor* (GnSAF), has been postulated to be physiologically involved in the control of luteinizing hormone (LH) secretion during the menstrual cycle. This factor appears to be distinct from the inhibin family of peptides and is produced by medium-sized antral follicles. It may function during the follicular phase of the cycle to prevent a premature LH surge.

Quite unexpectedly, the ovary has been found to produce peptides of the proopiomelanocorticotropin (POMC) family including β-endorphin, adrenocorticotropin (ACTH), and α-melanocyte-stimulating hormone (α-MSH). The ovary also produces vasopressin and oxytocin. These two peptides are synthesized in luteal cells, and at least one of them, oxytocin, is secreted into the bloodstream. Within the ovary, they appear to exert paracrine effects.

Pituitary Control of Ovarian Hormone Formation

Steroids

The production of ovarian steroids is under the control of two main hormones secreted by the anterior hypophysis, LH and FSH. In rodents, prolactin and growth hormone (GH) have also been shown to act directly on the ovary. Experiments in rats demonstrated that, depending on its level, prolactin may either inhibit or support the stimulatory effect of LH on ovarian steroidogenesis through modulation of the number of LH receptors. In contrast, GH has been found to facilitate FSH actions in rats by a mechanism involving local production of IGF-I.

Although the secretion of progesterone can be stimulated by both LH and FSH, the secretion of androgens is enhanced only by LH. The formation of estradiol, conversely, depends on both LH and FSH. While LH stimulates production of androgens, FSH directly activates the aromatase enzyme complex that catalyzes the conversion of androgens to estrogens.

The LH receptors are found on steroidogenic cells of the stroma, corpus luteum, and thecal cells of the follicles, all of which produce progesterone and androgens. When the follicles become antral, the granulosa cells acquire LH receptors. As these cells have limited 17,20-lyase activity, their exposure to LH results primarily in increased production of progesterone and little, if any, androgen production. Thus, although granulosa cells are endowed with substantial aromatase activity, LH cannot stimulate estrogen formation unless androgens are provided by another cell type. The same holds true for FSH. Its receptors are located exclusively on granulosa cells, which respond to FSH with estrogen formation if they are provided with an adequate supply of androgens.

These interactions have formed the basis for the formulation of a *two-cell, two-gonadotropin* hypothesis to explain the gonadotropic control of ovarian steroidogenesis. According to this hypothesis, the follicular theca, under the influence of LH, produces androgens that, on diffusion to the granulosa cell compartment of the follicle, are converted to estrogens via an FSH-supported aromatization reaction (Fig. 9-3).

Peptide Hormones

Both LH and FSH help to regulate the production of inhibin. While FSH always stimulates the secretion of this peptide, the role of LH is more complex. Inhibin production in preovulatory follicles decreases sharply soon after the preovulatory surge of gonadotropins (see below, Dynamics of the Hypothalamic–Pituitary–Ovarian Relationship). This decrease appears to be brought about by LH, which, however, simultaneously increases inhibin production in smaller follicles not destined to ovulate in that cycle. It also appears that formation of POMC peptides, vasopressin, and oxytocin is under gonadotropin control. While gonadotropins stimulate the formation of oxytocin and β-endorphin, they decrease the production of vasopressin.

Mechanism of Action of Gonadotropins

Both LH and FSH act on the ovary by first binding to high-affinity, low-capacity–specific membrane receptors. Follicle-stimulating hormone initiates its actions by binding to a seven-transmembrane domain G protein–coupled receptor. The receptor is a glycoprotein with a predicted molecular weight of 75,000 encoded by a single gene that maps to chromosome 2 in the human genome. Although the LH receptor maps to the same chromosome, it is not located in the same region of the chromosome. The human FSH receptor protein is encoded by an open reading frame of 2085 nucleotides, which generates a 678-amino acid mature protein with a predicted molecular mass of ~75,000. Expression of the receptor is highly specific, as it can be found only in Sertoli cells of the testis and granulosa cells of the ovary. Binding of FSH results in cAMP formation and calcium mobilization. It is not clear whether the calcium mobilization is a consequence of the increase in cAMP formation or a cAMP-independent phenomenon. It is known, however, that cAMP activates protein kinase A, which, in turn, induces the phosphorylation of several downstream proteins involved in regulating the expression of cAMP-responsive genes.

The LH receptor is also a seven-transmembrane, G protein–coupled receptor. Its amino acid sequence shows significant homology to the FSH receptor, particularly in the transmembrane domain. The mature protein is a polypeptide of 674 amino acids with a predicted molecular mass of 75,000. Its short intracellular domain contains a number of potential sites for phosphorylation. Interestingly, although activation of the LH receptor causes a clear increase in cAMP levels, the intracellular domain of the receptor contains weak consensus sequences for cAMP-dependent protein kinase–mediated phosphorylation.

Actions of Ovarian Steroids

Ovarian steroids exert intra- and extraovarian actions. The best-known intraovarian actions are those exerted on follicular development. Among the extraovarian actions are those exerted on the hypothalamic–pituitary unit (negative and positive feedback on gonadotropin secretion), on reproductive tissues such as fallopian tubes, uterus, vagina, and mammary gland, and on other tissues such as bone, kidney, and liver.

Intraovarian Actions

Estrogens. Estradiol (E_2) induces proliferation of the granulosa cells, increases E_2 receptors in these cells, and facilitates the action of FSH.

Androgens and Progestins. Testosterone and progesterone have been shown to affect ovarian steroidogenesis through binding to their respective receptors, which are present in granulosa cells. Progesterone inhibits FSH-induced estradiol production. Androgens, in contrast, enhance both the progesterone and estradiol secretion induced by FSH.

A very important intraovarian action of progesterone is in the ovulatory process. Mice lacking the progesterone receptor fail to ovulate despite having preovulatory follicles. This failure appears to be related to the inability of the follicle to produce proteolytic enzymes necessary for rupture of the follicular wall (see below).

Extraovarian Actions

The Uterus. The endometrium or uterine mucosa consists of a superficial layer of epithelial cells and a deeper stromal layer. The epithelial layer is interrupted by tubular invaginations or glands that penetrate into the stromal layer and that are lined by both epithelial cells and columnar secretory cells. The stroma is permeated by blood vessels (spiral arteries) and contains characteristically spindle-shaped cells.

During the first half of the menstrual cycle (i.e., before ovulation), estrogen stimulates proliferation of both the epithelial and stromal layers. The thickness of the endometrium increases three- to fivefold and the uterine glands become enlarged, but they maintain their straight shape. The spiral arteries also elongate. Because of such changes, this has been called the *proliferative phase* of the endometrium.

The uterine cervix contains endocervical glands that elaborate a mucus, which, under the influence of estrogen, changes from a scanty, viscous substance to a much more abundant, watery material. The elasticity of the mucus, usually referred to as *spinnbarkeit,* is greatly increased, a change that can be easily determined by stretching a small drop of mucus between two fingers. When estrogen production is maximal, that is, close to the time of ovulation, the elasticity of the cervical mucus is such that the drop can be stretched maximally without rupture. If a drop of such mucus is spread on a slide and allowed to dry, the mucus forms a typical palm-leaf arborization or ferning pattern.

Under the influence of progesterone, which is produced in increasing amounts after ovulation, proliferation of the endometrium decreases and the uterine glands lose their straight configuration, becoming tortuous. Glycogen accumulates in large vacuoles at the basal portion of the cells. As the corpus luteum becomes firmly established, the glycogen vacuoles move toward the apical end of the cells and the secretory activity of the gland increases significantly. The stroma becomes edematous, and the elongating spiral arteries become coiled. These transformations establish the secretory phase of the endometrium. Coinciding with the loss of corpus luteum function and the resulting decline in plasma levels of estrogen and progesterone the endometrium undergoes focal necrosis, probably because of vasospasm of the spiral arteries. The areas of necrosis increase progressively and the mucosa exfoliates, with loss of all superficial cells except those lining the base of the glands. Because necrosis also affects the endometrial blood vessels, blood loss occurs as menstrual bleeding.

Vasospasm of the endometrial blood vessels is believed to be mediated by prostaglandins, in particular prostaglandin $F_{2\alpha}$. It appears that the loss of luteal progesterone and estrogen destabilizes the lysosomal membranes of endometrial cells, which enhances phospholipid hydrolysis and subsequently prostaglandin formation. Reinitiation of follicular growth during menstruation is accompanied by increased production of estrogen, stimulating the endometrium to proliferate again.

In addition to its effects on the endometrium, progesterone decreases both the quantity and the elasticity of the cervical mucus and inhibits its ferning pattern.

The Vagina. The human vagina is lined by a stratified, multilayered squamous epithelium that consists of superficial, intermediate, inner parabasal, and basal layers. In the presence of low levels of estrogen, such as before puberty or at menopause, the vaginal epithelium is thin, dry, and more susceptible to infections. Estrogens induce both proliferation and keratinization of the epithelium. As a result, mucosa thickness increases and there is increased exfoliation of superficial cells that can be readily identified under the microscope because of their acidophilia and pyknotic nuclei. Interestingly, the epithelium that lines the urethra is also sensitive to ovarian steroids. Thus, examination of urethral cells collected from a fresh urinary sediment can be used to assess alterations in circulating estrogen and progesterone levels in both prepubertal and mature women.

In general, progesterone has an effect on the vaginal epithelium that is opposite to that of estrogen. Under its influence the number of cornified cells decreases and the number of polymorphonuclear leukocytes increases.

The Mammary Gland. The human breast is composed of several lactiferous duct systems that are embedded in adipose and connective tissue. Each duct system contains thousands of sac-like milk-secreting alveoli, which are surrounded by myoepithelial cells and which drain into an increasingly large milk-transporting system comprised of ductules, ducts, lactiferous sinuses, and a single ampulla that opens into the nipple at the center of the areola. At puberty, when estrogen secretion rises, growth of the ducts accelerates and the size of the areola increases. Furthermore, estrogen causes selective accumulation of adipose tissue around the lactiferous duct systems, and this contributes significantly to the overall growth of the breast.

While estrogen stimulates the development of the duct system, progesterone induces the formation of secretory alveoli, an effect more clearly observed during pregnancy. Progesterone also facilitates the proliferating effect of estrogen on the duct epithelium. However, in the absence of priming by estrogen, progesterone has little effect on the mammary gland.

Metabolic Effects. One of the best-known metabolic effects of estrogen is to increase the amount of plasma proteins produced by the liver that bind estradiol, testosterone, cortisol, progesterone, and thyroxine. Estrogens also increase the plasma proteins that bind iron and copper, as well as the levels of high-density lipoproteins (HDL) and very-low-density lipoproteins (VLDL). The latter results in increased circulating levels of triglycerides, which are the lipids preferentially associated with these lipoproteins. In contrast to these effects, estrogen lowers the circulating levels of cholesterol and LDL. Estrogen also exerts appreciable effects on electrolyte balance because of its stimulatory effects on the formation of angiotensinogen and aldosterone. Awareness of these metabolic effects has been heightened by the use of oral contraceptives that, as will be discussed later, are a combination of estrogen and progesterone.

Progesterone itself has little effect on plasma triglycerides. However, some synthetic progestins used in oral contraceptives have been shown to decrease triglyceride levels. More important, progesterone increases the levels of cholesterol and LDL and decreases the level of HDL. Progesterone can also transiently increase sodium excretion in the urine owing to its capacity to antagonize aldosterone action.

The best-known metabolic effect of progesterone is to increase basal body temperature. This is observed after ovulation and can serve as an indicator that ovulation has occurred.

Effects on Nonreproductive Tissues. We have already mentioned the effect of estrogen on the liver. Two additional target tissues are the bone and the kidney. Estrogen acts on bone both to accelerate linear growth and to induce closure of the epiphyseal plates. In addition, it prevents bone resorption. The importance of this effect becomes clearly evident at menopause. At this time, estrogen secretion decreases, resulting in osteoporosis and bone fragility in some women. It is now clear that at least part of this supportive effect of estrogen is exerted directly via binding of the steroid to specific receptors.

In the kidney, estradiol enhances the reabsorption of sodium from the renal tubules.

THE MENSTRUAL CYCLE

Reproductive function in the female is cyclic. A series of functional interrelationships among the hypothalamus, the anterior pituitary, and the ovaries leads to the monthly rupture of an ovarian follicle and extrusion of an ovum (i.e., *ovulation*), which is then transported to the fallopian tubes to be fertilized. Should fertilization fail to occur, menstruation ensues within 14 days and the hormonal and morphological events that led to ovulation are repeated. This coordinated series of events is known as the *menstrual cycle*. The normal menstrual cycle has an average duration of about 30 days, with a range from 25 to 35 days. It can be divided into four phases: menstruation, which lasts about 4–5 days; a follicular phase of the ovary, which corresponds to the proliferative phase of the endometrium and lasts for 10–16 days; an ovulatory phase, which lasts for about 36 hours; and a luteal phase, which corresponds to the secretory phase of the endometrium. The last is usually very constant, lasting for about 14 days; thus, the length of the menstrual cycle is determined by the follicular phase, which can be highly variable. The greatest variability occurs during the few years that follow the first menstruation (menarche) and during the years preceding the loss of reproductive function (menopause).

An understanding of the menstrual cycle requires knowledge of the functional components responsible for its occurrence. These are (1) the gonadotropin-releasing system and its neural (hypothalamic) control; (2) the ovarian follicle, including its rupture at ovulation and its subsequent transformation into a corpus luteum; and (3) the ovarian negative and positive feedback control of gonadotropin secretion.

The Gonadotropin-Releasing System and Its Neural Control (Fig. 9-4)

As discussed in Chapter 6, the adenohypophysis has a population of cells—the gonadotrophs—that secretes LH and FSH. Some cells secrete only LH, others FSH, and still others secrete both hormones.

Release of LH and FSH to the bloodstream is pulsatile. This is particularly noticeable in the case of LH, which has episodes of release every 70–100 minutes. Because the interpulse intervals are about an hour long, this rhythm has been called *circhoral*. The LH pulses are less frequent during the luteal phase of the menstrual cycle than during the follicular phase, presumably because of an inhibitory effect of progesterone, which is secreted in large amounts by the corpus luteum.

In addition to this circhoral rhythm, LH secretion exhibits a sleep-related rhythm. This mode of secretion is not clearly manifested in adult women, but it constitutes a fundamental feature at the onset of puberty. At this time, an increased amount of LH is released during sleep, the first overt neuroendocrine manifestation of the initiation of puberty (see p. 209).

Both types of release (circhoral and diurnal) are a function of luteinizing hormone-releasing hormone (LHRH), the hypothalamic peptide responsible for the control of gonadotropin secretion. Experiments performed in rats, sheep, and monkeys have demonstrated that LHRH is released into the portal circulation, and hence reaches the adenohypophysis, in a pulsatile fashion.

In nonhuman primates, surgical isolation of the medial basal hypothalamus fails to disturb the circhoral release of LH, indicating that the rhythm originates within this area of the brain. Lesion of the arcuate nucleus, which is located in the foremost ventral portion of the medial basal hypothalamus, abolishes basal release of both LH and FSH, indicating that the most essential neural center controlling gonadotropin secretion resides within the arcuate nucleus of the hypothalamus. It is also clear, however, that the function of this *pulse generator* is subject to modifying influences emanating from both extra- and intrahypothalamic loci. An increase in electrical activity in the arcuate nucleus area precedes, with astounding regularity, the discharge of LH into the bloodstream.

As discussed in Chapter 6, there are several neurotransmitter systems involved in the control of LHRH secretion. The most important appear to be those that utilize excitatory amino acids and γ-aminobutyric acid (GABA) as neurotransmitters.

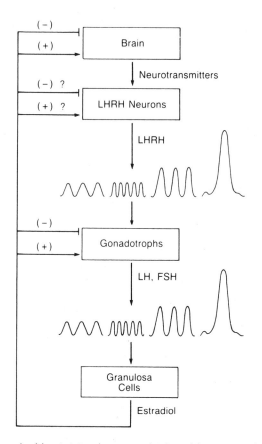

Fig. 9-4 The control of luteinizing hormone (LH) and luteinizing hormone-releasing hormone (LHRH) secretion by ovarian estradiol. Both LH and LHRH are released in pulses. Estrogen (and combinations of estrogen plus progesterone) can alter the frequency and/or amplitude of the pulses by acting at both the hypothalamus and the anterior pituitary. Within the brain, estradiol may inhibit (−) or stimulate (+) the activity of neurotransmitters that affect LHRH secretion. It is not clear whether estradiol can act directly on LHRH neurons (?). Estradiol can also induce a large preovulatory surge of LH and LHRH secretion. FSH, follicle-stimulating hormone.

While excitatory amino acids (predominantly glutamate) stimulate LHRH secretion, GABAergic neurons exert a powerful inhibitory influence. This inhibition, however, is not directly exerted on LHRH neurons. Other stimulatory neurotransmitters include the catecholamine norepinephrine (NE) and the peptide neuropeptide Y (NPY). Neurotransmitters, such as the amines dopamine (DA) and serotonin, can either stimulate or inhibit LHRH secretion, depending on the prevalent steroid milieu present.

In addition to GABA, opioid peptides are also able to inhibit LHRH release. β-Endorphin, synthesized in neurons of the medial basal hypothalamus, is a prominent example of this class of inhibitory inputs to LHRH neurons. If naloxone, a blocker of opioid receptors, is administered during the luteal phase of the menstrual cycle, the frequency of LH discharges increases to levels similar to those seen during the early follicular phase. Because progesterone increases β-endorphin production in the hypothalamus, it has been suggested that the inhibitory effect exerted by progesterone during the luteal phase on LH pulse frequency is mediated by β-endorphin.

Despite the complexity of the transsynaptic control of LHRH secretion, it is becoming increasingly evident that most of the above-mentioned neuronal networks play roles secondary to that of the glutamate–GABA regulatory systems. Recent experiments in rodents and nonhuman primates have implicated glial cells as an additional component of the regulatory complex controlling LHRH secretion. Glial cells of the astrocytic lineage were shown to affect LHRH release via production of trophic molecules, which, acting in a paracrine–autocrine fashion, stimulate the glial secretion of neuroactive substances able to stimulate LHRH release. The epidermal growth factor (EGF)-like peptides transforming growth factor-α (TGFα) and neuregulins have been identified as some of these glial regulatory molecules.

Follicular Development, Ovulation, and Atresia (Fig. 9-5)

Follicular Development

The primordial germ cells originate in the endoderm of the yolk sac, allantois, and hindgut of the embryo. By 5–6 weeks of gestation they migrate to the genital ridge and begin to multiply rapidly, so that by 24 weeks of gestation the total number of oogonia is about 7 million. They concentrate mostly within the cortical portion of the primitive gonad. As multiplication of the oogonia proceeds, some of them reach the prophase stage of meiosis and are called *primary oocytes*. Many others degenerate and die, so that at birth only 2 million primary oocytes remain, a number that

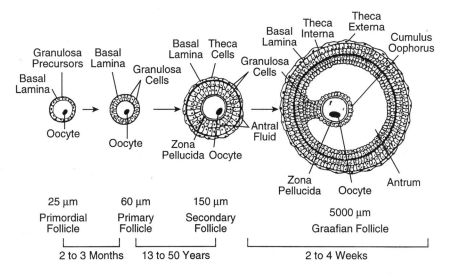

Fig. 9-5 Schematic representation of the development of an ovarian follicle (not to scale). (Redrawn and modified from Berne RM and Levy MN: *Physiology*, Mosby, St. Louis, p. 1092, 1983, with permission.)

is further reduced before puberty to about 400,000. The first meiotic division is not completed until the moment of ovulation; at this time, the oocyte has grown from 10–25 μm to 150 μm in diameter. The mechanisms underlying the long suspension of oocytes in meiotic prophase are incompletely understood, but they appear to involve the presence of high cAMP levels in the oocyte. These high levels may be maintained by a factor(s) originated in either follicular cells or the oocyte itself.

Primordial follicles are formed when a single layer of flattened epithelial cells surrounds a primary oocyte. These cells, which will later generate the granulosa cells, provide nutrients to the oocyte via protoplasmic processes that reach the oocyte's plasma membrane. The primordial follicle becomes separated from surrounding spindle-shaped mesenchymal cells by a basement membrane called the *basal lamina.* When the flattened epithelial cells become cuboidal, the follicle becomes a primary follicle. The oocyte secretes a mucoid substance rich in glycoproteins that forms a band separating the oocyte from the granulosa cells. This band is called the *zona pellucida.*

The granulosa cells located next to the zona pellucida continue to extend protoplasmic processes to the oocyte, presumably to maintain a nutrient flow and chemical signals to the growing oocyte. As these changes occur, the stromal cells adjacent to the basal lamina become differentiated in concentric layers around the primary follicle, constituting the follicular theca. The portion of the theca contiguous to the basal lamina is called the *theca interna;* the outer portion is called the *theca externa.* It is now known that the assembly of primordial follicles requires a transcription factor called *factor in the germ line, alpha* (FIGα) and that the subsequent growth of primary follicles requires both an oocyte-derived growth factor known as *growth differentiation factor-9* (GDF-9) and *kit ligand* (KL), a growth-promoting polypeptide produced by granulosa cells. Very recently, the neurotrophic factors, *nerve growth factor* (NGF), *neurotrophin 4/5* (NT-4/5), and *brain-derived neurotrophic factor* (BDNF) have also been implicated in the facilitatory control of early follicular growth.

Development of primary follicles is a very slow process lasting for several years. At puberty and throughout the reproductive years, cohorts of primary follicles enter into a new phase of development that is completed in approximately 3 weeks. During this phase, granulosa cells proliferate more rapidly, and some of the cells of the theca interna become cuboidal and filled with lipid droplets, indicative of enhanced steroidogenesis. In addition, the theca interna is invaded by the capillaries that terminate at the basal lamina. In some follicles the continuity of the granulosa cell layers is disrupted by the appearance of spaces filled with fluid. Gradually, these spaces become confluent, forming a single central cavity called the *antrum.* The follicles with these characteristics are known as *antral follicles.* As they grow further, their antrum is greatly expanded. These follicles are known as *graafian follicles.* At this stage, the oocyte reaches its maximum size (150 mm).

The antrum is filled with a fluid that contains steroids and local growth factors at concentrations several times greater than those in plasma. As the granulosa cells continue to proliferate and the antrum enlarges, the oocyte is displaced from the center of the follicle and becomes surrounded by a hillock of granulosa cells called the *cumulus oophorus.* By the end of this stage, the antral follicle has reached a diameter of 5 mm. Because the granulosa cells and the oocyte are surrounded by the basal lamina throughout follicular development, they remain avascular; hormones, neurotransmitters, and blood-borne nutrients must reach them by diffusion.

During the second half of the follicular phase, one follicle becomes dominant and undergoes further growth so as to finally expel its oocyte at ovulation. The factors responsible for the selection of a single follicle (from a cohort of 6 to 10 follicles that become antral) in every cycle remain to be identified.

Ovulation

As discussed below, a large increase in plasma levels of gonadotropins takes place at the end of the follicular phase. This surge greatly enhances the production of antral fluid in the dominant follicle; the follicle enlarges, reaching a diameter of 10–20 mm in 48 hours. The granulosa become less cohesive and the cumulus oophorus loosens. Studies in the rabbit have shown that the first morphological changes in the thecal compartment of the ovulatory follicle occur by 4 hours after the initial gonadotropin stimulation. The theca interna begin to develop edema, and the fibroblastic cells of this region begin to dissociate. Thereafter, no major morphological changes occur until the last hour before rupture; at this time, the fibroblasts and collagenous matrix of the apical portion of the follicular wall undergo dissociation. Simultaneously, there is extravasation of blood cells into the extracellular space of the follicular wall, which deteriorates at a specific site on its surface called the *stigma*. Formation of the stigma begins with a local decrease of blood flow, followed by a gradual thinning and depolymerization of the connective tissue in the area and reorganization of the vasculature around the edge of the stigma. Sixteen to 24 hours after the gonadotropin surge, the follicular wall at the stigma becomes exceedingly thin and finally appears to dissolve, allowing the extrusion of the oocyte surrounded by the cumulus oophorus.

It is now clear that ovulation requires the functional integrity of at least two effector proteins: the progesterone receptor (PR) and the cyclooxygenase enzyme COX-2, which catalyzes the formation of prostaglandins from arachidonic acid. Null mutation of the genes encoding these proteins results in ovulatory failure, clearly establishing the absolute requirement for each of these molecules in the ovulatory process. Both genes are expressed in granulosa cells and are induced by the preovulatory LH surge. While COX-2 is predominantly induced in granulosa cells of the cumulus oophorus, PR is mostly induced in mural granulosa cells, that is, those adjacent to the basal lamina of the follicle. In addition to COX-2 and PR, a transcription factor known as C/EBPβ (for CCAAT/enhancer binding protein) is strongly induced by LH in granulosa cells. Mice lacking this factor fail to ovulate, indicating that C/EBPβ is an essential early downstream signal used by LH to induce ovulation. However, C/EBPβ does not act by activating PR or cyclooxygenase expression. On the one hand, it does not bind to the PR promoter; on the other hand, mice lacking C/EBPβ exhibit persistently elevated levels of cyclooxygenase instead of a decrease.

While the signaling mechanisms underlying the induction of PR by LH remain to be identified, recent studies have implicated the oocyte-derived growth factor GDF-9 in the process by which LH induces COX-2 synthesis in cumulus cells. Activation of prostaglandin synthesis results in dissociation of these cells; this phenomenon, known as *cumulus expansion,* is an essential early event of ovulation.

Mice lacking the *COX-2* gene fail to show cumulus expansion in response to LH and do not ovulate.

The downstream signals used by prostaglandins to effect cumulus expansion and PR activation to cause ovulatory rupture are also beginning to be identified. Thus, COX-2 seems to be required for the expression of *TSG-6* (tumor necrosis factor-stimulated gene-6), an inflammation-related gene in cumulus cells. On the other hand, activation of PR expression in mural granulosa cells induces expression of two proteases, ADAMTS-1 (a disintegrin and metalloproteinase, with thrombospondin-like motifs) and cathepsin L (a lysosomal cysteine protease), suggesting the involvement of these proteases in the mechanism of follicular rupture. Notwithstanding the progress made, much more needs to be done to clarify the cellular and molecular mechanisms underlying the ovulatory process.

The first meiotic division is completed at the time of ovulation. The first polar body is eliminated, and the secondary oocyte is captured by the fimbria of the oviduct, which is closely applied to the surface of the ovary. The oocyte is then transported to the ampulla of the oviduct via ciliary movements. The second meiotic division occurs at the time of fertilization, yielding the ovum with a haploid number of chromosomes and a second polar body that is discarded.

Atresia

Because the human female has approximately 30 years of reproductive life, only 300–400 follicles reach maturity within a lifetime. The rest undergo a degenerative process called *atresia.* Atresia occurs via a regulated form of cell death known as *apoptosis,* a physiological process that occurs in all tissues throughout development. During apoptotic death, very distinct morphological and molecular changes take place that allow one to follow the demise of the cell as it occurs. Within the nucleus there is an initial condensation of chromatin, followed by disruption of the nuclear membrane and fragmentation of the nucleus into pieces that form a dense structure known as the *pyknotic nucleus.* During apoptosis the DNA is cleaved between nucleosomal units by calcium/magnesium–dependent endonucleases; if the DNA of cells undergoing apoptosis is isolated and analyzed on a gel, it will show a characteristic *ladder* pattern with fragments of sizes made of multiples of about 200 base pairs. The cytoplasm of an apoptotic cell also undergoes a series of characteristic changes: aggregation and disintegration of organelles; shrinkage of the plasma membrane; and finally, cell fragmentation followed by phagocytosis by neighboring macrophages.

Atresia occurs in both germ cells and follicles. Apoptosis of germ cells is initiated during fetal life, during both migration and after arrival at the ovary, while they proliferate. In rodents, germ cells (termed *oogonia* after they reach the ovary) enter meiosis shortly before birth but remain arrested at the diplotene stage of prophase until near ovulation (see above). Within a few hours after birth, some germ cells (now called *oocytes*) become surrounded by epithelial pregranulosa cells to form the primordial follicles. Many oocytes fail to be enclosed and undergo atresia. Only a small fraction (less than 10%) of the germ cells become finally encapsulated into a follicular structure. Thus, atresia of germ cells is massive before formation of the follicles.

Follicular atresia occurs at all stages of antral follicular development. The follicles to die are those that fail to be supported by survival factors. The FSH is the most critical of these factors; if a follicle receives sufficient FSH support during development, it will escape atresia and reach the preovulatory stage. In addition, LH and GH are also antiapoptotic but less potent than FSH. The signaling pathway utilized by gonadotropins (FSH and LH) to prevent apoptosis involves the activation of cAMP formation. Gonadotropins can also exert survival effects indirectly by stimulating the production of IGF-I, interleukin-1 (IL-1), estrogen, and both EGF and basic fibroblast growth factor (bFGF), all of which are produced by the ovary. Atresia occurs mainly in granulosa cells. In marked contrast, thecal cells lose their differentiated condition and, instead of dying, return to the pool of interstitial cells not associated with follicles. The atretic follicle, in contrast, is invaded by fibroblasts and becomes an avascular, nonfunctional scar.

Factors that induce follicular atresia (atretogenic factors) include the cytokine tumor necrosis factor-α (TNFα) and a still unidentified ligand that activates a death domain–containing receptor known as Fas. It is now clear that TNFα acts via a signaling pathway that involves the production of ceramide, a lipid second messenger. Additional atretogenic factors are IL-6, a cytokine produced in granulosa cells, and androgens.

The signaling pathways utilized by survival and atretogenic factors involve the activation of an array of genes encoding antiapoptotic and proapoptotic protein molecules, respectively. The former group includes genes encoding proteins related to the apoptotic-suppressing protein Bcl-2. Intraovarian expression of Bcl-2 via a transgenic approach results in the development of many more follicles to the preovulatory stage and formation of germ cell tumors, indicating that prolonged survival of granulosa cells leads to tumorigenesis. The antiapoptotic Bcl-2 protein (*Mcl-1*, myloid cell lymphoma gene-1) and a Bcl-2–related proapoptotic protein (termed Bok, Bcl-2–related ovarian killer) have been identified as principal components of the molecular process governing follicular atresia.

The Corpus Luteum

Following ovulation the collapsed follicle becomes reorganized to form the corpus luteum, consisting of *luteinized* granulosa cells, as well as thecal cells, fibroblasts, and capillaries that invade the new structure. Luteinization of the granulosa cells involves the appearance of lipid droplets in the cytoplasm, development by the mitochondria of a dense matrix with tubular cristae, and hypertrophy of the endoplasmic reticulum. The outer portion of the corpus luteum is made up of thecal cells that are also luteinized. The basal lamina of the follicle, however, regresses. Should fertilization fail to occur, the corpus luteum remains functional for 13–14 days and then undergoes luteolysis. The luteal cells become necrotic, progesterone secretion ceases, and the corpus luteum is invaded by macrophages and then by fibroblasts. Endocrine function is rapidly lost, and the corpus luteum is replaced by a scar-like tissue called the *corpus albicans.*

Ovarian Feedback Control of Gonadotropin Secretion

The ovary regulates the secretion of gonadotropins through two basic mechanisms: an inhibitory or negative feedback effect and a stimulatory or positive feedback loop (Fig. 9-4). The former is produced mainly by estrogen, although other steroids, such as progesterone and androgens, and the gonadal protein inhibin also play a role. Positive feedback is exerted by estradiol, although progesterone can amplify the E_2

effect. In addition to these hormones, the FSH-releasing protein activin has a physiological role to play in maintaining FSH secretion.

Negative Feedback

Ablation of the ovaries produces a prompt increase in plasma levels of LH and FSH. Conversely, administration of estradiol returns the levels toward normal values. Estradiol acts on both the hypothalamus and the anterior pituitary to inhibit gonadotropin secretion. At the hypothalamus it suppresses LHSH secretion; at the pituitary it inhibits the release of LH induced by LHRH. The course of action of estrogen is fairly rapid. Within minutes of its intravenous injection, LH levels begin to decline. However, FSH levels are not normalized by administering estradiol to ovariectomized women. This is because the secretion of FSH is also under the inhibitory control of inhibin. Inhibin controls the secretion of FSH via a direct inhibitory action on the pituitary gonadotrophs.

The mechanism by which estradiol inhibits LHRH secretion in the hypothalamus appears to involve activation of inhibitory neurotransmitter systems coupled to the LHRH neuronal network. The GABA neurons have been implicated as a major inhibitory neuronal group mediating the negative feedback effect of estradiol on LHRH secretion. At the pituitary level, estradiol decreases gonadotropin synthesis by suppressing gene expression of the LH β-subunit and, to a lesser extent, that of the FSH β-subunit (for an understanding of gonadotropin structure, see Chapter 6).

Positive Feedback

Like negative feedback, positive feedback is for the most part estrogen dependent. Progesterone, however, can markedly potentiate the stimulatory effect of estradiol on gonadotropin release when given several hours after estradiol. In contrast to negative feedback, which occurs within minutes, the positive effect of estradiol has a latency of several hours. Typically, administering estradiol results in a rapid decline in plasma LH levels that lasts for at least 24 hours (negative feedback); this is followed by an abrupt, marked increase in the secretion of both LH and FSH (positive feedback). During the normal menstrual cycle, this discharge of gonadotropins is a consequence of increases in plasma estrogen levels produced by the growing follicles (see below); the gonadotropin surge at the end of the follicular phase is essential for ovulation.

The anatomical site(s) where estradiol exerts its stimulatory effect have been a matter of controversy, but it is now clear that the steroid acts on the hypothalamus to elicit LHRH release and on the adenohypophysis to increase the sensitivity of the gonadotrophin to LHRH. Whereas the stimulatory effect of estradiol on LHRH release appears to be mediated by the activation of stimulatory neurotransmitter systems functionally coupled to LHRH neurons (glutamatergic, noradrenergic, and NPY neurons), at the pituitary level estradiol may act by both increasing the releasable pool of gonadotropins and by stimulating the expression of the β-subunit genes. This stimulation occurs only in the presence of LHRH.

Dynamics of the Hypothalamic–Pituitary–Ovarian Relationship

Hormonal changes occurring during the menstrual cycle are depicted in Figure 9-6. During menstruation and the early follicular phase, plasma FSH levels are

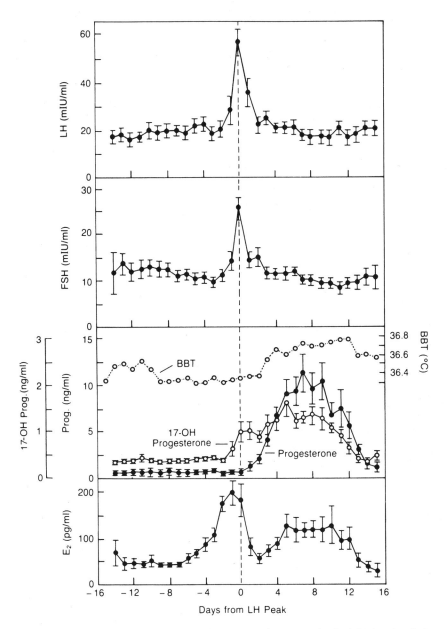

Fig. 9-6 Changes in plasma levels of luteinizing hormone (LH), follicle-stimulating hormone (FSH), progesterone, estradiol, and 17-hydroxy-progesterone (17-OH) during the human menstrual cycle. The day of the LH peak is considered as day 0. Changes in basal body temperature (BBT) induced by progesterone are also represented. (Redrawn from Thorneycroft IH et al: Am J Obstet Gynecol 111:950, 1971, and from Ross GT et al: Recent Prog Horm Res 26:19, 1970, with permission.)

1.5- to 2-fold higher than at the end of the preceding luteal phase. The LH values are low. Thereafter, plasma FSH falls and LH increases moderately, so that by the end of the follicular phase the LH/FSH ratio has increased to about 2. The increase in mean plasma LH appears to be due mainly to an increased frequency of episodic LH discharges.

Estrogen levels (estradiol and estrone) increase very little during the first half of the follicular phase, while progesterone, 17α-hydroxyprogesterone, and the aromatizable androgens, androstenedione and testosterone, remain essentially unchanged. During the second half of the follicular phase, and as follicles grow, plasma estrogen levels begin to rise, a change that becomes more pronounced toward the ovulatory phase, at which time estrogen levels rise up to ninefold over basal values. Estradiol is produced directly by the ovaries, but most of the circulating estrone originates from peripheral conversion of estradiol and androstenedione. Progesterone and 17α-hydroxyprogesterone levels remain unchanged until the ovulatory phase begins; they are mostly derived from the ovary. Indeed, the concentration of progesterone in the follicular fluid increases markedly during the second half of the follicular phase, but not sufficiently to alter the systemic levels. Plasma androstenedione and testosterone also remain at relatively constant levels throughout the follicular phase. Normally, circulating androgens derive from both the ovary and the adrenal gland. The relative contribution of these glands, however, varies both during the day and during the cycle.

The initiation of the ovulatory phase is characterized by elevated estrogen levels that trigger an abrupt discharge of gonadotropins. This preovulatory gonadotropin surge is more pronounced in the case of LH than FSH and lasts for about 24 hours. As gonadotropin levels begin to rise, there is a concomitant increase in 17α-hydroxyprogesterone and a smaller rise in testosterone and androstenedione. Progesterone, in contrast, increases transiently during the LH surge, but not to the same extent as 17α-hydroxyprogesterone. Although LH and FSH are still elevated, there is a precipitous fall in circulating estrogen levels. Plasma levels of progesterone and androgens also decline, but this occurs after gonadotropin levels have returned to basal values.

Ovulation occurs 16–20 hours after the peak of the gonadotropin surge. At this time gonadotropins, estrogen, progesterone, and androgen levels have fallen. In contrast, 17α-hydroxyprogesterone values remain elevated.

Both LH and FSH remain at low levels during the luteal phase. At the beginning of this phase the frequency of episodic LH discharges decreases, but they have a greater amplitude. Later on there is a progressive decrease in both the amplitude and frequency of the LH pulses. A sustained elevation of progesterone and 17α-hydroxyprogesterone secreted by the corpus luteum becomes a predominant feature of this phase. Estrogens and androstenedione of luteal origin are also increased throughout the luteal phase. After about 8–10 days, progesterone values begin to decrease, falling rapidly thereafter, so that by day 14 after ovulation they have reached very low levels and menstruation ensues.

There is little doubt that the selective elevation in FSH levels observed during the early follicular phase plays a decisive role in initiating the growth of secondary follicles, that is, with at lest two layers of granulose cells. Although the formation of primordal and primary follicles is independent of the pituitary, development of these follicles to the antral stage cannot proceed in the absence of FSH. The first wave of follicular development is initiated by the midcycle preovulatory surge of FSH. On reaching the antral stage, however, these follicles undergo atresia in the midst of the luteal phase. A second crop of follicles that is recruited by the elevation of FSH levels at the beginning of the follicular phase progresses to the large antral stage, but only one of them, the *dominant* follicle, reaches the ovulatory condition.

As the follicular phase progresses, aromatase activity increases under FSH control. As more estradiol is produced, the steroid further facilitates the proliferation of granulosa cells, enhances synthesis of its own receptor, and synergizes with FSH to amplify the stimulatory effect of the hormone on granulosa cell differentiation. More specifically, it facilitates the ability of FSH to stimulate estrogen secretion and to induce the formation of both FSH and LH receptors. A gradual increase in plasma LH levels promotes the differentiation of thecal cells and induces the synthesis of the 17,20-lyase enzyme, thereby increasing available androgens for estrogen biosynthesis.

At the end of the follicular phase, estrogen secretion is further increased as the dominant follicle reaches the preovulatory stage. Plasma FSH levels are depressed, perhaps as a consequence of the increase in estrogen and inhibin secretion (stimulated by FSH itself). Pituitary responsiveness to LHRH increases as a consequence of estrogen action, and within 48 hours the preovulatory surge of gonadotropins occurs.

It was previously mentioned that during the second half of the follicular phase a follicle is selected to reach the ovulatory stage. The factors involved in this selection are unknown; however, recent findings demonstrating the presence of noradrenergic and peptidergic nerves in the ovary of several species, including the human, raise the possibility that selection of a dominant follicle may have a neural component.

Once this selection has been made, the rest of the growing follicles undergo atresia. An important characteristic of follicles undergoing atresia is their increased androgen content and reduced estrogen and progesterone levels in comparison with healthy graafian follicles. This is associated with a decreased concentration of FSH and an increased level of prolactin in the follicular fluid. It seems evident, therefore, that the fate of follicles is individually determined by the action of local factors (see above). After ovulation, loss of the oocyte from the ruptured follicle appears to initiate luteinization of the granulosa cells. However, the LH discharge itself contributes significantly to the process. The mechanisms involved in maintaining the function of the corpus luteum for 14 days and in precipitating its regression at the end of this period are incompletely understood. It is clear, however, that in humans LH is luteotropic—that is, it maintains the functional and morphological integrity of the corpus luteum. Prolactin has been found to be luteotropic in rodents, but its role in humans is unclear. The capacity of LH to maintain corpus luteum function declines as the luteal phase progresses. This phenomenon may be related to the influence of luteolytic factors that acquire predominance as the corpus luteum becomes older. Among these factors, estrogen, oxytocin, and prostaglandin $F_{2\alpha}$ deserve mention. The luteolytic effect of both estrogen and oxytocin appears to be mediated at least in part by local formation of prostaglandin $F_{2\alpha}$.

DEVELOPMENT AND MAINTENANCE OF REPRODUCTIVE FUNCTION

Acquisition of reproductive competence is a long and extraordinarily complex process that takes an average of 12–14 years in the human female. Understanding of this process necessitates knowledge of both the initiation and progression of the neuroendocrine changes within the hypothalamic–pituitary–ovarian axis that lead to adult reproductive function.

Fetal, Neonatal, and Infantile Phases

The Hypothalamic–Pituitary Unit

The fetal pituitary gland synthesizes both FSH and LH as early as the fifth week of gestation, and circulating levels of these two hormones are detected by the end of the third month (the earliest fetus studied). The pituitary content of both LH and FSH rises from this gestational age, reaching maximum levels at 25–29 weeks, and then declines as pregnancy progresses. Newborn infants have two to five times less pituitary gonadotropin content than fetuses at 25–29 weeks.

Serum gonadotropins, and in particular FSH, begin to increase at around the third month of gestation, reaching very high values (in the castrate range) by 150 days, that is, before the peak in pituitary gonadotropins. From then to birth, serum levels fall.

This pattern of gonadotropin release is related to the maturation of the negative feedback mechanism produced by gonadal steroids. In the absence of this inhibitory feedback, FSH and LH secretion is relatively unrestrained. Later in fetal development the inhibitory feedback mechanism matures and becomes operative, leading to suppression of the synthesis and release of FSH and LH.

After birth, serum FSH (and to a lesser extent LH) levels increase again and remain elevated for at least the first 2 postnatal years. Part of this increase seems to result from the loss of placental steroids, which greatly contributes to the inhibition of fetal gonadotropin release during the second half of pregnancy. It is unclear, however, why FSH levels remain elevated for such a long period after birth when the infantile ovary is capable of producing estrogens, which can keep gonadotropin secretion restrained. In fact, in ovariectomized neonatal nonhuman primates or agonadal patients, plasma gonadotropin levels are markedly increased (Fig. 9-7).

Two to 4 years after birth, gonadotropin secretion begins to decline and remains low throughout childhood (Fig. 9-7). This reduced output of gonadotropins is most likely due to events that occur within the central nervous system. A loss of excitatory inputs coupled with an increase of inhibitory influences on LHRH neurons may be an important factor determining the decline in gonadotropin secretion that characterizes the juvenile period.

By the eighth to tenth year of life, gonadotropin secretion begins to increase. The FSH levels rise before LH levels do and attain adult values while LH levels are still increasing. In fact, mean plasma LH may not increase noticeably until secondary sexual development is quite advanced. As before, the mechanism responsible for the pubertal reactivation of gonadotropin release is of central nervous system origin and independent of the ovary (see pp. 212–214).

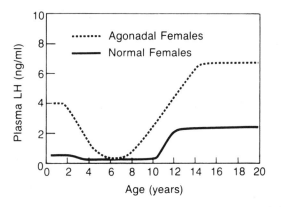

Fig. 9-7 Changes in circulating gonadotropin levels during postnatal development in normal and agonadal human females. Notice that gonadotropin levels in the agonadal subjects decrease during childhood and increase at puberty, similar to the pattern in normal subjects, indicating that these changes occur independently of the ovary. LH, luteinizing hormone. (Redrawn from Grumbach MM: The neuroendocrinology of puberty. In: *Neuroendocrinology*, DT Krieger and JC Hughes, eds., Sinauer, Sunderland, MA, p. 252, 1980, with permission.)

The Ovaries

The prepubertal ovary shows morphological signs of activity such as follicular maturation to the stage of graafian follicle development and subsequent atresia. The cellular residue of atretic follicles contributes substantially to the mass of the human ovary, which increases rectilinearly from birth to puberty.

Ovarian steroidogenic capability is present from birth. Estradiol is the major ovarian secretory product, although estrone, androstenedione, testosterone, and other steroids are also produced. Umbilical artery levels of estradiol, reflecting fetal production of the steroid, are more than 100 times higher than those in adult females despite considerable metabolism of estrogen by the fetus. Estrogen levels decline rapidly in the first postnatal week and remain at less than 10 pg/ml until the onset of puberty.

Puberty

Hormonal Changes

The first endocrine manifestation of the onset of puberty is amplification of a sleep-related pattern of LH release. During childhood, LH is secreted in a pulsatile manner, but the magnitude of the pulses is small. In addition, greater LH levels are seen during sleep than during waking hours. At the end of childhood, before mean gonadotropin levels begin to increase, the difference in LH secretion becomes more pronounced and the magnitude of the LH pulses is enhanced (Fig. 9-8). These changes not only reflect the initial activation of the central mechanism governing LH secretion, but are also believed to be the initial event leading to the attainment of puberty.

As puberty progresses and plasma gonadotropin levels increase, there is a wide range of serum LH and FSH values, probably reflecting superimposed menstrual

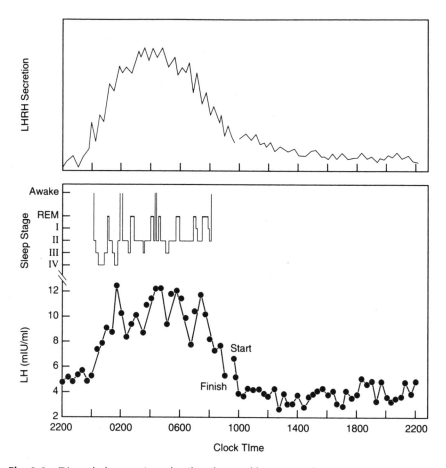

Fig. 9-8 Diurnal changes in pulsatile release of luteinizing hormone (LH) at puberty. The upper panel depicts the hypothetical changes in luteinizing hormone-releasing hormone (LHRH) secretion assumed to occur during puberty at night. This increase in LHRH secretion does not require the presence of the gonads and is thought to be responsible for the nocturnal increase in LH secretion depicted in the lower panel. REM, rapid eye movement. (Redrawn from Boyar RM et al: N Engl J Med 287:583, 1972.)

cyclicity. Episodic increases in LH levels (ovulatory spikes) have occasionally been recorded in girls within several months of the first menstruation. A short rise in progesterone levels following these LH peaks has also been found in these girls, suggesting that a corpus luteum is formed after ovulation but that the luteal phase is shortened. Accordingly, the infertility of the young adolescent girl may be related either to anovulatory cycles or to inadequate corpus luteum function.

The rising levels of plasma gonadotropins stimulate the ovary to produce increasing amounts of estradiol. Estradiol is responsible for the development of secondary sexual characteristics, that is, growth and development of the breasts and reproductive organs, fat redistribution (hips, breasts), and bone maturation. Using an ultrasensitive assay for estradiol, evidence has been provided that in childhood, plasma estradiol levels, though very low, are higher in girls than in boys. This difference may contribute to the earlier onset of puberty in girls. As puberty approaches, plasma estradiol levels fluctuate widely, probably reflecting successive waves of follicular development that fail to reach the ovulatory stage. The uterine endometrium is affected by these changes and undergoes cycles of proliferation and regression until a point is reached when substantial growth occurs so that withdrawal of estrogen results in the first menstruation. This is called *menarche*. Plasma testosterone levels also increase at puberty, although not as markedly as in boys. In contrast, plasma progesterone remains at low levels, even if secondary sexual characteristics have appeared. A rise in progesterone after menarche indicates, in general, that ovulation has occurred.

Menarche occurs at an average of 12 years of age. However, the first ovulation does not take place until 6–9 months after menarche because the positive feedback mechanism of estrogen is not developed. A single estrogen injection to premenarchial subjects fails to induce LH release. However, experiments with rhesus monkeys have shown that if *priming* doses of estradiol are given, the surge mechanism can be activated shortly after menarche.

Somatic Changes

Somatic changes during puberty include a rapid general increase in the growth rate of skeleton, muscles, and viscera, known as the *adolescent growth spurt,* a sex-specific increase in hip width and changes in body composition caused by an increase in muscle and in fat tissue, the latter being more pronounced in girls than in boys. The large increase in fat (120%) between growth spurt initiation and menarche in both early- and late-maturing girls may have a secondary significance. The mean fat for both early and late maturers at menarche is about 11 kg, which is equivalent to 99,000 calories. The number of calories estimated to sustain a pregnancy is 80,000. Thus, although speculative, it is possible that one of the main functions of the adolescent growth spurt in females might be the storage of energy to sustain pregnancy and lactation. Figure 9-9 shows schematically the sequence of events at

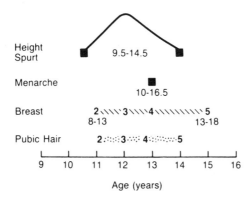

Fig. 9-9 Schematic sequence of somatic events during female puberty. The age range at which each event occurs is indicated at the beginning and end of each event. The numbers 2–5 correspond to the different stages of puberty as defined by Tanner. (Redrawn from Tanner JM: In: *The Control of the Onset of Puberty,* MM Grumbach, GD Grave, and FE Mayer, eds., Wiley, New York, p. 460, 1974, with permission.)

puberty in females. The development of the breasts is known as *thelarche,* and the growth of axillary and pubic hair is known as *pubarche.*

The age at which these morphological changes occur varies from individual to individual. A classification that is widely used by clinicians to assess the normalcy of pubertal progression divides the pubertal process into five stages based on the degree of breast development, age at peak velocity of linear growth, and growth and distribution of pubic hair.

In addition to estrogens and androgens, GH may play a role in inducing pubertal growth. Plasma GH levels are low but pulsatile in peripubertal subjects. Immediately on falling asleep, there is an increase in GH release; usually several episodes of GH secretion can be detected during the sleep period. The magnitude of these episodes reaches a maximum in advanced puberty.

Metabolic Signals

Earlier studies demonstrated that the mean weight of girls at the beginning of the adolescent growth spurt (around 30 kg), at the time of peak velocity of weight gain (around 39 kg), and at menarche (around 47 kg) is very similar in early- and late-maturing girls. This led to the notion that the attainment of a critical weight causes a change in metabolic rate per unit mass (or per unit of surface area), which, in turn, may affect hypothalamic ovarian feedback by decreasing the sensitivity of the hypothalamus to gonadal steroids so that gonadotropin release increases, triggering the pubertal process.

The hypothesis of a critical weight was later modified to state that a particular ratio of fat to lean mass is normally necessary for puberty and the maintenance of female reproductive ability. Experiments conducted to test this hypothesis did not confirm it, but suggested that there may be metabolic signals used by peripheral tissues to influence the time of puberty. Two of these signals have been identified, namely, IGF-I and leptin, the former produced mainly in the liver, the latter by white adipose tissue. Although both peptides can act centrally to stimulate LHRH release and to accelerate the initiation of puberty, neither appears to initiate the pubertal process in the absence of other hormonal changes, an activity that seems essential for a substance to be considered a metabolic trigger of puberty.

In addition, experiments with nonhuman primates have demonstrated that LH pulsatile release is dramatically decreased by underfeeding and activated by administration of calorie-rich food, suggesting that caloric intake may be a mechanism by which the diet could affect the timing and/or progression of puberty. It seems clear that undernutrition delays the onset of puberty and disrupts menstrual cyclicity.

Mechanisms Involved in the Regulation of the Onset of Puberty (Fig. 9-10)

Change in the Setpoint of the Negative Feedback Mechanism. As previously discussed, the negative feedback of gonadal steroids is poorly developed during fetal life but becomes fully operative during childhood. Several years ago, from experiments in rats, the concept was advanced that a decrease in hypothalamic sensitivity to circulating sex steroids (*resetting of the gonadostat*) results in the increased gonadotropin secretion seen at puberty. It is now clear that this event is not the cause of puberty but rather a consequence of it.

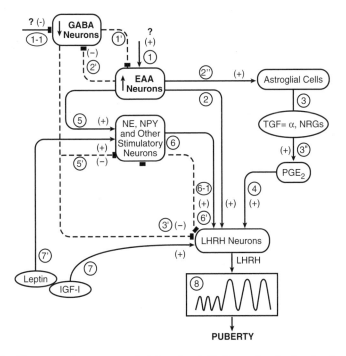

Fig. 9-10 The central events underlying the initiation of puberty. An increase in episodic luteinizing hormone-releasing hormone (LHRH) secretion is activated by an integrative mechanism involving both neuron-to neuron and glia-to-neuron communication processes. The neuron-to-neuron (transsynaptic) component involves the simultaneous activation of excitatory transsynaptic inputs and a reduction in inhibitory inputs to LHRH neurons. The main excitatory transsynaptic input affecting LHRH release is postulated to be provided by neurons that use excitatory amino acids (EAA) as neurotransmitters. Noradrenergic (NE)- and neuropeptide Y (NPY)–containing neurons provide a complementary facilitatory input to the LHRH neuronal network. The chief inhibitory neuronal input restraining LHRH release is provided by GABAergic neurons (γ-aminobutyric acid, GABA). The glia-to-neuron component of the process involves the production of the epidermal growth factor (EGF)-related peptides, transforming growth factor-α (TGF-α) and neuregulins (NRGs), by astroglial cells and the stimulatory effect of these peptides on the glial production of neuroactive substances, such as prostaglandin E_2, which act directly on LHRH neurons to elicit LHRH secretion. Current evidence suggest that an increase in EAA neurotransmission (1) may be primarily responsible for the pubertal activation of pulsatile LHRH secretion in the rat, whereas a decrease in inhibitory GABAergic tone (1-1) may be the initial transsynaptic event underlying the process in the rhesus monkey. Evidence collected in rodents indicates that EAA can act directly on LHRH neurons (2) to enhance LHRH release and on GABA neurons (2') to inhibit GABA neurotransmission. It is also possible, however, that a primary decrease in GABA release (1') triggers the pubertal increase in EAA neurotransmission. Excitatory amino acids acting on astroglial cells (2") appear to facilitate the glial production of TGF-α/NRGs (3). While the decrease in GABA transmission begins to release LHRH neurons from GABAergic inhibitory control (3'), the increased production of EGF-related glial peptides stimulates the formation of prostaglandin E_2 (3"), which acts directly on LHRH neurons to elicit LHRH release (4), amplifying the stimulatory effect of EAA (2) and magnifying the loss of GABAergic inhibitory control (3').

(Figure legend continues on next page)

Fig. 9-10 continued   On the initiation of these changes, a further increase in EAA stimulation (5) and a further decrease in GABAergic inhibitory tone (5') lead to activation of NE and NPYneuronal systems (6). Both NE and NPY would then contribute to the progression of the pubertal process by stimulating LHRH secretion (6'). There is also evidence that an inhibitory NPY influence (6-1) on LHRH release is lifted at the end of juvenile development and thus contributes to the initiation of the pubertal process. The metabolic signals, leptin and insulin-like growth factor-I (IGF-I), further the process by stimulating LHRH secretion either directly (7) or via functionally connected neuronal networks (7'). The resulting increase in pulsatile LHRH secretion (8) then results in the initiation of puberty. (−), inhibition; (+), stimulation. (Modified from Ojeda SR and Bilger M: In: *Neuroendocrinology in Physiology and Medicine,* PM Conn and ME Freeman, eds., Humana Press, Totowa, NJ, p. 218, 1999, with permission.)

Activation of the Hypothalamic Pulse Generator.   As discussed above, pulsatile release of LH becomes more prominent at the end of childhood. If juvenile monkeys are treated with LHRH delivered in a pulsatile manner for several weeks, they show repetitive, normal ovulatory cycles. These cycles cease on removal of the LHRH treatment. Direct measurement of LHRH released from the mediam eminence of the hypothalamus in nonhuman primates demonstrated that LHRH secretion does indeed increase as puberty approaches. These and other observations have led to the concept that the onset of puberty is determined by the enhancement of endogenous pulsatile LHRH release (Fig. 9-10). Such activation drives the pituitary to secrete larger amounts of LH, particularly during sleep, and puberty is initiated.

The pubertal activation of LHRH release appears to be brought about by the coordinated interplay of transsynaptic inputs and glial influences on LHRH neurons. According to this concept, LHRH release increases as a consequence of an activation of stimulatory transsynaptic inputs (glutamate, but also NE and NPY), a decrease in GABA inhibition, and a growth factor–dependent increase in glial production of neuroactive substances such as prostaglandins.

Another factor that operates at the time of puberty is enhanced pituitary responsiveness to LHRH. The release of LH following the administration of LHRH is minimal in prepubertal children but increases markedly at puberty and is even greater in adult males. There is a sex difference in the rise of serum FSH: prepubertal and pubertal females release more FSH than do males at all stages of sexual maturation.

This increased gonadotropin response to LHRH is probably due to the elevated circulating levels of gonadal and adrenal steroids present at that time. As the response can be elicited before the development of secondary sex characteristics in both girls and boys, this change in pituitary responsiveness probably plays an important role in the progress of the pubertal process.

The Adrenal Gland and Puberty

Circulating levels of aromatizable androgens such as dehydroepiandrosterone and its sulfate, and androstenedione, are mostly of adrenal origin. Their concentrations in the bloodstream begin to increase at about 7–8 years of age, reaching maximum values by ages 13–15. This phenomenon is called *adrenarche*. It begins before the rise in gonadotropin secretion. Adrenal androgens are responsible to a significant extent for the growth of pubic and axillary hair; however, they do not appear to play a decisive role in determining the initiation of puberty. Premature adrenarche is not associated with advancement of gonadarche (i.e., the activation of the hypothalamic–pituitary–gonadal axis). Conversely, gonadarche occurs in the absence of adrenarche in children with chronic primary adrenal insufficiency and in children with true idiopathic precocious puberty. It is evident, therefore, that adrenarche and gonadarche are separately controlled albeit temporally associated phenomena.

Reproductive Cyclicity (Fig. 9-11)

This reproductive phase has already been discussed. Basically it entails the orderly repetition of the menstrual cycle, a sequence that may be interrupted by pregnancy. It begins with the first ovulation at puberty and extends on average to about 50 years of age.

Menopause

Menopause can be defined as the time at which the final menstrual bleeding occurs. Like *puberty,* however, the term *menopause* is used in a much broader sense and describes a period of the female climacteric during which reproductive cyclicity gradually disappears. The menstrual cycles become irregular, and the intervals between menses become shorter because of a reduction in the duration of the follicular phase.

Menopause is regarded as the result of the loss of ovarian function. There is an exhaustion of ovarian follicles, mainly due to the repeated cycles of atresia that occur twice in every menstrual cycle. Histologically, the stroma hypertrophies and primordial follicles disappear. Ovarian weight declines as menopause progresses, and plasma gonadotropin levels increase when estradiol production falls as follicles fail to mature (Fig. 9-11). The loss of estrogen is accompanied by atrophic changes of the breasts, uterus, and vagina, vasomotor instability (hot flashes), and, in many instances, osteoporosis.

The occurrence of hot flashes is temporally related to pulses of LH secretion. Because such pulses appear to be the consequence of an increase in noradrenergic impulses arriving at hypothalamic LHRH neurons, the inference has been made that hot flashes are caused by a change in hypothalamic noradrenergic activity.

THE MAMMARY GLAND

Lactation is an evolutionarily conserved mammalian physiological function. The offspring of placental mammals are entirely dependent in early postnatal life on nutrients provided by the mother through the secretion of milk. The mammary gland replaces the nourishing function of the placenta after birth.

Development and Hormonal Control

During early fetal development, epithelial cells cluster in areas that will later give rise to the areola of the breast and proliferate to form cord-like structures that penetrate the underlying mesenchyme. These epithelial cords give origin to the duct

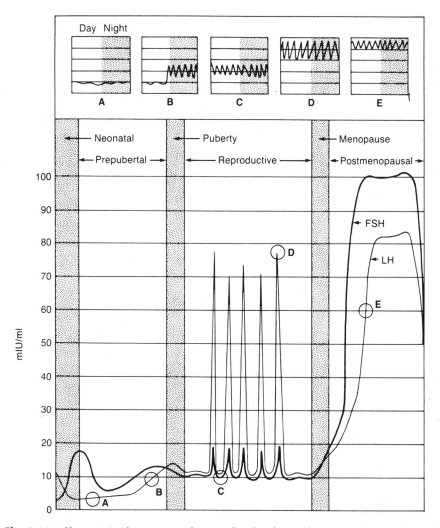

Fig. 9-11   Changes in the pattern of serum levels of gonadotropins during postnatal life in the human female. During neonatal and prepubertal phases, follicle-stimulating hormone (FSH) levels are greater than luteinizing hormone (LH) levels and pulsatile LH secretion is minimal (A). As puberty approaches, LH secretion increases during sleep (B). When puberty is completed, LH secretion is greater than FSH secretion (C) and cyclic gonadotropin release occurs (D). At menopause, cyclic gonadotropin release ceases (E) and plasma levels of both gonadotropins increase. (Redrawn from Yen SSC: In: *Neuroendocrinology,* DT Krieger and JC Hughes, eds., Sinauer, Sunderland, MA, p. 260, 1980, with permission.)

system of the mammary gland that converges into a single ampulla that opens to the nipple. During the last part of gestation, the distal portion of the fetal ducts develops into alveolar structures that at birth are able to secrete. This secretion, known as *witch's milk,* can be observed in most infants by the first week of postnatal life and lasts for 4–6 weeks. Once the effect of placental steroids subsides, the secretory alveoli regress so that in children only scattered ducts without alveoli are observed embedded in stromal tissue.

As previously indicated, when estrogen secretion increases at puberty, breast development is markedly stimulated. When the ovulatory cycles begin and the corpus luteum secretes progesterone, the estrogen-dependent branching and lengthening of the ducts are enhanced and alveolar development is accelerated.

During pregnancy the mammary gland undergoes further growth under the concerted influence of estrogen, progesterone, glucocorticoids, prolactin, and human placental lactogen (hPL). The duct system develops markedly, the alveoli form clusters called *lobules,* and their epithelial cells acquire vacuoles indicative of intense secretory activity. Actual secretion of milk (lactation) does not occur, however, until after birth due to an inhibitory effect of placental estrogen and progesterone. Following delivery of the placenta, estrogen and progesterone levels drop precipitously and secretion of milk begins.

A pituitary hormone that plays a critical role in the process of breast development during pregnancy is prolactin. In combination with estrogen, prolactin causes primarily ductal but also lobuloalveolar growth. In the presence of progesterone its effect on alveolar growth is greatly enhanced. Prolactin not only induces cell proliferation but also controls the synthesis of key components of milk such as casein and α-lactoalbumin. Prolactin (PRL) initiates its biological actions by binding to a membrane-anchored receptor. The PRL receptor shows structural similarity to the GH receptor; it belongs to the class 1 cytokine receptor superfamily, which also includes the receptors for leukemia-inhibiting factor, granulocyte colony-stimulating factor, leptin, and erythropoietin, among others. The PRL receptor has a single transmembrane domain encoded by an mRNA transcript that can be alternatively spliced to produce multiple isoforms, referred to as *long, intermediate,* and *short,* according to their size. Binding of PRL to its receptor results in phosphorylation of the receptor itself and of several other cellular proteins. Upon PRL binding, the receptor interacts with JAK2, a member of a family of protein tyrosine kinases known as *JAK kinases,* which transmit cytokine-initiated signals into the cell. Activation of JAK2 occurs within 1 minute of PRL stimulation and leads to receptor tyrosine phosphorylation. The phosphorylated tyrosines recruit a cytoplasmic protein known as Stat 5, which become part of the PRL receptor–JAK2 kinase complex and is phosphorylated by the kinase. The phosphorylated Stat protein is then released and dimerizes with other Stat molecules, and the dimer is translocated into the nucleus, where it binds to the DNA to activate the transcription of PRL-responsive genes. Mice lacking the *PRL* gene fail to become pregnant, have reduced ovulation and stunted follicular development, and are unable to sustain preimplantation development. Heterozygotic animals are unable to lactate after the first, but not after subsequent, pregnancies, possibly because of the activation of compensatory mechanisms. One of the hormones that may replace PRL under these conditions is GH.

Growth hormone produced by the anterior pituitary shares many of the actions of PRL, and, in fact, is as effective as PRL in inducing duct development. Nevertheless, its presence is not essential for breast development or lactation to occur. The human placenta produces hPL, which has actions similar to those of GH.

Insulin and glucocorticoids are also required for most phases of breast development. Their function, however, is permissive rather than regulatory in nature.

Lactation

Lactation can be divided into four stages: (*1*) milk synthesis, which is initiated during the last part of pregnancy by PRL and hPL action; (*2*) lactogenesis, which comprises the synthesis of milk by the alveolar cells and its secretion into the alveolar lumen—it is initiated by the loss of placental steroids after birth; (*3*) galactopoiesis, or maintenance of established lactation, which is mainly controlled by PRL, whose release increases because of suckling by the infant; and (*4*) milk ejection, which is controlled by the neurohypophyseal hormone oxytocin and comprises the passage of milk from the alveolar lumen to the duct system, its collection in the ampulla and larger ducts, and its delivery to the infant (see below).

Oxytocin and PRL play fundamental roles in the maintenance and dynamics of lactation. The act of nursing itself is a powerful stimulus for oxytocin release. Sensory impulses arising from the nipple travel via the spinal cord through a multisynaptic pathway to the hypothalamic neurons that produce oxytocin and evoke its release. Oxytocin then reaches the mammary gland via the bloodstream and induces the contraction of the myoepithelial cells that surround the alveoli and the ducts. Contraction of these cells mobilizes milk from the alveoli and duct system to the nipple, producing the sensation of *milk let-down* in the mother. Oxytocin release is also induced by audiovisual stimuli, such as seeing the baby or hearing its cry, or even by the anticipation of nursing.

Prolactin secretion is stimulated by suckling (Fig. 9-12) but not by audiovisual or psychological stimuli. Throughout the lactational period, plasma PRL levels vary

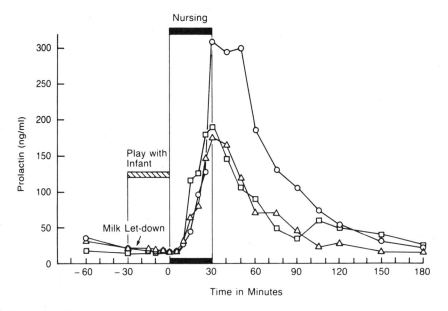

Fig. 9-12 Changes in plasma prolactin levels during anticipation of nursing and nursing itself in women. The women played with their infants for 30 minutes before suckling began. Milk let-down, which results from an action of oxytocin on the breast, occurred before suckling. (Redrawn from Noel GL et al: J Clin Endocrinol Metab 38:416, 1974, with permission.)

as follows: basal values are quite high during the first few weeks postpartum, and each nursing episode further elevates the levels. After about 2 months of lactation, basal PRL levels return to normal (10–20 ng/ml), but nursing is still able to elicit a rise in PRL levels. Such a response persists for many months following birth. It is clear that episodes of PRL secretion are important for the maintenance of lactation, as PRL-inhibiting drugs such as ergot alkaloids (see below) result in cessation of lactation.

The mechanism by which nursing increases PRL release involves both secretion of PRL-releasing substances from the hypothalamus into the portal vasculature (see Chapter 6) and suppression of DA release from the tuberoinfundibular dopaminergic neuronal system. Because DA itself is a PRL-inhibiting factor, suppression of its release enhances the secretion of PRL.

Major Milk Components

The major milk proteins are casein, α-lactalbumin, and β-lactoglobulin. The protein content in the human colostrum (the first milk secreted at parturition) is 2.7 g/dl compared to 1.2 g/dl in mature milk. The major carbohydrate is lactose (5.3 g/dl in the colostrum, 6.8 g/dl in mature milk). Milk is also rich in fat (2.9 vs. 3.8 g/dl) and contains many other substances including minerals (calcium, magnesium, phosphorus, iron), electrolytes (chloride, potassium, sodium), all vitamins with the exception of vitamin B_{12}, iron-binding proteins (transferrin), immunoglobulins (IgMs, IgEs, and particularly IgAs), and growth factors such as EGF and IGF-I.

CLINICAL ASSESSMENT OF REPRODUCTIVE FUNCTION

A thorough history and physical examination are essential in the assessment of female reproductive function. Valuable information includes the age of first menstruation, the presence of secondary sexual characteristics such as breast development, and the presence of regular, cyclic menses. The last implies that ovulation is occurring, that the secretion of gonadotropins and ovarian steroids is adequate, and that the outflow reproductive tract is intact. Should the symptoms be ambiguous, both plasma gonadotropin and steroid concentrations can be determined by radioimmunoassay.

As stated in Chapter 10, a reasonable assessment of plasma gonadotropin values can be obtained by drawing multiple blood samples every 20 minutes for 2 hours and pooling the samples to obtain a mean value. This is usually not necessary in women. There are cases (e.g., precocious puberty and delayed puberty), however, in which each blood sample must be analyzed individually, and the sequential sampling needs to be extended for several hours.

Plasma estradiol levels can also be measured by sensitive immunoassays, but because of the normal variations in circulating levels of the steroid during the menstrual cycle, it is preferable to use other, less direct but more informative tests. For example, adequate estrogen production can be inferred by the presence of a moist vagina and a copious, clear cervical mucus that shows a high degree of elasticity on stretching and an arborization (ferning) pattern on spreading on a glass slide. A test commonly used to assess the estrogen status is the progesterone withdrawal test. Administration of progesterone followed by menstrual bleeding on termination of the treatment is indicative of adequate estrogen priming to allow the withdrawal bleeding.

The occurrence of ovulation can be assessed by measuring plasma progesterone by radioimmunoassay. A functional test that can be employed to assess the progesterone status is the increase in basal body temperature associated with normal luteal function. If such an increase occurs and is maintained for 2 weeks, progesterone secretion and corpus luteum function can be considered to be adequate.

One very important diagnosis is that of pregnancy. Again, the history and physical examination are critical for a correct diagnosis. In this case, however, the laboratory measurement of the placental product hCG is recommended because of its reliability and sensitivity.

DERANGED REPRODUCTIVE FUNCTION

There are many forms of reproductive dysfunction. Only the most common one will be considered.

Sexual Precocity and Delayed Puberty

Early advent of sexual maturity can be isosexual, that is, feminization in girls and virilization in boys, or heterosexual, that is, feminization in boys and virilization in girls.

Isosexual Precocity

Isosexual precocity can be manifested in three forms: true precocious puberty, precocious pseudopuberty, and incomplete isosexual precocity.

True precocious puberty is characterized by an early but normal sequence of pubertal development, including the initiation of menstrual cycles in girls. In 90% of cases the factors determining the early advent of sexual maturation are unknown; the syndrome is called *constitutional* or *idiopathic precocious puberty.* Prompt treatment is essential and usually relies on the use of LHRH agonists. These analogs act by down-regulating pituitary LHRH receptors and desensitizing the gland to LHRH.

Precocious pseudopuberty is defined as a dysfunction in which girls feminize but fail to ovulate. In general, precocious pseudopuberty is caused by an enhanced secretion of estradiol, which in most cases originates from granulosa-theca cell tumors of the ovary. These tumors can be detected by rectoabdominal examination, sonography, or laparoscopy.

Incomplete isosexual precocity is defined as the premature development of a single clinical pubertal event. This event may be breast enlargement before the age of 7, known as *premature thelarche,* or the appearance of axillary and pubic hair, known as *premature pubarche.* The former is thought to be caused by a transient increase in estrogen levels or to a heightened breast sensitivity to normal plasma levels of estrogen. The latter is caused by a premature increase in androgens of adrenal origin. Neither syndrome requires treatment because in both cases these changes are transient and often regress, the patient entering puberty at the normal age.

Heterosexual Precocity

Heterosexual precocity of girls—that is, virilization—is usually caused by congenital adrenal hyperplasia (see Chapter 8) or androgen-secreting tumors of the ovary or adrenal.

Delayed Puberty

Delayed puberty is much less common in girls than in boys. The onset of puberty may be regarded as delayed if breast development has not begun by age 13. The progression of puberty is regarded as delayed if menses have not occurred 5 years after the onset of breast development. Delayed puberty may be due to disorders of the ovary or the hypothalamic–pituitary unit. In the former case, gonadotropin levels are elevated because of the absence or insufficiency of steroid secretion. The syndrome is called *hypergonadotropic hypogonadism;* the most common form in girls is gonadal dysgenesis, known as *Turner syndrome* (see Chapter 8). The term *hypogonadotropic hypogonadism* is applied to disorders of the hypothalamic–pituitary unit that result in decreased secretion of gonadotropins. These conditions must be differentiated from a constitutional delay in the onset of puberty that is characterized by a pattern of slow maturation but an otherwise normal attainment of puberty at a late age. Patients with hypogonadotropic hypogonadism do not reach puberty owing to their inability to produce gonadotropins. Because failure of gonadotropin secretion is usually the only pituitary hormone deficiency observed in these patients, the syndrome is termed *isolated gonadotropin deficiency;* it is the result of defective synthesis or release of hypothalamic LHRH or the absence of LHRH neurons in the hypothalamus (see also Chapter 10).

Abnormal Uterine Bleeding

Abnormal uterine bleeding is a disorder of the menstrual cycle that may be associated with either ovulatory or anovulatory cycles. In the first case, abnormal bleeding may occur in the presence of regular cycles, but it deviates from normal menstruation because it is too abundant and prolonged (hypermenorrhea) or too light and interrupted (hypomenorrhea). Hypermenorrhea may be caused by polyps, submucus myomas, or adenomyosis of the uterus. Hypomenorrhea may result from obstruction of the uterine cervical lumen. Bleeding may also occur between normal menstruations and is usually due to cervical and/or endometrial lesions.

Uterine bleeding associated with anovulatory cycles is painless bleeding that is unpredictable with respect to onset, amount, and duration. The syndrome is called *dysfunctional uterine bleeding* and is caused by alterations of ovarian function rather than by abnormalities of the uterus. As previously discussed, the sequential changes in estradiol and progesterone secretion during the menstrual cycle determine both the cyclic pattern of endometrial activity and the onset of menses on their withdrawal.

Dysfunctional uterine bleeding may result from three different mechanisms. (*1*) Estrogen withdrawal bleeding results from interruption of ovarian estrogen production in the absence of progesterone. For example, if estrogen is given to a postmenopausal woman and the treatment is then interrupted, bleeding will occur. (2) Estrogen breakthrough bleeding occurs when the corpus luteum fails to form (or function), so that progesterone levels are low and the uterus is chronically exposed to continuous estrogen. It is the most common type of dysfunctional uterine bleeding. (3) Progesterone breakthrough bleeding occurs when the progesterone/estrogen ratio to which the endometrium is exposed is abnormally high, as in women taking continuous progesterone-only contraceptives (see below).

Amenorrhea

Amenorrhea is the failure to menstruate. It may be classified as primary amenorrhea (i.e., complete absence of menses) or secondary amenorrhea (i.e., menses that occurred but then ceased). Operationally, amenorrhea has been defined as the failure of menarche by age 16, irrespective of the presence of secondary sexual characteristics, or the absence of menstruation for 6 months in a woman with previous periodic menses.

Amenorrhea may result from anatomical defects (e.g., pseudohermaphroditism, congenital defects of the vagina, imperforate hymen), ovarian failure (the most frequent being gonadal dysgenesis in which the ovary does not develop normally), or chronic anovulation with or without estrogen present. More than 80% of all amenorrhea is the result of chronic anovulation. This disorder is characterized by the failure to ovulate spontaneously with the possibility of ovulating with therapy. In the most common type of chronic anovulation, estrogen is present. Women with this condition have withdrawal bleeding after progesterone administration, indicating the prior presence of estrogen. However, most of the estrogen produced is estrone formed by peripheral aromatization of androstenedione. In most cases the ovaries are sclerotic and show a thick capsule, multiple follicular cysts, and hyperplastic thecal and stromal tissue. The disorder is known as *polycystic ovarian disease* and is usually characterized by increased plasma levels of androgens, hirsutism, obesity, and amenorrhea. Its etiology is complex, but it may be caused by both a defect in pulsatile LH secretion and alterations in the ovarian microenvironment (e.g., growth factor dysfunction).

Galactorrhea

A common abnormality of breast function is galactorrhea—the persistent discharge of milk in the absence of parturition or beyond 6 months postpartum in a nonnursing mother. In most of these cases, plasma PRL levels are elevated, and imaging of the pituitary occasionally reveals the presence of microadenomas. Most of these patients suffer from reproductive malfunction ranging from ovulatory failure to amenorrhea—that is, failure to menstruate.

The discovery that ergot alkaloids such as bromocriptine are potent suppressors of PRL release provided a useful tool in the treatment of hyperprolactinemia. Bromocriptine treatment not only suppresses PRL secretion but often results in significant regression of the pituitary PRL-secreting tumor. Ergot alkaloids suppress PRL release because they are DA agonists.

Hirsutism

Hirsutism, or excessive growth of hair, is the result of an abnormally high production of androgens. The androgens may be produced by neoplastic tissue; in this case, the onset of hair growth is rapid. They may also have an adrenal origin in the absence of a tumor; in most such cases, the excessive androgen production results from heritable defects in adrenal steroidogenesis (congenital adrenal hyperplasia), which can occur as *late-onset* forms. An excess of circulating androgens may also result from intake of some drugs or steroids with androgenic capacity.

A more common cause of hirsutism, however, is ovarian hyperandrogenism and, in particular, polycystic ovarian disease. Its pubertal onset is associated with chronic anovulation.

The treatment of hirsutism depends on the source of excessive androgen production. If it is a tumor, the tumor should be removed. If it is the ovary, suppression of ovarian function is attempted by administering oral contraceptives; adrenal hyperfunction is reduced by suppressing ACTH secretion with dexamethasone.

FERTILITY CONTROL

There are several methods of contraception, including (*1*) natural rhythm, (*2*) withdrawal, (*3*) barriers such as condoms, foams, and diaphragms, (*4*) intrauterine devices (IUDs), (*5*) sterilization, (*6*) abortion, and (*7*) oral and subdermal steroid contraceptives.

The most effective preventive method is the use of oral and subdermal contraceptives. The least effective are the rhythm and withdrawal methods. Barrier methods are much more effective than the *natural* methods but not as efficient as IUDs, which have a success rate of more than 95%.

Use of an IUD, however, carries significantly greater health risks than barrier methods. It is believed that IUDs prevent pregnancy by inducing a chronic inflammation of the endometrium, which then becomes unable to allow implantation of the blastocyst. The most serious side effect of the IUD is pelvic infection.

Oral contraceptives are the most widely used method of fertility control. When properly used, their success rate is more than 99%. They are easy to administer, and in general the incidence of side effects is low. Oral contraceptives prevent pregnancy by inhibiting ovulation through suppression of gonadotropin secretion.

There are three types of oral contraceptive pills: a combination of estrogen–progestin, phasic estrogen–progestin, and progestin-only pills. The combination pill consists of a synthetic estrogen (mestranol or ethinyl estradiol) and a synthetic progestin (such as norethindrone or norgestrel). The pills are taken continuously for 21 days followed by 7 days of rest. During these 7 days the person may discontinue taking the pill altogether or—as some manufacturers recommend—take a placebo pill for 7 days. Phasic pills consist of different concentrations of estrogen plus progesterone, which vary throughout a 21-day treatment schedule followed by 7 days of placebo. Progesterone-only pills are taken continuously on a daily basis.

The ideal combination pill has the least amount of steroids necessary to prevent pregnancy but a sufficient amount to avoid breakthrough bleeding. Oral contraceptives are not free of side effects. Users of progesterone-only pills have a high incidence of breakthrough bleeding. Combination pills may in some patients increase the risk of deep vein thrombosis, pulmonary embolism, thromboembolic stroke, and hemorrhagic stroke. Because of the stimulatory effect of estrogen on liver protein synthesis, including the renin substrate angiotensinogen, use of contraceptive pills results in a small rise in blood pressure. In some women, however, hypertension may develop after several years of use. As previously indicated, estrogen increases both HDL and VLDL levels and decreases cholesterol and LDL concentrations. Progestins increase cholesterol and LDL levels and decrease HDL. However, their combination in pills usually has minimal effects in the low doses used today. In some women glucose tolerance changes, manifested by elevated plasma insulin and glucose levels after a glucose load. Because of all these possible side effects, oral contraceptives are contraindicated in women with diabetes mellitus, abnormal liver function tests, hypercholesterolemia, hypertension, or heavy smoking habits. Oral contraceptives do not appear to increase the incidence of uterine, cervix, breast, or ovarian cancer.

Although oral contraceptives are contraindicated in a small fraction of the population, they are the most reliable and effective method of birth control available to women throughout the world.

An alternative system of steroid administration is the subdermal implantation of the progestin levonorgestrel (Norplant). Implantation of six silicone capsules in the inside part of the lower arm provides continuous contraception for 5 years. The progestin acts by inhibiting ovulation. It may be used by women who cannot take estrogens or by women who cannot use any other form of contraception. The main problem with this system is the surgery it requires; it also causes irregular menstrual bleeding and headaches in some patients.

An alternative form of contraception that provides a safe and efficient means of abortion is the antiprogestin mifepristone (known as RU486). When RU486 administration is followed 48 hours later by prostaglandin $F_{2\alpha}$ given orally, intravaginally, or by injection, abortion occurs in almost 100% of the cases. Mifepristone in combination with prostaglandin $F_{2\alpha}$ can be used to induce abortion in case of fetal death or for the voluntary termination of pregnancy during the first trimester of pregnancy.

SUGGESTED READING

Bole-Feysot C, Goffin V, Edery M, and Binart N: Prolactin (PRL) and its receptor: actions, signal transduction pathways and phenotypes observed in PRL receptor knockout mice. Endocr Rev 19:225–268, 1998.

Buffet NC, Djakoure C, Maitre SC, and Bouchard P: Regulation of the human menstrual cycle. Front Neuroendocrinol 19:151–186, 1998.

Carr BR and Griffin JE: Fertility control and its complications. In: *Williams Textbook of Endocrinology,* 9th ed., JD Wilson, DW Foster, HM Kronenberg, and PR Larsen, eds., Saunders, Philadelphia, pp. 901–926, 1998.

DiZegera GS and Hodgen GD: Folliculogenesis in the primate ovarian cycle. Endocrinol Rev 2:27–49, 1981.

Fink G: Neuroendocrine regulation of pituitary function. In: *Neuroendocrinology in Physiology and Medicine,* PM Conn and ME Freeman, eds., Humana Press, Totowa, NJ, pp. 107–133, 1999.

Grumbach MM and Styne DM: Puberty: ontogeny, neuroendocrinology, physiology, and disorders. In: *Williams Textbook of Endocrinology,* 10th ed., PR Larsen, HM Kronenberg, S Melmed, and KS Polonsky, eds., Saunders, Philadelphia, pp. 1115–1286, 2003.

Hirshfield AN: Development of follicles in the mammalian ovary. Int Rev Cytol 124:43–101, 1991.

Kaipia A and Hsueh AJW: Regulation of ovarian follicle atresia. Annu Rev Physiol 59: 349–363, 1997.

Kellie AE: Structure and nomenclature. In: *Biochemistry of Steroid Hormones,* HLJ Makin, ed., Blackwell Scientific, Oxford, pp. 1–19, 1984.

Knobil E and Neill JD: *The Physiology of Reproduction,* Vols. 1 and 2, Raven Press, New York, 1994.

Matsuk MM, Burns KH, Viveiros MM, and Eppig JJ: Intercellular communication in the mammalian ovary: oocytes carry the conversation. Science 296:2178–2180, 2002.

Ojeda SR and Terasawa E: Neuroendocrine regulation of puberty. In: *Hormones, Brain and Behavior,* D Pfaff, ed., Academic Press-Elsevier Science (USA), San Diego, pp. 589–659, 2002.

Parker KL and Schimmer BP: Steroidogenic factor 1: a key determinant of endocrine development and function. Endocr Rev 18:361–377, 1997.

Richards JS: Perspective: the ovarian follicle—a perspective in 2001. Endocrinology 142: 2184–2193, 2001.

Schwartz NB: Neuroendocrine regulation of reproductive cyclicity. In: *Neuroendocrinology in Physiology and Medicine,* PM Conn and ME Freeman, eds., Humana Press, Totowa, NJ, pp. 135–145, 1999.

Stocco DM and Clark BJ: Regulation of the acute production of steroids in steroidogenic cells. Endocr Rev 17:221–244, 1996.

Tucker HA: Neuroendocrine regulation of lactation and milk ejection. In: *Neuroendocrinology in Physiology and Medicine,* PM Conn and ME Freeman, eds., Humana Press, Totowa, NJ, pp. 163–180, 1999.

10

Male Reproductive Function

JAMES E. GRIFFIN

Like the ovaries, the testes are the source of both germ cells and hormones important for reproductive function. The production of both sperm and steroid hormones is under complex feedback control by the hypothalamic–pituitary system.

STRUCTURAL ORGANIZATION OF THE TESTIS AND THE MALE REPRODUCTIVE TRACT

The testis consists of a network of tubules for the production and transport of sperm to the excretory ducts and a system of interstitial or Leydig cells that contain the enzymes necessary for the synthesis of androgens. The spermatogenic or seminiferous tubules are lined by a columnar epithelium composed of germ cells and Sertoli cells and surrounded by peritubular tissue made up of collagen, elastic fibers, and myofibrillar cells (Fig. 10-1). Tight junctions between Sertoli cells at a site between the spermatogonia and the primary spermatocyte form a diffusion barrier that divides the testis into two functional compartments, basal and adluminal. The basal compartment consists of the Leydig cells surrounding the tubule, the peritubular tissue, and the outer layer of the tubule containing the spermatogonia. The adluminal compartment consists of the inner two-thirds of the tubules including primary spermatocytes and more advanced stages of spermatogenesis. The base of the Sertoli cell is adjacent to the basement membrane of the spermatogenic tubule (Fig. 10-1), with the inner portion of the cell engulfing the developing germ cells so that spermatogenesis actually takes place within a network of Sertoli cell cytoplasm. The mechanism by which spermatogonia pass through the tight junctions between Sertoli cells to begin spermatogenesis is not known. The close proximity of the Leydig cell to the Sertoli cell with its embedded germ cells is thought to be critical for normal male reproductive function.

The seminiferous tubules empty into a network of ducts termed the *rete testis*. Sperm are then transported into a single duct, the epididymis. Anatomically, the epididymis can be divided into the caput, the corpus, and the cauda regions. The caput epididymidis consists of 8 to 12 ductuli efferentes, which have a larger lumen tapering to a narrower diameter at the junction of the ductus epididymidis. The diameter then remains constant through the corpus, or body, of the epididymis. In the

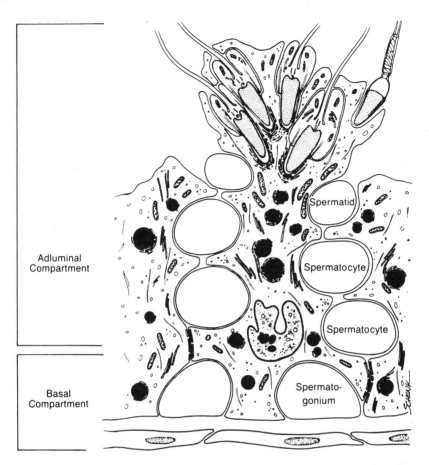

Fig. 10-1 Diagram of a Sertoli cell showing the relation between Sertoli cell cytoplasm and developing spermatocytes. (From Griffin JE and Wilson JD: In: *Williams Textbook of Endocrinology,* 8th ed., JD Wilson and DW Foster, eds., Saunders, Philadelphia, p. 802, 1992.)

cauda epididymis the diameter of the duct enlarges substantially, and the lumen acquires an irregular shape. The entire epididymal length is 5 to 6 cm. The epithelium exhibits regional differences of ciliated and nonciliated cells with evidence of a blood–epididymis barrier.

The vas deferens is a tubular structure about 30 to 35 cm in length beginning at the cauda epididymis and terminating in the ejaculatory duct near the prostate. In cross section there is a middle circular muscle layer surrounded by inner and outer longitudinal muscle layers. The pseudostratified epithelium lining the lumen of the vas deferens is composed of basal cells and three types of tall, thin columnar cells, all three of which have cilia.

The normal adult prostate weighs about 20 g. The gland is composed of alveoli that are lined with tall columnar secretory epithelial cells. The acini of these alveoli drain into the floor and lateral surfaces of the posterior urethra. The alveoli and the ducts draining them are embedded with a stroma of fibromuscular tissue. The seminal vesicles are paired pouches 4–5 cm long that join the ampulla of the distal vas deferens to form the ejaculatory ducts. The seminal vesicles are composed of tubular alevoli containing viscous secretions. The ejaculatory ducts pass through the prostate and terminate within the prostatic urethra.

ANDROGEN PHYSIOLOGY

Testosterone Formation

The pathway of testosterone synthesis from cholesterol and the conversion of testosterone to active androgen and estrogen metabolites are depicted in Figure 10-2. Cholesterol, the precursor steroid, can be either synthesized *de novo* or derived from the plasma pool by receptor-mediated endocytosis of low-density lipoprotein particles. In contrast to the ovary, which uses lipoprotein-derived cholesterol as its major source of substrate for steroid hormone formation (see Chapter 9), the testis appears to derive about half of the cholesterol required for testosterone formation from *de novo* synthesis. The rate-limiting process in testosterone synthesis is the delivery of cholesterol to the inner mitochondrial membrane by the steroidogenic acute regulatory protein (StAR) (see Chapter 9). This protein and the enzymes involved in testosterone formation are stimulated by luteinizing hormone (LH). Five enzymatic steps are involved in the conversion of cholesterol to testosterone: side-chain cleavage enzyme (CYP11A1), 3β-hydroxysteroid dehydrogenase 2 (3β-HSD2), 17α-hydroxylase (CYP17), 17,20-lyase (CYP17), and 17β-hydroxysteroid dehydrogenase 3 (17β-HSD3). The initial reaction in the process is the side-chain cleavage of cholesterol in mitochondria to form pregnenolone. The remaining four enzymes in the pathway of testosterone synthesis are located in the microsomes. The 3β-hydroxysteroid dehydrogenase–isomerase enzyme complex oxidizes the A ring of the steroid to the D4-3-keto configuration. Evidence indicates that the 17α-hydroxylase and 17,20-lyase activities are accomplished by a single cytochrome P450 enzyme, CYP17. Whereas the first four enzymatic activities in the pathway of testosterone synthesis are also common to the adrenals, the 17β-hydroxysteroid dehydrogenase activity is present primarily in the testes.

Although testosterone is the major secretory product of the testis, some of the precursors in the pathway, as well as small amounts of dihydrotestosterone and estradiol, are also directly secreted by the testis. The major sites of formation of dihydrotestosterone and estradiol are androgen target tissues and adipose tissue, respectively (see below). Concentrations of testosterone in testicular lymph and testicular venous blood are similar; however, because of its greater flow, the major route of testosterone secretion is via the spermatic vein. About 25 mg of testosterone is present in the normal testes, so that the total hormone content must turn over several hundred times each day to provide the 5–10 mg of testosterone secreted daily.

Testosterone Transport and Tissue Delivery

Testosterone circulates in the plasma largely bound to plasma proteins, primarily albumin and sex hormone-binding globulin (SHBG, also called *testosterone-*

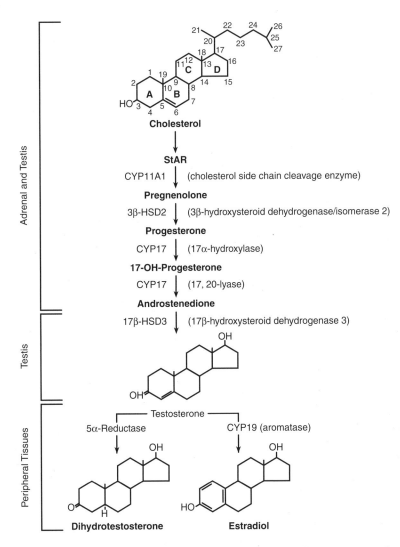

Fig. 10-2 Pathway of testosterone formation in the testis and the conversion of testosterone to active metabolites in peripheral tissues. (Redrawn from Griffin JE and Wilson JD: Disorders of the testes. In: *Harrison's Principles of Internal Medicine*, 15th ed., E Braunwald, AS Fauci, DL Kasper, SL Hauser, DL Longo, and JL Jameson, eds., McGraw-Hill, New York, p. 2144, 2001.)

binding globulin [TeBG]). Plasma SHBG and its testicular counterpart, androgen-binding protein (ABP), have an identical primary structure and are encoded by the same gene on chromosome 17. Sex hormone-binding globulin is a β-globulin homodimer with a size of 95,000 Da containing 30% carbohydrate. It has sequence homology to the coagulation factor protein S, laminin, and the growth arrest–specific gene 6 (*GAS6*). The unliganded SHBG can apparently interact with a cell surface receptor.

In normal men, only about 2% of testosterone is unbound in *in vitro* tests of peripheral blood, whereas 44% is bound to SHBG and 54% is bound to albumin and other proteins. Albumin has about 1000-fold lower affinity for testosterone than does SHBG, but albumin has an approximately 1000-fold greater binding capacity than does SHBG, so that the capacity 3 affinity product is similar. The proportion of testosterone (or estradiol) bound to the SHBG fraction in serum is directly proportional to the SHBG concentration. As discussed in Chapter 5, we now know that debinding of steroid hormones occurs in the microcirculation *in vivo* and that tissue availability of steroid hormones is greater than the *free* fraction measured *in vitro*. The amount of hormone available for entry into cells depends on the given organ as a function of capillary transit time, dissociation rate from the given binding protein, and endothelial membrane permeability. In studies of *in vivo* tissue delivery, nearly all of the albumin-bound testosterone is available for brain uptake, while the SHBG-bound testosterone is not significantly transported into the brain. (Brain is used as a representative nonhepatic organ.) Although capillary transit time in liver is longer than in brain, it is still short in relation to the half-time of dissociation from SHBG so that testosterone available for transport into hepatocytes is similar to that in brain or about 40%–50% of the total plasma testosterone in normal men (i.e., the free plus the albumin-bound fraction). In contrast, because estradiol dissociates more rapidly from SHBG, both albumin-bound and SHBG-bound estradiol are available for transport into liver cells.

This difference between testosterone and estradiol delivery to certain tissues from SHBG increases the significance of changes in SHBG levels. The SHBG levels in men are one-third to one-half those in women, and they decrease from the prepubertal level to the lower level in normal adult men as a result of sexual maturation and the associated testosterone secretion. Decreased SHBG levels occur in hypothyroidism, and thyroid hormone excess increases SHBG levels, possibly because of increased estrogen formation. (The increased estrogen levels of normal pregnancy increase the SHBG levels by 5- to 10-fold.) In men with an intact hypothalamic–pituitary–testicular axis, increases or decreases in SHBG levels do not affect tissue delivery of testosterone in the steady state because of temporary compensatory changes in testosterone formation. However, as the level of plasma estradiol is not directly regulated in men (see below), changes in SHBG levels may have a more profound effect on estradiol tissue delivery. Because SHBG binds to estradiol less avidly than testosterone or dihydrotestosterone, increases in SHBG amplify the amount of estradiol cleared by the liver relative to the amount of testosterone. For example, increases in SHBG cause decreased hepatic clearance of testosterone but have no effect on the hepatic clearance of estradiol. Thus, even in normal men, changes in SHBG levels can produce alterations in the ratios of androgens to estrogens that persist even when androgen levels themselves are not permanently altered.

Metabolism of Androgens

Testosterone and its metabolites are excreted primarily in the urine. About half of the daily turnover is recovered in the form of urinary 17-ketosteroids (androsterone and etiocholanolone) and the other half in polar metabolites (diols, triols, and conjugates). These excretory metabolites are thought to be largely inactive. A small fraction of testosterone metabolism is initially to two types of active metabolites, which in turn mediate many androgen actions. These metabolites are formed in peripheral tissues, and in this regard testosterone serves as a prohormone (Fig. 10-2). The first category of active metabolites is 5α-reduced steroids, primarily dihydrotestosterone, that mediate many androgen actions in target tissues. The second category of active testosterone metabolites is estrogens formed by the aromatization of androgens in a number of peripheral tissues. Estrogens in some instances act in concert with androgen to affect physiological processes, but they may also exert independent effects or oppose the actions of androgens. Each of these reactions to form active metabolites (5α-reduction and aromatization) is physiologically irreversible; furthermore, 5α-reduced androgens cannot be converted to estrogens. Thus, physiological actions of testosterone are the result of the combined effects of testosterone itself plus those of estrogen and the active androgen metabolites. In some instances these metabolites are active only in the tissues in which they are formed, whereas in other cases the 5α-reduced and estrogen metabolites reenter the circulation to act in other tissues.

5α-Reductase accepts a number of Δ^4-3-ketosteroids as substrate and requires reduced nicotinamide adenine dinucleotide phosphate (NADPH) as cofactor. There are two steroid 5α-reductase isozymes. Enzyme 1 is encoded by a gene on chromosome 5, and enzyme 2 is encoded by a gene on chromosome 2. 5α-Reductase has a distinct tissue localization, with the most activity found in the accessory organs of reproduction, liver, and skin. In skin the highest activity is in the genital skin, but hair follicles from all anatomical sites contain the enzyme. 5α-Reductase 2 has a lower K_m for testosterone and is primarily localized in androgen target tissues. In normal men, about 6%–8% of the total testosterone produced is metabolized to dihydrotestosterone by 5α-reductase. Testosterone can also be converted to 5β-reduced metabolites in the liver; however, these 5β-reduced metabolites do not have androgenic activity. A key observation in the history of androgen physiology was the discovery in 1968 that 5α-dihydrotestosterone was the main intracellular androgen and the predominant androgen concentrated in the nucleus of the rat prostate. These findings, together with the observation that dihydrotestosterone is about twice as potent as testosterone in most bioassay systems, indicated that dihydrotestosterone is a major cellular mediator of androgen action. The importance of dihydrotestosterone in normal androgen physiology has been confirmed by studies of human mutations in which the steroid 5α-reductase 2 enzyme responsible for dihydrotestosterone formation is defective (see Chapter 8).

The aromatization of androgens to estrogens in testes and in extraglandular tissues of men is accomplished by the same enzyme complex present in placenta and ovary, CYP19. Estrogen formation involves sequential hydroxylation, oxidation, and removal of the C-19 carbon and aromatization of the A ring of the steroid. Three moles of NADPH and 3 moles of oxygen are required to convert each mole of androstenedione or testosterone to estrone or estradiol, respectively. The oxidations are of the mixed function type (see Chapter 9) involving a specific cytochrome P450 (CYP19). The enzymes involved appear to be bound in a microsomal complex that includes NADPH–cytochrome P450 reductase as well as cytochrome. Of the 45 mg of estradiol produced per day on average in normal young men, only about 10%–

15% comes from direct secretion by the testes, while the remaining 85%–90% is derived from peripheral aromatization of secreted androstenedione (via estrone) and testosterone. Estrogen formation in the testes is enhanced by increased levels of LH or human chorionic gonadotropin (hCG). The rate of overall aromatase in nongonadal tissue does not appear to be influenced by gonadotropins but rises with advancing age.

Androgen Action

Androgens exert their actions predominant by acting through a classical nuclear receptor that affects transcription of genes. In addition, like the other classes of steroid hormones, androgens have been shown to have nongenomic actions that are rapid and mediated by interaction with classical steroid receptors or G protein–coupled receptors located within the plasma membrane (see Chapter 3). The current concepts of androgen action in target cells are diagrammed in Figure 10-3. Among the major functions of androgen are regulation of gonadotropin secretion by the hypothalamic–pituitary system, stimulation of spermatogenesis, formation of the male phenotype during sexual differentiation, and promotion of sexual maturation at puberty. Inside the cell, testosterone can be converted to dihydrotestosterone by either steroid 5α-reductase 1 or 2; steroid 5α-reductase 2 is the predominant isozyme in most androgen target tissues. Either testosterone or dihydrotestosterone then binds to the androgen receptor protein. The androgen receptor is coded by a gene on the long arm of the X chromosome and has a size of about 110,000 Da. It is similar to other members of the steroid–thyroid–retinoid family of receptors with distinct hormone-binding, DNA-binding, and functional domains (see Chapter 3).

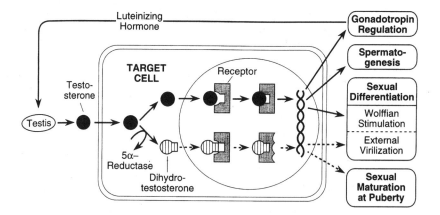

Fig. 10-3 Normal androgen physiology. Testosterone, secreted by the testis, binds to the androgen receptor in a target cell, either directly or after conversion to dihydrotestosterone. Dihydrotestosterone binds more tightly than testosterone, and the complex of dihydrotestosterone and the androgen receptor can bind more efficiently to the chromatin. The major actions of androgens, shown on the right, are mediated by testosterone (solid arrows), or by dihydrotestosterone (broken arrows). (Redrawn from Griffin JE: N Engl J Med 326:612, 1992.)

The androgen receptor is predominantly in the nucleus in the unbound state. The binding of androgen to the hormone-binding domain of the receptor to form the hormone–receptor complexes is a prerequisite to the transformation reaction in which the hormone–receptor complexes acquire increased affinity for nuclear components. The DNA-binding domains of the receptors then bind to androgen response elements (AREs) in the promoter region of target genes activating transcription. Estradiol, as discussed above, may be either secreted directly by the testis or formed in peripheral tissues. The mechanisms by which estrogens augment or block androgen action are not fully understood.

Based on studies in humans and animals, it appears that the testosterone–receptor complex is responsible for gonadotropin regulation, stimulation of spermatogenesis, and the virilization of the wolffian ducts during sexual differentiation, whereas the dihydrotestosterone–receptor complex is responsible for external virilization during embryogenesis and for most male secondary sexual characteristics of the adult (see below). Androgen receptor concentrations are highest in the accessory organs of male reproduction that depend on androgens for their growth. Other tissues such as skeletal muscle, liver, and heart have smaller amounts of the receptor. In the testis, androgen receptors are present both in isolated Sertoli cells and in interstitial cells. Whether the presence of androgen receptors identifies a tissue as androgen responsive is not clear, although androgen receptors are present in greater numbers in tissues known to respond to androgen. Single-gene mutations in humans and animals (see Chapter 8) indicate that a single androgen receptor binds both testosterone and dihydrotestosterone and that the receptor protein is coded by a locus on the X chromosome. Dihydrotestosterone formation appears to be required for normal androgen action even though there is only a single receptor. In the case of the human androgen receptor, a partial explanation for this requirement of dihydrotestosterone may be the severalfold greater affinity of the receptor for dihydrotestosterone than for testosterone. Dihydrotestosterone may also facilitate transformation of the receptor for transactivation more efficiently (Fig. 10-3). Thus, a difference in the interaction of the two hormones with the androgen receptor may serve as an amplifying mechanism for androgen action in certain target tissues.

SPERMATOGENESIS, SEMINAL FLUID FORMATION, AND CAPACITATION

Stages of Spermatogenesis

After migration of the germ cells to the gonadal ridges during embryogenesis (see Chapter 8), the total number of germ cells is approximately 3×10^5 per gonad. This number increases to about 6×10^6 spermatogonia per testis by the time of puberty. With sexual maturation, sperm production of about 2×10^8 sperm per day develops. As depicted in Figure 10-4, each spermatogonium undergoing differentiation gives rise to 16 primary spermatocytes, each of which enters meiosis and gives rise to four spermatids and ultimately four spermatozoa. Thus, 64 spermatocytes can develop from each spermatogonium. It appears that contiguous groups of spermatogonia begin the differentiation process simultaneously, resulting in certain typical cellular associations in seminiferous tubules.

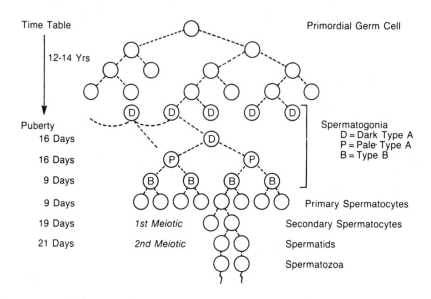

Fig. 10-4 Cell divisions during spermatogenesis. (From Griffin JE and Wilson JD: In: *Williams Textbook of Endocrinology,* 8th ed., JD Wilson and DW Foster, eds., Saunders, Philadelphia, p. 810, 1992.)

The conversion of the round spermatid to the mature spermatozoa (spermiogenesis) requires reorganization of the nucleus and cytoplasm and development of a flagellum. The nucleus comes to occupy an eccentric position near what will become the head of the spermatozoon and is covered by an acrosomal cap. The cilial structure that serves as the core of the sperm tail consists of nine outer fibers and two inner fibers. The mitochondria form a helix around this cilia in the middle piece of the spermatozoon, and most of the cytoplasm is lost. The differentiation of the spermatocyte to a motile sperm takes about 70 days, and the transport of the sperm through the epididymis to the ejaculatory ducts takes about 14 days. Sperm maturation occurs during passage through the epididymis, as evidenced by the development of a capacity for sustained motility. The mechanism of sperm motility is believed to involve the sliding action of microtubules (fibers) contained in the axial structure of the tail. The microtubules are attached to each other by dynein arms that contain the protein dynein, an adenosine triphosphatase (ATPase). The energy for the process is derived from hydrolysis of ATP generated in the mitochondrial sheath.

Regulaton of Spermatogenesis

Normal spermatogenesis requires follicle-stimulating hormone (FSH), testosterone, and normal Sertoli cell function. Follicle-stimulating hormone binds to the surface of Sertoli cells, stimulating adenylyl cyclase and thus activating protein kinase. One of the products of the Sertoli cell stimulated by FSH is androgen-binding protein

(ABP), which serves as a binding protein for testosterone in the seminiferous tubule lumen, maintaining the high androgen levels all the way to the epididymis. Testosterone interacts with androgen receptors in Sertoli cells to activate specific genes necessary for the differentiation process. Testosterone may also act indirectly by stimulating peritubular cells to produce peritubular factors that modulate Sertoli cell function (P-Mod-S). These factors are yet-to-be-purified proteins. Following removal of the pituitary gland in the adult, no spermatocytes are formed. Spermatogenesis can be restored by treatment with the combination of hCG and human menopausal gonadotropin (hMG), which contains FSH, and once restored, spermatogenesis can be maintained by hCG alone. This might seem to imply that FSH is required for initiation of spermatogenesis but not for its maintenance. But in studies of normal men in whom FSH is selectively suppressed by the sequential administration of exogenous testosterone followed by hCG, FSH administration is required for quantitatively normal spermatogenesis. Thus, it is likely that both FSH and luteinizing hormone (LH) play a continuing role in human spermatogenesis.

Based on animal studies, it appears that at least three other factors in addition to FSH and testosterone play an essential role in modulating spermatogenesis: vitamin A, c-*fos*, and stem cell factor. Rats fed on a vitamin A–deficient diet develop defective spermatogenesis with germ cell arrest. The nuclear protooncogene c-*fos* was found to be necessary for spermatogenesis by studies of mice homozygous for germline mutations at the locus. Stem cell factor is the ligand for c-*kit*. Stem cell factor is made in Sertoli cells, and the c-*kit* receptor is present in germ cells. Mutations in either stem cell factor or c-*kit* genes result in abnormal spermatogenesis. The cyclic adenosine monophosphate (cAMP)-response element modulator (CREM) is a protein that accumulates in large amounts during spermiogenesis, and mice carrying homozygous deletions of the CREM gene have a block in spermatogenesis.

A number of other factors have been studied *in vitro* and postulated to have paracrine/autocrine roles in modulating spermatogenesis. These include transferrin, insulin-like growth factor (IGF)-I, fibroblast growth factor (FGF), nerve growth factor (NGF), interleukin (IL)-1, opioids, transforming growth factors (TGF), growth hormone-releasing hormone (GHRH), inhibin/activin (see below), and others.

Seminal Fluid Formation

During the approximately 12 days of transit through the epididymis, sperm undergo maturation with development of the capacity for sustained motility, modification of the structural state of the nuclear chromatin and tail organelles, and loss of the remnant of spermatid cytoplasm. The epididymis also serves as a reservoir for sperm. After transport of the sperm and secretory products of the testis and epididymis through the vas deferens, the fluid reaching the ejaculatory ducts is enriched by the secretions from the seminal vesicles. The seminal vesicles are the source of seminal fluid fructose and prostaglandins and contribute about 60% of the total volume of the seminal fluid. Approximately 20% of the total seminal fluid volume is derived from prostatic secretions added to the semen when the ejaculatory ducts terminate in the prostatic urethra. The prostatic fluid is the source of seminal fluid spermine, citric acid, zinc, and acid phosphatase.

Capacitation

Fertilization normally takes place within the fallopian tube. Spermatozoa usually require a period in the female reproductive tract before they can fertilize. This functional change, termed *capacitation,* is thought to have at least two components: (*1*) an increased rate of flagellar beat and acceleration of sperm movement and (2) an acrosome reaction in sperm that allows the underlying plasma membrane of the sperm to fuse with the ovum. The time required for optimal capacitation of normal sperm may vary from 2 to more than 6 hours. Whether capacitation is an absolute requirement in the human or serves only to enhance fertilizing capabilities has not been established.

The elements of the capacitation reaction that promote motility may include a change in the intracellular concentration or metabolism of calcium or cAMP. The acrosome reaction appears to be more complex but also involves calcium. Neither the fallopian tube nor the egg itself appears to be essential for this process. The acrosome reaction involves fragmentation and loss of the acrosome with release of a variety of hydrolytic enzymes and proteases allowing the sperm to penetrate and fuse with the ovum. Understanding of the mechanism of sperm penetration is largely based on studies of fertilization of human eggs *in vitro.* Ovulated eggs are surrounded by layers of cumulus cells embedded in a matrix of hyaluronic acid. The mechanism by which spermatozoa tunnel through the cumulus is not known. Possibly hyaluronidase is released by the degenerating acrosome, and the mechanical agitation of the flagellum may disperse cumulus cells (see Chapter 11).

THE HYPOTHALAMIC–PITUITARY–TESTICULAR AXIS

Luteinizing Hormone-Releasing Hormone and Gonadotropins and Their Actions

As discussed in detail in Chapter 6, peptidergic neurons in the hypothalamus secrete luteinizing hormone-releasing hormone (LHRH, also called *gonadotropin-releasing hormone* [GnRH]). The LHRH is transported to the pituitary by a portal vascular system and interacts with cell surface receptors on pituitary gonadotrophs to stimulate the release of LH and FSH (Fig. 10-5). The LHRH is a decapeptide that is widely distributed in the central nervous system and may also be present in other tissues. However, a physiological role for LHRH in sites other than the pituitary has not been established. The amount of LH and FSH released in response to LHRH depends on age and hormonal status. In a primate model, the sensitivity of the gonadotrophs to LHRH is high during the first few months of life and then declines and remains low until the onset of puberty, when it increases and attains an adult level of response. The secretion of FSH in response to LHRH is relatively greater than that of LH before puberty.

Both LH and FSH are secreted by the same basophilic cells in the pituitary. Like thyrotropin (TSH) and hCG, LH and FSH are glycoproteins consisting of two polypeptide chains designated α and β. The α-subunit of each of the four hormones is identical, and distinct immunological and functional characteristics are determined

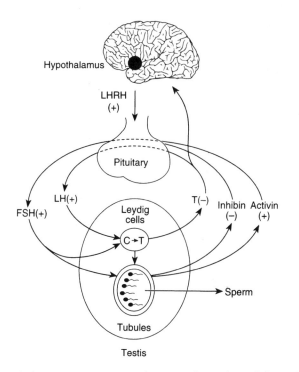

Fig. 10-5   Hypothalamic–pituitary–testicular interrelationships. Schematic diagram indicating the feedback relationship of testosterone, inhibin, and activin produced by testes on gonadotropin secretion by the hypothalamic–pituitary complex and the site of action of follicle-stimulating hormone (FSH) and luteinizing hormone (LH) on testis. C, cholesterol; T, testosterone; LHRH, LH-releasing hormone. (From Griffin JE and Wilson JD: In: *Harrison's Principle of Internal Medicine,* 13th ed., KJ Isselbacher, E Braunwald, JD Wilson, JB Martin, AS Fauci, and DL Kasper, eds., McGraw-Hill, New York, p. 2008, 1994.)

by unique β-subunits. The turnover of FSH is slower than that of LH. The receptors for FSH and LH are typical seven-transmembrane domain G protein–coupled receptors. Luteinizing hormone interacts with specific high-affinity cell surface receptors on Leydig cells and utilizes a cAMP second messenger (see Chapter 3). Activation of Leydig cell protein kinase via unspecified intermediates eventually results in stimulation of testosterone formation (see above). The rate of testosterone synthesis correlates more closely with the degree of occupancy of the regulatory subunits of the protein kinase by cAMP than with the total amount of cAMP in the cells. Whether the LH–receptor complex undergoes internalization for degradation or receptor recycling is unclear.

In the intact testis and in cultured Leydig cells, the receptors for LH decrease in number following administration of LH or hCG. This down-regulation of LH receptors is maximal at 24 hours and is followed by return to control levels several days later. It is associated with a decreased responsiveness to subsequent LH administration, but this desensitization is not due solely to a decreased receptor number. Rather, the diminished steroidogenic response appears to be due to inhibition of some postreceptor event since cAMP is ineffective in overcoming the desensitization. In fact, the desensitization can be produced by cAMP stimulation of steroidogenesis under conditions that do not alter LH receptor number. The diminished response of the Leydig cell to LH that follows LH administration appears to be a component of an intratesticular control system for regulating testosterone production.

As mentioned above, the second messenger for FSH action following its binding to receptors on the basal aspects of Sertoli cells is also cAMP. Follicle-stimulating hormone is known to stimulate the rate of synthesis of ABP and the aromatase enzyme complex in Sertoli cells. Also, FSH may play a role in steroidogenesis by influencing Leydig cell maturation and modifying the effects of LH on steroidogenesis by stimulating paracrine–autocrine factors. Based on *in vitro* studies, IGF-I, TGF-β, epidermal growth factor (EGF), TGF-α, FGF, inhibin/activin, cytokines, GHRH, corticotropin-releasing hormone (CRH), arginine vasopressin (AVP), endothelin, and other agents have been postulated to have effects on Leydig cells. Their physiological significance is unclear.

Regulation of Secretion of Luteinizing Hormone-Releasing Hormone and Gonadotropins

The secretion of LHRH is episodic, resulting in the intermittent secretion of both immunoreactive and bioactive LH in 8–14 pulses/24 hours in adult men. Pulsatile secretion of FSH also occurs but is of smaller amplitude, in part because of the longer half-life of FSH in the circulation. The rate of LH secretion is controlled by the action of sex steroids on the hypothalamus and pituitary. The control of LH in men operates primarily by negative feedback since normal levels of gonadal steroids inhibit secretion (Fig. 10-5). Both testosterone and estradiol can inhibit LH secretion. Testosterone and its metabolites act on the central nervous system to slow the hypothalamic pulse generator and consequently decrease the frequency of LH pulsatile release. Testosterone can be converted to estradiol in the brain and pituitary, but the two hormones are thought to act independently. The fact that the testosterone metabolite dihydrotestosterone, which cannot be converted to estrogen, exerts negative feedback on LH secretion suggests that testosterone does not require conversion to estradiol to inhibit LH secretion. Testosterone also appears to have a negative feedback on LH secretion at the pituitary level, since moderate elevations of plasma testosterone levels result in a diminished LH response to acute LHRH stimulation in the presence of normal levels of plasma estradiol. In normal men, endogenous estrogens also act to restrain tonically the hypothalamic release of LHRH.

The negative feedback inhibition of testicular hormones on FSH secretion is less well understood. Serum FSH levels increase selectively in proportion to the loss of germinal elements in the testis. A nonsteroidal inhibitor of FSH is present in the testis, semen, and cultured Sertoli cells, and a similar material is present in ovarian follicular fluid. The inhibitor is termed *inhibin*. Inhibin is a heterodimeric protein consisting of α- and β-polypeptide subunits connected by disulfide bonds (see Chapter 9). Interestingly, significant structural homology of the β-subunit of inhibin to a subunit of human TGF-β has been found. As discussed in Chapter 12, TGFs may not only affect tumor growth in an autocrine manner but also participate in the regulation of nonneoplastic processes. There are two different forms of the β-subunit of inhibins βA and βB. Thus, the α-subunit can combine with the β-subunit to form either inhibin A (α-βA) or inhibin B (α-βB). Inhibin B is the physiologically important form of inhibin in the human male; an inverse relationship between inhibin B and FSH has been shown across a wide range of FSH concentrations in normal and infertile men. The level of inhibin B correlates with the presence of germ cells in early spermatogenesis in adult men rather than with the presence of Sertoli cells (as seen before puberty; see below). An additional hormone identified during the purification of inhibin, activin, is formed by the dimerization of the inhibin β-subunits. Activin A (βA-βA), activin B (βB-βB), and activin AB (βA-βB) stimulate FSH secretion from anterior pituitary cells in culture. Sertoli cells are the site of inhibin production, and inhibin production is enhanced by FSH and androgen.

Studies of pituitary cells cultured with purified bovine inhibin indicate that inhibin acts to block LHRH-stimulated FSH release. Whether inhibin also has effects at the hypothalamic level is not known. Testosterone and estradiol also have direct effects on FSH secretion, and a decrease in the pulse frequency of LHRH release may produce a selective increase in FSH. A primate model has been useful in defining the relative importance of inhibin and gonadal steroids in physiological feedback control of FSH secretion. When episodic gonadotropin secretion was maintained by chronic, intermittent LHRH infusion, neither circulating testosterone nor estradiol could account for the testicular inhibition of FSH, implying by exclusion that inhibin must be the gonadal hormone of greatest importance for feedback control at the level of the pituitary.

DEVELOPMENT AND MAINTENANCE OF REPRODUCTIVE FUNCTION

The development and maintenance of reproductive function in the male can be correlated with alterations in plasma testosterone. During embryogenesis testosterone levels rise in the late first trimester in association with male sexual differentiation (see Chapter 8).

Neonatal Period

In the first 6 months of life, the testosterone level rises to about half of adult levels, falling back to low levels before age 1 year. The concentration of testosterone remains low until the onset of puberty, when it rises again. This neonatal surge in testosterone secretion results from a rise in plasma LH levels, but the function of the temporary increase in testosterone secretion is not well understood. Inhibin B levels also rise during this neonatal activation of the hypothalamic–pituitary–gonadal axis. Inhibin B levels actually exceed normal adult levels during this period and decrease more gradually than testosterone levels, remaining measurable during childhood. Inhibin B is stimulated by FSH during childhood and is thought to be produced by Sertoli cells. The first year of life is associated with an increase in the number of Sertoli cells and with changes in Leydig and germ cell numbers

as well. Thus it is postulated that this neonatal gonadotropin surge may be important for testicular development. Support for this concept has been provided by studies of a nonhuman primate in which temporary inhibition of the pituitary–testicular
axis in the neonate has been shown to be associated with impaired testicular function at puberty.

Puberty

Plasma gonadotropins and testosterone are low during the prepubertal years. In boys
around age 6 or 7 there is an increased secretion of adrenal androgens termed
adrenarche. This increased section of dehydroepiandrosterone and androstenedione
is probably under the control of corticotropin (ACTH) and is in part responsible for
the prepubertal growth spurt and the initial development of axillary and pubic hair.
These adrenal androgens are thought to act via the androgen receptor after conversion to testosterone. Total plasma testosterone increases only slightly during this
time, and plasma LH levels are low but show some low-amplitude pulsations. However, the low levels of gonadotropins in prepubertal boys are under feedback control by the prepubertal testis and low levels of plasma testosterone (5–20 ng/dl),
since castration elevates both gonadotropins. The degree of elevation of gonadotropins in the absence of gonadal feedback is less during the late childhood
years than at other times, suggesting that more than exquisite sensitivity of the
hypothalamic–pituitary system to feedback inhibition is involved in the low gonadotropin levels of normal prepubertal boys (see also Chapter 9).

The pituitary hormonal changes associated with the onset of puberty are sleep-
associated surges in LH secretion. Later, as puberty advances, the increased plasma
gonadotropin levels are present throughout the day and are accompanied by increased plasma levels of testosterone. Inhibin B levels rise early in puberty. The increase in gonadotropin secretion is thought to result from both increased LHRH secretion and enhanced responsiveness of the pituitary to LHRH. Plasma levels of
bioactive LH increase even more than those of the immunoreactive hormone. Thus,
it appears that with sexual maturation the hypothalamic–pituitary system becomes
less sensitive to the feedback inhibition of testosterone on gonadotropin secretion.
Before puberty there is a positive correlation between inhibin B and FSH levels.
However, by early puberty, there is a negative correlation between the two hormones. This change appears to be correlated with the shift in inhibin B production
from Sertoli cells to germ cells.

The changes in the testes at puberty include the maturation of Leydig cells and
the initiation of spermatogenesis. The anatomical changes characteristic of puberty
are a result of testosterone secretion. Usually the first sign of male puberty is testis
enlargement, with some reddening and wrinkling of the scrotal skin. Pubic hair
growth begins first at the base of the penis. On average, this initiation of pubertal
development occurs between ages 11 and 12, but occasionally it takes place as early
as age 9 or as late as age 13 or 14. About a year after the onset of testis growth,
the penis begins to increase in size. The prostate, seminal vesicles, and epididymis
increase in size over a period of several years. Characteristic hair growth includes
development of mustache and beard, regression of the scalp line, appearance of body

and extremity hair, and extension of pubic hair upward into the upper pubic triangle. The larynx enlarges and the vocal cords become thickened, resulting in a lower pitch of the voice. There is an enhanced rate of linear growth, resulting in a height spurt somewhat later in puberty to a rate of about 3 inches per year. At this time the androgen-sensitive muscles of the pectoral region and the shoulder also increase in their characteristic male pattern, the hematocrit increases, and libido and sexual potency develop. These various maturation processes take place over about 4 years and reach some normal limit for the individual based on genetic and nutritional factors. Linear growth is halted by fusion of the epiphyses, which requires normal estrogen formation and action. The genetic evidence for this important role of estrogen in skeletal maturation in men came from the observation that men with mutations impairing the function of the aromatase enzyme or the estrogen receptor had persistent linear growth with failure of epiphyseal fusion. Administration of excess exogenous androgens has little effect on the parameters of sexual development once puberty is completed.

Adulthood

At the completion of puberty, usually between ages 16 and 18, plasma testosterone levels are in the adult range of 300–1000 ng/dl, sperm production is normal, and plasma gonadotropins are in the 1–15 mIU/ml range. Most anatomical changes are completed at this time except for androgen-mediated hair growth, which is usually not maximal until the mid- to late 20s. Some effects of androgens, such as the development of the larynx, are permanent and do not reverse if androgen production decreases. Other effects of androgen, such as stimulation of erythropoietin, reverse with androgen deprivation. Beard growth slows following postpubertal androgen deficiency but usually does not completely cease. Two results of postpubertal androgen deficiency are clear-cut. There is a negative nitrogen balance probably resulting from regression of accessory organs of reproduction and to a certain extent skeletal muscle. Complete androgen deficiency is followed by a progressive decline in male sexual drive so that most such men are unable to have intercourse after a few years.

Old Age

Men have a gradual decrease in free plasma testosterone levels and an increase in SHBG levels beginning around age 40. In elderly men there is a decrease in total plasma testosterone levels, a decrease in the ratio of androgen to estrogen, and some elevation in plasma LH and FSH. Sperm production decreases about 30% between the ages of 50 and 80. It is likely that any decline in sexual activity with age is the result of nonendocrine factors. Healthy elderly men commonly maintain a healthy sex life and reproductive capacity. Whether the changes in body composition that accompany aging—that is, decreased bone density and lean body mass and increased fat mass—are related to the fall in testosterone is under investigation. Inhibin B levels also decline about 25% in older men.

CLINICAL ASSESSMENT OF REPRODUCTIVE FUNCTION

History and Physical Exam

The assessment of androgen status should include an inquiry about defects of the urogenital tract at birth, sexual maturation at puberty, rate of beard growth, and current libido, sexual function, strength, and energy. If Leydig cell failure occurs before puberty, sexual maturation will not occur. In contrast, the detection of Leydig cell failure beginning after puberty requires a high index of suspicion of androgen deficiency and, usually, laboratory assessment. Many men without hormonal abnormalities complain of decreased sexual function. In addition, even when Leydig cell function is impaired, the rate of beard growth may not decrease for many months or even years.

The prepubertal testis measures about 2 cm in length and increases in size to a range of 4.0–5.5 cm in length in the normal adult. When damage to the seminiferous tubules occurs before puberty, the testes are small and firm. Following postpubertal damage the testes are characteristically small and soft. However, considerable damage must occur before the overall size is decreased below the lower limits of normal. Breast enlargement is the most consistent feature of feminizing states in men and may be an early sign of androgen deficiency.

Gonadotropins, Testosterone, and Inhibin B

Because of the pulsatile secretion of LH, the consequent pulsatile secretion of testosterone, and the need to interpret the LH level in light of the testosterone level, it is usually appropriate to measure gonadotropins and testosterone on a pool formed by combining equal quantities of blood obtained from three or four samples at 15- to 20-minute intervals. The normal plasma immunoreactive LH and FSH values must be established for each laboratory based on the antibody and standard used. The normal range for plasma testosterone in adult men is 300–1000 ng/dl. Free testosterone concentrations can be estimated by equilibrium dialysis, but as discussed above, a more accurate assessment of available testosterone *in vivo* can be obtained by measuring the non-SHBG-bound fraction (or the free plus albumin-bound fraction). The non-SHBG-bound testosterone (or bioavailable testosterone) can either be measured by precipitating the SHBG with ammonium sulfate or calculated by the known binding affinities if the albumin and SHBG concentrations are measured. Measurement of inhibin B is not routine in the evaluation of adult men.

Leydig cell function may be assessed before puberty by measuring the response to hCG administration. Single or multiple injections of hCG may be given. The testosterone response increases at the start of puberty, peaking in early puberty. Inhibin B may serve as a childhood serum marker for testicular activity. In boys without palpable testes, the finding of normal serum levels of inhibin B signals the presence of undescended but likely otherwise normal testes, whereas undetectable inhibin B levels suggest anorchia or gonadal dysgenesis. A single normal basal inhibin B level in a prepubertal subject with apparently undescended testes reliably predicts a testosterone response to hCG stimulation. In contrast to the adult, childhood inhibin B production is independent of the presence of germ cells. Thus boys with a disorder in which there are only Sertoli cells in the testis have normal inhibin B levels before puberty but undetectable levels after puberty.

In certain circumstances, the change in plasma LH after the administration of LHRH is measured to assess the functional integrity of the hypothalamic–pituitary–Leydig cell axis. When 100 mg of LHRH is given subcutaneously or intravenously to normal men, there is, on average, a four- to fivefold increase in LH, with the peak level at 30 minutes. However, the range of response is broad, some normal men having less than a doubling of LH levels. In general, the peak LH following a single LHRH injection correlates with basal levels. In patients with primary testicular failure, measurement of basal LH is usually sufficient, and measurement of the LHRH response adds little to the diagnosis. Men who have either pituitary or hypothalamic disease may have either a normal or abnormal LH response to an acute dose of LHRH. Therefore, a normal response is of no diagnostic value, whereas a subnormal response is of value in determining that an abnormality exists, even though the site is not known. Men with secondary hypogonadism and a subnormal response to an acute infusion of LHRH who develop a normal response to an acute dose after daily infusion of LHRH for a week usually have a hypothalamic cause of the hypogonadism (see Chapter 5 and Fig. 5-5).

Seminal Fluid Examination

Routine evaluation of seminal fluid is largely dependent on tests that do not assess the functional capacity of sperm. Seminal fluid should be obtained after masturbation into a clean glass or plastic container. The volume of the normal ejaculate is 2–6 ml. The specimen should be analyzed within an hour. Estimation of motility is made by examining a drop of undiluted seminal fluid and recording the percentage of motile forms. Normally 60% or more of the sperm should be motile with forward progression. Sperm density can be determined by diluting seminal fluid 20-fold with an appropriate solution and estimating its density in a hemocytometer or with the aid of an electronic particle counter. The normal value is usually considered to be greater than 20 million/ml with total sperm per ejaculate of greater than 60 million.

After the first 2 days, the total sperm in the ejaculate per the number of days since the last ejaculation is relatively constant in normal men who ejaculate daily. Random sampling of sperm density in men is complicated by variable extragonadal sperm reserves and by effects of toxic factors such as hot baths, acute febrile illnesses, and unknown medications. The net result is that it is difficult to define the minimally adequate ejaculate. Ordinarily, three ejaculates are required to establish inadequacy of sperm number or cytology.

Seminal cytology is a useful index of fertility, and the seminal fluid smear is prepared in the same way as a blood smear but with special stains. Some abnormal spermatozoa are present in all semen. The best correlations between histological abnormalities and infertility are seen when a single anomaly is found in a large percentage of the sample. It is generally believed that 60% or more of the spermatozoa should have a normal morphology. When it is available, the details of sperm structure can be studied by electron microscopy. Such studies are useful in identifying the abnormalities in immotile sperm.

DERANGED REPRODUCTIVE FUNCTION

Abnormalities of male reproductive function may occur at any stage of life from embryogenesis through old age. Disorders of testicular function during embryogenesis result in abnormalities of sexual differentiation (see Chapter 8). This section will consider examples of deranged reproductive function occurring at puberty and in adulthood.

Deficient Puberty: Isolated Gonadotropin Deficiency

Deranged reproductive function related to pubertal events in boys more commonly involves delayed or deficient puberty rather than sexual precocity. This is not so in girls (see Chapter 9). It is often difficult to decide whether puberty is merely being delayed or is actually incomplete or deficient. A common cause of deficient puberty is isolated gonadotropin deficiency, which occurs in both sporadic and familial forms. It is second only to Klinefelter's syndrome (see Chapter 8) as a cause of hypogonadism in men. The disorder was originally described as a familial syndrome associated with an impaired sense of smell (Kallmann's syndrome). The defect in most affected individuals is detected because of a failure to undergo puberty. Subsets of patients, particularly familial cases, have associated congenital defects commonly involving midline facial and head structure. There is no sense of smell because of defective development of the olfactory bulbs. Less severely affected individuals may have a negative family history (half of all subjects with the disorder) and only partial defects in FSH and/or LH secretion. Such individuals may undergo partial sexual maturation, develop partial testicular enlargement, and not come to medical attention until adulthood.

The underlying defect is at the hypothalamic level: absence or inadequate release of LHRH. A defect in a neural adhesion molecule may be responsible for abnormal migration of neurons leading to both the impaired sense of smell and defective LHRH release. Randomly obtained gonadotropin levels might be undetectable, low, or apparently normal in the face of a low testosterone level. The fact that the underlying defect is at the hypothalamic level was established when LHRH became available; following short-term administration of LHRH, plasma LH and FSH increase in about half of subjects. After repetitive infusion of LHRH for 5 days or longer, plasma gonadotropins rise to the normal range in virtually all affected patients but not in individuals with panhypopituitarism.

One group of investigators has attempted to define some of the clinical heterogeneity in patients with isolated gonadotropin deficiency by studying the patterns of LHRH secretion, as inferred by frequent measurements of plasma LH. Men with isolated gonadotropin deficiency displayed several abnormal patterns of LHRH secretion. Whereas the majority of men had an apulsatile pattern of LH release, other individuals demonstrated episodic LH secretion only during sleep (as in normal pubertal subjects). In these latter subjects a history of early but arrested pubertal development was often obtained, and testicular size was larger than in those subjects with an apulsatile pattern of LH release. In other families, the defect appears to impair LH pulse amplitude or pulse frequency. These findings imply that maintenance of a physiological amplitude and frequency of endogenous LHRH secretion appear to be essential for normal reproductive function.

Other mutations that cause gonadotropin deficiency involve a variety of different mechanisms. A mutation of the *DAX1* gene (see Chapter 8) leads to an X-linked form of gonadotropin deficiency associated with adrenal insufficiency. Mutations in the LHRH receptor can cause an autosomal recessive form of isolated gonadotropin deficiency not associated with anosmia. Finally, mutations in the LH β gene or the FSH β can also lead to hypogonadism.

Adult Reproductive Failure: Infertility

Approximately 15% of couples attempting their first pregnancy are unsuccessful. Couples who have been unable to achieve a pregnancy after 1 year of unprotected intercourse are usually considered to have primary infertility. In approximately one-third of such cases a significant abnormality impairing fertility is thought to be in the man alone, and in an additional fifth of couples, both the man and the woman have some abnormality. Thus, in about half of infertile couples, some abnormality in the male is in part responsible for the failure to conceive. Any man who has been unsuccessful in achieving fertility with a regularly menstruating woman after 1 year should be considered potentially subfertile.

Infertility in men can be an isolated problem with normal androgen production or one manifestation of an abnormality of testicular function that involves both Leydig cells and seminiferous tubules. In contrast, because sperm production depends on normal Leydig cell function, disorders that primarily affect androgen formation or action are usually associated with infertility. Therefore, it is essential to exclude the presence of subtle Leydig cell dysfunction in every man with infertility.

Adult abnormalities of testicular function can be due to hypothalamic–pituitary defects, testicular disorders, or abnormalities in sperm transport. The hypothalamic–pituitary defects include not only the isolated gonadotropin deficiency mentioned above, but also a variety of destructive and infiltrative lesions in the pituitary and functional impairments of gonadotropin secretion resulting from excess prolactin, glucocorticoids, or endogenous or exogenous androgens.

Testicular disorders known to be associated with infertility can be grouped into several categories. Developmental and structural defects include Klinefelter's syndrome and its variants (see Chapter 8), deletions or mutations in one of the azoospermia factor regions on the long arm of the Y chromosome, abnormal testicular descent, and a structural defect of sperm tails leading to immotile sperm. Acquired testicular defects include viral and other infections, trauma, radiation, drugs including alcohol and marijuana, and self-directed immune responses affecting the entire testis or primarily sperm. Systemic diseases may be associated with testicular abnormalities, as in chronic liver disease, renal failure, and certain neurological disease. Finally, androgen resistance due to a receptor defect may be manifested by underandrogenization with infertility or infertility alone in men with normal development of the external genitalia.

Disorders of sperm transport lead to infertility associated with normal Leydig cell function. The abnormality can be unilateral or bilateral, congenital or acquired.

In men with unilateral obstruction, infertility might be due to antisperm antibodies. Obstruction at the level of the epididymis may occur in association with chronic infections of the paranasal sinuses and lungs. Or the vas deferens might be congenitally absent in association with an absence of the seminal vesicles.

Unfortunately, the above elaboration of the known causes and of conditions associated with male infertility does not account for the problem in the majority of men. When a large series of consecutive patients seen by referral groups is evaluated, more than half of such men are classified as having *idiopathic* infertility. Because as many as 1 in 20 men are infertile, this represents a major area for improvement in medical knowledge.

FERTILITY CONTROL

Vasectomy

Other than the condom, the only proven effective means of fertility control in men is surgical interruption of the vas deferens (vasectomy). In the United States, about 50% of couples adopting surgical sterilization for fertility control choose vasectomy, and about 1 million vasectomy procedures are performed each year. Bilateral partial vasectomy is a relatively simple operative procedure usually performed with local anesthesia. Vasectomy is considered successful when sperm cannot be demonstrated in the semen on two consecutive specimens. On average, this takes 24 ejaculations following vasectomy. In less than 1% of men, the procedure fails due to recanalization, which occurs at a median time of 6 months. The changes in the testis following occlusion of the vas have been studied in animals. In the primate, spermatogenesis continues following vasectomy, with the sperm being resorbed or stored in distended ducts and cysts. Testicular volume does not change after vasectomy in men. There appear to be no significant changes in peripheral hormone levels following vasectomy as assessed by measuring plasma testosterone and gonadotropins. Moreover, Leydig cell reserve, as assessed by the response to hCG, is normal several years later. Vasectomy has no deleterious effects on potency or sexual performance. Antisperm antibodies do develop following vasectomy, and the presence of these antibodies may limit the success of attempted vasectomy reversal. Thus, vasectomy reversal (or vasovasostomy) has a success rate for appearance of sperm in the ejaculate of 80%–90%, but the associated pregnancy rate is only 30%–40%.

Search for a Male Contraceptive

Whereas the oral contraceptive is effective and relatively safe in controlling ovulation and fertility in women (see Chapter 9), there is no readily reversible and effective pharmacological contraceptive for men. One explanation for this is that it intuitively seems easier to prevent the production of only one ovum per month in the female than to prevent the production of millions of sperm each day in the male. In addition, sperm migration, capacitation, fertilization, and implantation all take place in women. Thus, even some measures designed to affect the sperm can be used in women but not in men.

In searching for a male contraceptive, pharmacological and other methods have been directed at inhibiting hypothalamic–pituitary function, directly inhibiting spermatogenesis or inhibiting epididymal function. It was hoped that the injection of long-acting testosterone esters might suppress gonadotropin secretion, resulting in defective spermatogenesis and at the same time replacing endogenous testosterone. However, this proved successful in completely eliminating sperm from the ejaculate only in a little over half of men. The inhibition of spermatogenesis in men who responded was reversible. A contraceptive trial of men using weekly testosterone injections who achieved either absence of sperm in the ejaculate or severely decreased numbers (<3 million/ml) found a failure rate no greater than that seen with women using oral contraceptive pills. The requirement for weekly intramuscular injections in this and the regimens below is a hindrance to acceptance. Gonadotropin levels are decreased in men given injections of long-acting analogs of LHRH with a resultant decrease in testosterone levels and associated impaired sexual function. Combining testosterone injections with LHRH agonist treatment results in a return of testosterone levels to normal but inconsistent success in totally inhibiting spermatogenesis. Trials of LHRH antagonists with testosterone gave similar results.

A number of anticancer drugs and other relatively toxic compounds impair sperm production by direct effects on the testes. Most of these compounds produce additional unacceptable side effects. An antifertility agent in cottonseed oil discovered in China is a naphthalphenol termed *gossypol*. It has been given to more than 10,000 men in clinical trials over a decade. Administration of this compound orally for 60 days causes the sperm in the ejaculate to become immotile and to decrease in number. Because the drug affects motility, it may not be necessary to have absence of sperm for an antifertility effect. Unfortunately, significant toxicity in regard to lowering the serum potassium has been observed, and the reversibility of the effect of the drug is uncertain. Other drugs with antispermatogenic activity have been studied less extensively. Physical methods such as heat and ultrasound have been tried to a limited extent, and immunological methods with antibodies directed at various testicular components have an uncertain duration of action.

Selective inhibition of epididymal function to cause impairment of sperm maturation would theoretically control fertility without the risk of impaired testicular function. In addition, the time required to achieve an effect on fertility with such agents should be less than the 2 to 3 months necessary for agents affecting the pituitary or testis. Because the epididymis is a target organ for androgens, antiandrogens were used in an attempt to inhibit sperm maturation in the epididymis. Both cyproterone and the nonsteroidal antiandrogen flutamide appear to be ineffective in inhibiting epididymal function.

In summary, the search for a male contraceptive has not been rewarding.

SUGGESTED READING

Anderson AM and Skakkebaek NE: Serum inhibin B levels during male childhood and puberty. Mol Cel Endocrinol 180:103–107, 2001.

Anderson RA and Baird DT: Male contraception. Endocr Rev 23:735–762, 2002.

Baker HWG: Reproductive effects of nontesticular illness. Endocrinol Metab Clin North Am 27:831–850, 1998.

Baker HWG, Burger HG, de Kretser MD, and Hudson B: Relative incidence of etiological disorders in male infertility. In: *Male Reproductive Dysfunction,* RJ Santen and RS Swerdloff, eds., Marcel Dekker, New York, pp. 341–372, 1986.

Behr R and Weinbauer GF: cAMP response element modulator (CREM): an essential factor for spermatogenesis in primates? Int J Androl 24:126–135, 2001.

Bhasin S, Ma K, Sinha I, Limbo M, Taylor WE, and Salehian B: The genetic basis of male infertility. Endocrinol Metab Clin North Am 27:783–805, 1998.

Carr BR and Griffin JE: Fertility control and its complications. In: *Williams Textbook of Endocrinology,* 9th ed., JD Wilson, DW Foster, HM Kronenberg, and PR Larsen, eds., Saunders, Philadelphia, pp. 901–926, 1998.

Foresta C, Moro E, and Ferlin A: Y chromosome microdeletions and alterations of spermatogenesis. Endocr Rev 22:226-239, 2001.

Griffin JE and Wilson JD: Disorders of the testes and male reproductive tract. In: *Williams Textbook of Endocrinology,* 10th ed., PR Larsen, HM Kronenberg, S Melmed, and KS Polonsky, eds., Saunders, Philadelphia, pp. 709–769, 2003.

Hammes SR: The further redefining of steroid-mediated signaling. Proc Natl Acad Sci USA 100:2168–2170, 2003.

Hayes FJ, Hall JE, Boepple PA, and Crowley WF Jr: Differential control of gonadotropin secretion in the human: endocrine role of inhibin. J Clin Endocrinol Metab 83:1835–1841, 1998.

Hayes FJ, Seminara SB, and Crowley WF Jr: Hypogonadotropic hypogonadism. Endocrinol Metab Clin North Am 27:739–763, 1998.

Matsumoto AM, Karpas AE, and Bremner WJ: Chronic human chorionic gonadotropin administration in normal men: evidence that follicle-stimulating hormone is necessary for the maintenance of quantitatively normal spermatogenesis in man. J Clin Endocrinol Metab 62:1184–1192, 1986.

Matsumoto AM, Paulsen CA, and Bremner WJ: Stimulation of sperm production by human luteinizing hormone in gonadotropin-suppressed normal mem. J Clin Endocrinol Metab 59:882–887, 1984.

McLachlan RI, Wreford NG, O'Donnell L, de Kretser DM, and Robertson DM: The endocrine regulation of spermatogenesis: independent roles for testosterone and FSH. J Endocrinol 148:1–9, 1996.

Pardridge WM: Serum bioavailability of sex steroid hormones. Clin Endocrinol Metab 15:259–278, 1986.

Pescovitz H, Srivastava CH, Breyer PR, and Monts BA: Paracrine control of spermatogenesis. Trends Endocrinol Metab 5:126–131, 1994.

Plant TM and Marshall GR: The functional significance of FSH in spermatogenesis and the control of its secretion in male primates. Endocr Rev 22:764–786, 2001.

Riggs BL, Khosla S, and Melton LJ: Sex steroids and the construction and conservation of the adult skeleton. Endocr Rev 223:L279–L302, 2002.

11

Fertilization, Implantation, and Endocrinology of Pregnancy

BRUCE R. CARR
KHURRAM S. REHMAN

The complex and coordinated set of events leading to sperm and egg maturation and transport in the female genital tract that culminates in fertilization is one of the most remarkable phenomena in nature. This set of events is followed by the equally important unique processes of implantation, fetal maturation, and parturition. The hormonal changes that regulate these events are dependent on the close interaction of the fetal–placental–maternal unit.

FERTILIZATION AND IMPLANTATION

Ovum Maturation and Transport

Just before ovulation, the egg, which has been arrested in the diplotene stage, completes the first meiotic division and forms the first polar body. The second meiotic division starts at the time of ovulation but ends only after fertilization by a sperm.

The process of egg maturation is regulated through a closely interrelated set of hormonal events, most notably involving follicle-stimulating hormone (FSH), luteinizing hormone (LH), and estrogen. At the time of ovulation the fimbria of the oviduct are closely applied to the surface of the ovary. The extruded oocyte and adherent granulosa cells, known as the *cumulus oophorus*, is collected by the ciliated fimbrial end of the fallopian tube. The transport of the egg into the end of the fallopian tube occurs within minutes and is regulated primarily by ciliary action. The cumulus cells are able to communicate with one another via a network of intercellular bridges through the zona pellucida to the perivitelline space. The cumulus cells have also been reported to play a role in nutrition and maintenance of the ovum.

There are three different stages of passage of the ovum through the fallopian tube. The first stage includes the transfer of the ovum from the fimbriated end of the fallopian tube until the egg reaches and is retained at the ampullary–isthmic junction. The ampullary–isthmic junction is a functional block but is not a clearly defined anatomical structure. The ovum remains at this junction for 1–2 days, during which time fertilization occurs. The second stage begins soon after fertilization when the egg traverses the isthmic portion of the tube, where it again is retained at another functional block, the isthmic–utero or utero–tubal junction. The length of time from the process of ovulation until the release of the egg from the isthmus is species dependent and averages 3 days in women. The detection of the embryo at the utero–tubal junction appears to be influenced by ovarian steroid hormones, namely, estrogen and progesterone. During this stage, estrogen and progesterone also act on the endometrium to prepare it for implantation of the fertilized egg. The final stage of egg transportation occurs during the 3–4 days after ovulation when the fertilized egg leaves the isthmus and arrives in the uterine cavity (Fig. 11-1).

Sperm Transport and Capacitation

The sperm are required to traverse an even greater distance in the female genital tract than is the ovum. Spermatozoa leave the vagina after ejaculation and pass through the cervix, the entire length of the uterine cavity, the utero–tubal junction, the isthmus, and finally the ampullary–isthmic junction, where fertilization occurs. The process of sperm transport is very rapid in comparison to egg transport. Spermatozoa have been found in the distal end of the fallopian tube 5 minutes after ejaculation. However, the rate of attrition of sperm is high. Of an estimated 250 million sperm deposited in the vagina, only 50 or less ever reach the oviduct (Fig. 11-1). The principal mechanism controlling sperm transport is flagellar movement; thus, semen characterized by low sperm motility is usually associated with infertility.

In most species, the process of sperm capacitation requires sperm to reside in or be exposed to the female tract before they are capable of fertilizing an ovum. This process is not yet fully defined, but it includes the acrosome reaction that involves a breakdown and merging of the plasma membrane and acrosomal mem-

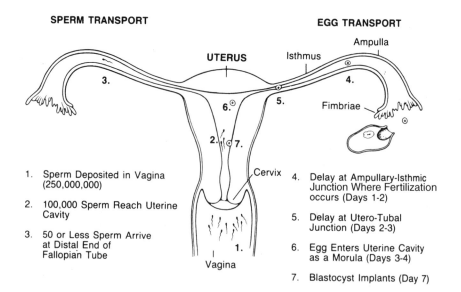

Fig. 11-1 The transport of sperm and the egg in the female reproductive tract.

brane of the sperm head. This reaction is stimulated by the oocyte zona pellucida glycoprotein ZP3. This is followed by a release of enzymes thought to play a role in sperm penetration. During the process of capacitation, the sperm also become hypermotile. Progesterone, found in both follicular and oviductal fluid, may play a role in the acrosome reaction and in promoting sperm motility. These effects appear to be mediated by cell membrane progesterone receptors rather than classical nuclear progesterone receptors.

Process of Fertilization

The first stage of fertilization requires the equatorial region of the sperm head to adhere to the zona pellucida surrounding the egg (Fig. 11-2). This is mediated by ZP3, which binds to specific receptors on the sperm surface. The molecular details of this binding are unclear and may involve more than one sperm surface protein. The sperm must then penetrate the zona, which requires 15–25 minutes. After passage through the zona pellucida, the sperm moves rapidly across the perivitelline space (in less than 1 second), where it attaches to the perivitelline membrane and penetrates it (in less than 1 minute).

After the sperm head penetrates the vitelline membrane, the male pronucleus is formed. The penetration of the vitelline membrane initiates two important events: the release of cortical granules into the perivitelline space, which prevents further penetration of the egg by other sperm, and the development of polyspermy. The second event is the triggering of the final stage of meiosis of the oocyte. The second polar body is extruded from the egg, and a haploid number of chromosomes (23) are present in the egg pronuclei just before fertilization.

The male and female pronuclei are visible about 2–3 hours after the sperm has penetrated the vitelline membrane. Within 4 hours, the sperm tail is incorporated within the egg. Within 24 hours, the two pronuclei have moved toward the center of the egg. Next, their respective haploid chromosomes replicate and a mitotic spindle forms. The fertilized egg then divides and forms two cells, or blastomeres.

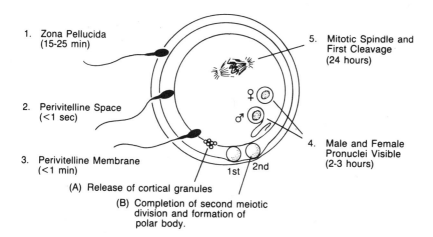

1. Zona Pellucida (15-25 min)
2. Perivitelline Space (<1 sec)
3. Perivitelline Membrane (<1 min)
    (A) Release of cortical granules
    (B) Completion of second meiotic division and formation of polar body.
5. Mitotic Spindle and First Cleavage (24 hours)
4. Male and Female Pronuclei Visible (2-3 hours)

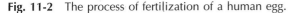

Fig. 11-2 The process of fertilization of a human egg.

The initial cleavages of the embryo occur in the fallopian tube, and the rate of cleavage remains remarkably constant in mammals. The rate of cleavage of fertilized human eggs has been determined primarily from *in vitro* studies. The timing of cleavage of the human embryo is as follows: two cells (38 hours), four cells (46–48 hours), eight cells (51–62 hours), morula formation (111–135 hours), and the formation of a blastocyst (123–147 hours).

The life span of an unfertilized egg is less than 20 hours following ovulation, after which it undergoes cell death and cytolysis. The life span of a sperm is about 24 hours after ejaculation.

In Vitro Fertilization

The first successful delivery of a live-born infant by the method of *in vitro* fertilization in 1978 stimulated further clinical and laboratory investigations. The knowledge and methods that were developed from these studies are now available for the treatment of infertile couples with a variety of disorders including damaged or blocked fallopian tubes, male factor infertility involving semen abnormalities, cervical factors, and even unexplained infertility.

In vitro fertilization and embryo transfer starts with the administration of exogenous hormones, consisting of purified human or recombinant FSH, and/or human menopausal gonadotropins (hMG, containing both FSH and LH), to stimulate growth and development of multiple ovarian follicles. A gonadotropin-releasing hormone (GnRH) agonist or antagonist is usually added to prevent an endogenous rise in LH levels from estrogen-positive feedback at the hypothalamus, which can decrease success rates. The GnRH agonists have a long half-life resulting in GnRH receptor down-regulation and thus function like antagonists. Transvaginal ultrasound is used to monitor follicular size, and when sufficient follicular growth has occurred, an injection of human chorionic gonadotropin (hCG), which mimics LH activity, is given to induce oocyte maturation. Thirty-six hours after the hCG injection, the ova are aspirated from ripe follicles by transvaginal ultrasonographic techniques. The eggs are then transferred to a culture system containing medium and serum.

Freshly ejaculated semen is washed in buffer and centrifuged to remove the seminal fluid. The sperm are preincubated in defined medium for 1–2 hours to initiate capacitation. Next, approximately 1 million sperm are added to each culture dish containing an ovum. Fertilization occurs within 6–8 hours. During the next 2–3 days, the embryos divide and reach the four- to eight-cell stage. Then, up to a maximum of four to six fertilized two- to eight-cell stage embryos are transferred by a catheter to the uterine cavity. Improved *in vitro* culture techniques now allow transfer of blastocysts at day 5 after fertilization, as an alternative to day 3 embryo transfer. The rest of the embryos that are not initially transferred may be frozen and placed in the uterus during a subsequent menstrual cycle.

If fertilization fails to occur or if the male demonstrates severe impairment in sperm number or motility, intracytoplasmic sperm injection (ICSI) is recommended, using microscopic guidance to directly inject a single sperm into each egg. The average pregnancy rate now exceeds 30% per embryo transfer cycle in women under 35, with a rate of live births of about 20%–30% per cycle worldwide. In addition, increasing availability of ovum donation allows women with diminished oocyte number or quality, often due to advanced age, to achieve 30%–40% live birth rates per treatment cycle.

Implantation and Placentation

In the human the embryo enters the uterine cavity as a morula on the third to fourth day after ovulation. The morula is transformed into a blastocyst during the fifth to sixth day after ovulation. At this stage of development, the embryo appears as a hollow sphere with two clearly distinguishable cell types: the outer cells, the trophectoderm cells that will form the placenta, and the inner cell mass from which the fetus will develop.

On the seventh day after ovulation, the blastocyst implants on the endometrial lining of the uterine cavity. The embryo attaches to the endometrium, with the embryonic pole facing the uterine cavity. The endometrium, under the influence of progesterone secreted by the corpus luteum, is transformed into a decidua. The decidua consists of large polyhedral endometrial cells that are laden with glycogen and lipid and are often multinucleated. In the absence of progesterone, the development of decidua and implantation fail to occur. Continued progesterone secretion ensures further development of the decidua and maintenance of pregnancy. The corpus luteum is the main source of progesterone during the first 6–8 weeks of pregnancy. During the remainder of gestation, the principal source of progesterone is the placenta. Decidual development also appears to respond to signals from the invading embryo, including hCG. Another important signal is corticotropin-releasing hormone (CRH) produced by the trophoblast, which promotes blastocyst implantation and facilitates immune tolerance of the early pregnancy by killing maternal activated T cells.

Next, endometrial cells begin to interdigitate with the microvilli of the trophectodermal cells. The layer of trophoblast cells develops into an inner cytotrophoblast layer and an outer syncytiotrophoblast layer. The syncytiotrophoblasts secrete proteolytic enzymes that erode the endometrium and allow the syncytiotrophoblast cells to invade further. The human embryo undergoes interstitial implantation in which the embryo is deeply embedded and enclosed by the endometrium by the eleventh day after ovulation (Fig. 11-3).

The placenta develops from the trophoblast. Lacunar spaces form among the syncytiotrophoblasts, and these spaces are contiguous with the maternal capillary circulation. Within these spaces the functional and structural compartment of the placenta, the chorionic villi, develops. In the absence of vascularization of the villi, further development into secondary and tertiary villi does not occur. Instead, the villi become cystic and fill with fluid (hydatidiform mole). Before ultrasound diagnosis was available, hydatidiform moles were often spontaneously aborted, which could result in extensive maternal hemorrhage and shock. Molar pregnancy is part of a spectrum of gestational trophoblastic neoplasia and may precede the development of invasive malignant trophoblastic disease known as *choriocarcinoma*.

Placental development varies widely among different animal species. The human placenta is *hemochorial*: fetal endothelium and fetal connective tissues are directly bathed by maternal blood. The maternal side of the placenta is composed of the decidual layer of the endometrium, which fuses with chorionic villi into sepa-

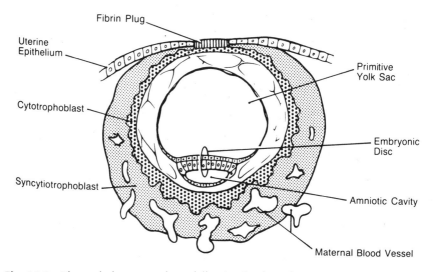

Fig. 11-3 The early human embryo following implantation.

rate lobes known as *cotyledons*. The cotyledons and their chorionic villi are exposed to maternal blood from the decidual spiral arterioles. The fetal side of the placenta is composed of the amnion and chorion. The amnion is a thin avascular membrane that surrounds the fetus and contains amniotic fluid. Adjacent to the amnion is the chorion tissue layer, and these cells are next to the decidua lining the uterine cavity. It has been proposed that hormones produced in the fetus, amnion, chorion, and decidua communicate information between each compartment. This information may play a role in the onset of parturition.

ENDOCRINOLOGY OF PREGNANCY

The Fetal–Placental–Maternal Unit

The hormonal change and maternal adaptation that occur during human pregnancy are extensive. During pregnancy the placenta, supplied with precursor hormones from the maternal–fetal unit, synthesizes large quantities of steroid hormones as well as various protein and peptide hormones, and in turn secretes these products into the fetal and maternal circulation. Near the end of pregnancy a woman is exposed daily to large quantities of estrogen, progesterone, mineralocorticoids, and glucocorticoids. The mother and, to a lesser extent, the fetus are also exposed to large quantities of human placental lactogen (hPL), hCG, prolactin (PRL), relaxin, prostaglandins, and smaller amounts of pro-opiomelanocortin (POMC)-derived peptides such as corticotropin (ACTH) and endorphin, gonadotropin-releasing hormone (GnRH), also called *luteinizing hormone–releasing hormone* (LHRH), thyroid-stimulating hormone (TSH), CRH, somatostatin, and other hormones.

Implantation, the maintenance of pregnancy, parturition, and finally lactation depend on a complex interaction of hormones in the maternal–fetal–placental unit.

In addition, protein and peptide hormones produced by the placenta act via a paracrine mechanism to regulate the secretion of placental steroid hormones.

Placental Compartment

In mammals, particularly humans, the placenta has evolved into a complex structure that delivers nutrients to the fetus, produces numerous steroid and protein hormones, removes metabolites from the fetus, and delivers them to the maternal compartment.

Progesterone

The main source of progesterone during pregnancy is the placenta. The corpus luteum, however, is the major source of progesterone secretion during the first 6–8 weeks of gestation. It is believed that the developing trophoblast takes over as the major source of progesterone secretion by 8 weeks' gestation, as removal of the corpus luteum before, but not after, this time leads to spontaneous abortion. After 8 weeks' gestation the corpus luteum of pregnancy continues to secrete progesterone, but the amount of progesterone secreted is only a fraction of that secreted by the placenta. The placenta of a term pregnancy produces approximately 250 mg of progesterone each day. Maternal progesterone plasma levels rise from 25 ng/ml during the late luteal phase to 150 ng/ml at term (Fig. 11-4). Most of the progesterone secreted by the placenta enters the maternal compartment.

Although the placenta produces large amounts of progesterone, under normal circumstances it has very limited capacity to synthesize cholesterol from acetate. Maternal cholesterol in the form of low-density lipoprotein (LDL) cholesterol is the principal source of precursor substrate for biosynthesis of progesterone in human pregnancy (Fig. 11-5). The LDL cholesterol attaches to its receptor on the trophoblast

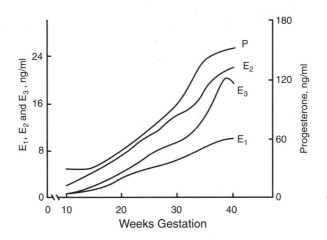

Fig. 11-4 Maternal serum levels of progesterone (P), estrone (E_1), estradiol-17β (E_2), and estriol (E_3) in normal pregnant women as a function of weeks of gestation. (Adapted from Parker CR Jr, Illingworth DR, Bissonnette J, and Carr BR: N Engl J Med. 314:557, 1986, and unpublished studies by Parker CR Jr.)

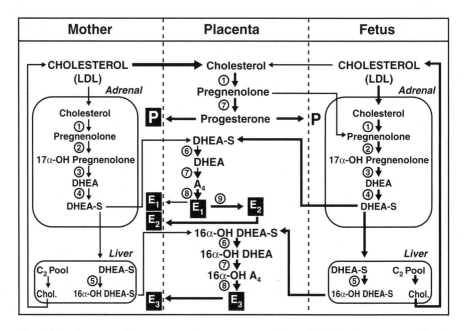

Fig. 11-5 Sources of estrogen and progesterone biosynthesis in the maternal–fetal–placental unit. LDL, low-density lipoprotein; Chol., cholesterol; C_2 pool, carbon–carbon units; DHEA, dehydroepiandrosterone; DHEA-S, dehydroepiandrosterone sulfate; A_4, androstenedione; E_1, estrone; E_2, estradiol-17β; E_3, estriol; P, progesterone. Enzymes: ① cholesterol side-chain cleavage (CYP11A), ② 17α-hydroxylase (CYP17), ③ 17,20 lyase (CYP17), ④ DHEA sulfotransferase, ⑤ 16α-hydroxylase, ⑥ sulfatase, ⑦ 3β-hydroxysteroid dehydrogenase type 1, ⑧ aromatase (CYP19), ⑨ 17β-hydroxysteroid dehydrogenase type 1.

and is taken up and degraded by the trophoblast to free cholesterol, which then is converted to progesterone and secreted.

A functioning fetal circulation is not important for the regulation of progesterone levels in the maternal unit. In fact, fetal death, ligation of the umbilical cord, and anencephaly, which are all associated with a decrease in estrogen production, have no significant effect on progesterone levels in the maternal compartment.

The physiological role of the large quantity of progesterone produced by the placenta has been an area of great interest. Progesterone binds to receptors in uterine smooth muscle, thereby inhibiting smooth muscle contractility and leading to myometrial quiescence and prevention of uterine contractions. It also inhibits prostaglandin formation, which is known to be critically involved in human parturition. Progesterone is essential for the maintenance of pregnancy in all mammals, possibly owing to its ability to inhibit T-lymphocyte cell–mediated responses involved in graft rejection. Because the fetus is a foreign body within the uterus, the high local levels of progesterone can block cellular immune responses to foreign antigens and may be important in giving immunological privilege to the pregnant uterus.

Estrogen

During human pregnancy the rate of estrogen production and the level of estrogens in plasma increase markedly (Fig. 11-4). The levels of urinary estriol (E_3) have been reported to increase 1000-fold during pregnancy. The corpus luteum is the principal source of estrogen during the first few weeks of pregnancy, but afterward nearly all of the estrogen formed is from the trophoblast of the placenta. However, the mechanism by which estrogen is produced by the placenta is unique. The placenta is unable to convert progesterone to estrogens because of a deficiency of 17α-hydroxylase/17,20 lyase enzyme (CYP17) (Fig. 11-5, ② and ③). Thus, the placenta has to rely on preformed androgens produced in the maternal and fetal adrenal glands. Estradiol-17β (E_2) and estrone (E_1) are synthesized by the placenta via conversion of dehydroepiandrosterone sulfate (DHEA-S), which reaches it from both maternal and fetal bloodstreams.

The placenta metabolizes DHEA-S to estrogens in the presence of the following enzymes: placental sulfatase, 3β-hydroxysteroid dehydrogenase type 1, and the aromatase enzyme complex (CYP19). Estriol is synthesized by the placenta from 16α-hydroxy DHEA-S formed in fetal liver from circulating DHEA-S secreted by the fetal adrenal gland. At least 90% of urinary estriol is ultimately derived from the fetal adrenal gland. The sources of estrogen and progesterone biosynthesis in the maternal–fetal–placental unit are presented in Figure 11-5. The major source of fetal adrenal DHEA-S is cholesterol circulating in fetal blood. A minor source of fetal adrenal DHEA-S is formed from pregnenolone secreted by the placenta. Only 20% of fetal cholesterol is derived from the maternal compartment. Because amniotic fluid cholesterol levels are negligible, the main source of cholesterol appears to be the fetus itself. As the fetal liver synthesizes *de novo* cholesterol at a high rate, and if one considers the size of the fetal liver, it can be computed that the fetal liver may supply sufficient cholesterol to the fetal adrenal to maintain steroidogenesis.

The measurement of estrogens, in particular urinary estriol, was historically utilized to monitor fetal well-being in high-risk pregnancies. There are several disorders that lead to low urinary excretion of estriol by the mother. The most notable of these conditions is *placental sulfatase deficiency*, also known as *steroid sulfatase deficiency syndrome*, which is an X-linked inherited metabolic disorder characterized during fetal life by decreased maternal estriol production due to deficient placental sulfatase (see Fig. 11-5). In this disorder, the placenta is unable to cleave the sulfate moiety from DHEA-S and, consequently, the levels of maternal estrogens, particularly estriol, are quite low. Placental sulfatase deficiency is also associated with prolonged gestation and difficulty of cervical dilatation at term, often requiring cesarean section. Steroid sulfatase deficiency is thought to occur in 1 out of every 2000–6000 newborns. The male offspring are, of course, sulfatase deficient and they have a characteristic scaling skin condition termed *ichthyosis*, which is first apparent after the first few months of life. Other conditions resulting in low estriol are aromatase deficiency, which reduces conversion of androgens to estrogens, mostly by the placenta (Fig. 11-5), fetal adrenal hypofunction, as occurs in the anencephalic fetus secondary to lack of pituitary ACTH production, and fetal demise.

The ultimate destination of estrogen and progesterone secretion by the placenta is primarily the maternal compartment. The physiological role of the large quantity of estrogen produced by the placenta is not completely understood. It has been proposed that estrogen may regulate or fine-tune the events leading to parturition, as pregnancies are often prolonged when estrogen levels in maternal blood and urine are low, as in placental sulfatase deficiency or anencephaly. Estrogen stimulates phospholipid synthesis and turnover, increases incorporation of arachidonic acid into phospholipids, stimulates prostaglandin synthesis, and increases the number of lysosomes in uterine endometrium. Estrogens are known to increase uterine blood flow and may also play a role in fetal organ maturation and development.

Human Chorionic Gonadotropin

Human chorionic gonadotropin is secreted by the syncytiotrophoblast of the placenta into both the fetal and maternal circulations. It is a glycoprotein with a molecular weight of about 38,000 that consists of two noncovalently linked subunits, α and β, and is similar to LH in structure and action. Human chorionic gonadotropin has been used extensively as a pregnancy test and can be detected in serum as early as 6–8 days following ovulation. Plasma levels rise rapidly in normal pregnancy, doubling in concentration every 2–3 days until they reach a peak between 60 and 90 days' gestation. Thereafter, the concentration of hCG in maternal plasma declines, plateauing at about 120 days before delivery. Changes in maternal serum hCG levels are shown in Figure 11-6. The levels of hCG are higher in multiple pregnancies, in pregnancies associated with rhesus isoimmunization, and in pregnant diabetic women; they are highest in pregnancies associated with hydatidiform moles and in women with choriocarcinoma.

There is some evidence that the regulation of the rate of secretion of hCG by the syncytiotrophoblastic cells may be a paracrine mechanism involving the release of GnRH by the cytotrophoblast. Activin and inhibin as well as the transforming growth factors α and β secreted by the trophoblastic cells also appear to regulate

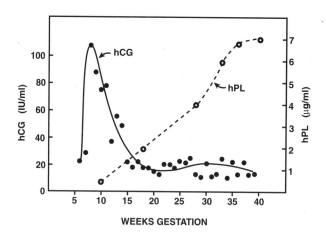

Fig. 11-6 Maternal serum levels of human chorionic gonadotropin (hCG) and human placental lactogen (hPL) in normal pregnant women. (Adapted from Pritchard JA, MacDonald PC, and Gant NF: *Williams Obstetrics*, 17th ed., Appleton-Century-Crofts, New York, p. 121, 1985, with permission.)

hCG secretion. Fetal concentrations of hCG reach a peak at 11–14 weeks' gestation and thereafter fall progressively until delivery.

Various theories have been proposed as to the functional role of hCG in pregnancy. The most widely accepted theory is that hCG maintains the early corpus luteum of pregnancy to ensure continued progesterone secretion by the ovary until this function is replaced by the growing trophoblast. Some investigators have demonstrated that hCG promotes steroidogenesis (namely, progesterone) by the trophoblast. It is most likely that a primary role for hCG in the fetus is to regulate the development and secretion of testosterone by the fetal testes. Male sexual differentiation occurs at an early but critical time in development when fetal serum hCG levels are high and fetal plasma LH levels are low. It has been suggested that hCG may affect fetal ovarian development as well. An additional role may be to give immunological privilege to the developing trophoblast. Finally, several investigators have demonstrated that the excess thyrotropic activity during the clinical development of hyperthyroidism observed in some women with gestational trophoblastic neoplasia, including hydatidiform moles, results from excessive hCG secretion. Both TSH and hCG have similar structures, and purified hCG inhibits binding to thyroid membranes and stimulates adenylate cyclase in thyroid tissues.

Human Placental Lactogen

Human placental lactogen is a single-chain polypeptide consisting of 191 amino acid residues that has a molecular weight of about 22,000. As its name suggests, hPL has both lactogenic and growth hormone (GH)–like activity and is also referred to as *chorionic growth hormone* or *chorionic somatomammotropin*. Human placental lactogen mainly exhibits lactogenic activity: it has only 3% or less of the growth-stimulating activity of GH. The structure and amino acid–base residues of hPL, PRL, and GH are quite similar.

Human placental lactogen is secreted by the syncytiotrophoblast and can be detected in serum by radioimmunoassay as early as the third week after ovulation. The plasma level of hPL continues to rise with advancing gestational age, unlike hCG, and appears to plateau at term (Fig. 11-6). The concentration of hPL in serum is closely correlated with increasing placental weight. Its half-life in serum is short. Although the level of hPL in serum before delivery is the highest of all the protein hormones secreted by the placenta, it cannot be detected in serum after the first postpartum day. The time sequence and peak of hPL secretion are significantly different from those of hCG, which suggests a different regulation for each hormone. This is interesting, as both are secreted by the syncytiotrophoblast rather than the cytotrophoblast.

Interestingly, hPL appears to be secreted primarily into the maternal circulation because very low levels are observed in cord blood of newborns. Thus, most of the proposed physiological roles of hPL have centered on its sites of action in maternal tissues. Human placental lactogen may have a major sparing influence on maternal glucose, providing adequate, continued nutrition for the developing fetus. It has been suggested that hPL exerts metabolic effects in pregnancy similar to those of GH. These effects include stimulation of lipolysis, resulting in increased circulating free fatty acids (which are available for maternal and fetal nutrition); inhibition of glucose uptake in the mother, resulting in increased maternal insulin levels;

development of maternal insulin resistance; and an inhibition of gluconeogenesis that favors transportation of glucose and protein to the fetus. However, these metabolic changes all predispose to the development of gestational diabetes mellitus, which may require maternal insulin treatment during pregnancy and can cause a range of maternal and fetal adverse effects including macrosomia (excessive fetal growth).

A *true* placental growth hormone has been shown to be produced by the syncytiotrophoblast of the placenta and secreted in parallel with hPL. This GH variant is now recognized to be the product of the *hGH-V* gene and differs from the major 22 kDa GH in 13 amino acid residues. A glycosylated variant of this GH form has also been described in an *in vitro* system, but it is not known if this form circulates. Because concentrations of the placental GH variant in maternal plasma correlate with plasma levels of insulin-like growth factor-I (IGF-I), it has been suggested that placental GH is involved in the control of serum IGF-I levels in normal pregnant women.

Other Placental Peptide and Protein Hormones

In addition to hCG and hPL, several other placental hormones similar or closely related with respect to biological and immunological activity to hypothalamic or pituitary hormones have been reported. These include human chorionic POMC peptides, CRH, growth hormone-releasing hormone (GHRH), human chorionic thyrotropin, and human chorionic gonadotropin-releasing hormone. Placental CRH will be discussed further in relation to parturition.

The regulation of the secretion of these hormones is not well understood, but classical negative feedback inhibition does not appear to exist. Furthermore, the function and significance of these hormones are incompletely understood. Most of these hormones are believed to enter primarily the maternal compartment.

Fetal Compartment

The regulation of the fetal endocrine system, like that of the placenta, is not completely independent but relies to some extent on precursor hormones secreted by the placenta or maternal tissues. As the fetus develops, its endocrine system gradually matures and becomes more independent, preparing the fetus for extrauterine existence. The following section summarizes our present understanding of the fetal endocrine unit and its relationship with the maternal–placental unit.

Fetal Hypothalamic–Pituitary Axis

The fetal hypothalamus begins to differentiate from the forebrain during the first few weeks of fetal life, and by 12 weeks hypothalamic development is well advanced. Most of the hypothalamic-releasing hormones, including GnRH, thyrotropin-releasing hormone (TRH), dopamine, norepinephrine, and somatostatin, as well as their respective hypothalamic nuclei, have been identified as early as 6–8 weeks of fetal life. The posterior pituitary, or neurohypophysis, is first detected at 5 weeks, and by 14 weeks the supraoptic and paraventricular nuclei are fully developed.

Rathke's pouch first appears in the human fetus at 4 weeks of fetal life. The immature anterior pituitary cells that develop from the cells lining Rathke's pouch are capable of secreting GH, PRL, FSH, LH, and ACTH *in vitro* as early as 7 weeks of fetal life. Recent evidence suggests that the intermediate lobe of the pituitary may be a significant source of POMC hormones. The intermediate pituitary lobe in the human fetus decreases in size after birth, with only remnants remaining in the adult.

The hypothalamo-hypophyseal portal system is the functional link between the hypothalamus and the anterior pituitary. Vascularization of the anterior pituitary starts by 13 weeks of fetal life, but a functioning intact portal system is not present until 18–20 weeks. Indirect evidence, however, shows that hypothalamic secretion of releasing hormones may influence anterior pituitary function before 18–20 weeks by simple diffusion as a result of their close proximity in early fetal development.

Fetal GH is detected in the human pituitary as early as 12 weeks; fetal pituitary GH content increases until 25–30 weeks' gestation and thereafter remains constant until term. In contrast, fetal plasma GH levels rise to a peak at 20 weeks of fetal life and thereafter fall rapidly until birth. Fetal plasma concentrations of GH, however, are higher than maternal concentrations at all ages. Maternal levels may be suppressed by the high circulating levels of hPL. The regulation of GH release in the fetus appears to be more complex than in the adult. To explain the high levels of fetal GH at midgestation and the fall thereafter, unrestrained release of GHRH or inhibition of somatostatin release leading to excessive release of GH at midgestation has been hypothesized. As the hypothalamus matures, somatostatin may increase and GHRH levels decline so that GH release also declines. The role of GH in the fetus is unclear as well. Considerable evidence indicates that GH is not essential to intrauterine somatic growth in primates. In newborns with pituitary agenesis, congenital hypothalamic hypopituitarism, or familial GH deficiency, birth weight and length are usually normal. However, a class of peptides known as *somatomedins*, in particular IGF-I and IGF-II, increase in fetal plasma, and IGF-I and IGF-II levels correlate better with fetal growth than do GH levels. Although GH is an important trophic hormone for somatomedin production in the fetus, somatomedin regulation may be independent of GH.

Prolactin is present in pituitary lactotropes by 19 weeks of life. Fetal PRL content in the pituitary increases throughout gestation. Fetal PRL plasma levels increase slowly until 30 weeks' gestation, after which the levels rise sharply until term and remain elevated until the third month of postnatal life. Both TRH and dopamine, as well as estrogens, appear to affect human fetal PRL secretion. Regulation of PRL secretion by dopamine in the fetus is supported by the observation that the dopamine agonist, bromocriptine, when ingested by the mother, crosses the placenta and inhibits PRL release from the fetal pituitary gland, lowering PRL levels in fetal blood. It has been suggested that PRL influences fetal adrenal growth, fetal lung maturation, and amniotic fluid volume.

Arginine vasopressin (AVP) and oxytocin are found in hypothalamic nuclei and in the neurohypophysis during early fetal development, but there have been relatively few studies of the regulation and secretion of these hormones in the fetus. The levels of AVP have been reported to be high in fetal plasma and newborn cord blood at delivery. The main stimulus to AVP release seems to be fetal hypoxia, although acidosis, hypercarbia, and hypotension also play a role. The elevated AVP level in fetal blood may lead to increased blood pressure, vasoconstriction, and the passage of meconium by the fetus. In contrast, oxytocin levels in the fetus are not affected by hypoxia but appear to increase during labor and delivery.

Fetal Thyroid Gland

Evidence suggests that the placenta is relatively impermeable to TSH and thyroid hormone so that the fetal hypothalamic–pituitary–thyroid axis appears to develop and function independently of the maternal system. However, some transfer of maternal thyroxine (T_4) does occur, and this hormone is detectable in human coelomic fluid in the first trimester, before the onset of fetal thyroid function.

By the end of the first trimester, the fetal thyroid has developed sufficiently to be able to concentrate iodine and synthesize iodothyronines. The levels of TSH and thyroid hormone are relatively low in fetal blood until midgestation (Fig. 11-7). At 24–28 weeks' gestation, serum TSH concentrations rise abruptly to a peak and decrease slightly thereafter until delivery. In response to the surge of TSH, T_4 levels rise progressively after midgestation until term. During this time, the pituitary becomes more responsive to TRH, and an increase in hypothalamic TRH content occurs. At birth there is an abrupt release of TSH, T_4, and triiodothyronine (T_3), followed by a fall in the levels of these hormones shortly thereafter. This brief thyroid

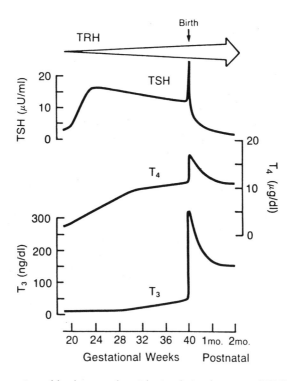

Fig. 11-7 Maturation of fetal serum thyroid-stimulating hormone (TSH), thyroxine (T_4), and triiodothyronine (T_3) during the second half of gestation and during early neonatal life. The increase in the effect or content of thyrotropin-releasing hormone (TRH) is also illustrated. (From Fisher DA: Clin Perinatol 10:615, 1983. Reproduced with permission of W.B. Saunders Company.)

excess is believed to facilitate thermoregulatory adjustments for extrauterine life. The abrupt increases in TSH and T_4 that occur at birth are thought to be stimulated by the cooling process associated with delivery. Finally, biologically inactive 3,3',5'-triiodothyronine (reverse T_3) levels are high during early fetal life, begin to fall at midgestation, and continue to fall after birth. The difference between the formation of T_3 and reverse T_3 is thought to be related to maturation of peripheral iodothyronine metabolism.

Fetal Gonads

Biologically active and immunoreactive GnRH has been detected in the fetal hypothalamus by 9–12 weeks of age. The hypothalamic content of GnRH has been reported to increase with fetal age, maximal content being noted between 22 and 25 weeks in females and between 34 and 38 weeks in males. The dominant gonadotropin fraction in the fetal pituitary is the α-subunit. However, the fetal pituitary is capable of secreting intact LH *in vitro* by 5–7 weeks. The plasma concentration of FSH in the human fetal plasma slowly rises and reaches a peak near the twenty-fifth week of fetal life and falls to low levels by term. Plasma FSH levels parallel the pituitary content of FSH with respect to sexual dimorphism, circulating FSH levels being higher in females than in males. The pattern of LH levels in fetal plasma parallels that of FSH. The fall in gonadotropin pituitary content and plasma concentration after midgestation is believed to result from the maturation of the hypothalamus. The hypothalamus also becomes more sensitive to feedback from sex steroids circulating in fetal blood, originating from the placenta.

In the male, the gene *SRY* (*S*ex determining *R*egion of *Y*) is critical for male differentiation of the gonad into a testis at 7 weeks of fetal life, encoding the testis determining factor (TDF). Fetal testosterone secretion begins soon after testicular differentiation, with the formation of Leydig cells at 8 weeks. Maximal levels of fetal testosterone are observed at about 15 weeks and decrease thereafter. The early secretion of testosterone is important in initiating sexual differentiation in the male (see Chapter 8). It is believed that the primary stimulus to the early development and growth of Leydig cells and the subsequent peak of testosterone is hCG. Thus, it appears that sexual differentiation of the male does not rely solely on fetal pituitary gonadotropins. However, fetal LH and FSH are still required for complete differentiation of the fetal ovary and testes. For example, male fetuses with abnormal brain formation (anencephaly), with low levels of circulating LH and FSH, secrete testosterone normally at 15–20 weeks because of adequate levels of hCG, but they have a decreased number of Leydig cells, exhibit hypoplastic external genitalia, and often have undescended testes. Likewise, male fetuses with congenital hypopituitarism often have small phalluses. These observations suggest that around and after midgestation, fetal pituitary gonadotropins affect testosterone secretion from the fetal testes.

The ovary develops from the bipotential gonad in the absence of *SRY*. The fetal ovary is involved primarily in the formation of follicles and germ cells. Although early follicular development in the ovary appears to be relatively independent of gonadotropins, the anencephalic female fetus with small ovaries and a decreased number of ovarian follicles suggests some pituitary involvement (however, the fetal ovaries do not contain hCG [LH] receptors, at least by 20 weeks' gestation). The ovaries appear to be relatively inactive with respect to steroidogenesis during fetal life but are capable of aromatizing androgens to estrogens *in vitro* as early as 8 weeks of gestation.

Fetal Adrenal Gland

Of all the endocrine glands in the human fetus, the adrenal has aroused the greatest interest. The human fetal adrenal gland secretes large quantities of steroid hormones, up to 200 mg of steroid daily near term. This rate of steroidogenesis may be five times that observed in the adrenal glands of adults at rest. The principal steroids found in the fetus are C-19 steroids (mainly DHEA-S), which serve as precursor substrate for estrogen biosynthesis in the placenta.

At the beginning of this century, investigators observed that the human fetal adrenal gland contained a unique *fetal zone* that accounts for the rapid growth of the fetal adrenal, and that this zone disappears during the first few weeks after birth. This fetal zone differs histologically and biochemically from the neocortex (also known as the *definitive* or *adult zone*). The uniqueness of a transient fetal zone has been reported in certain higher primates and some other rare species, but only humans possess the extremely large fetal zone that involutes after birth.

The cells of the adrenal cortex arise from coelomic epithelium. The cells comprising the fetal zone can be identified in the 8 to 10 mm embryo and before the appearance of the cells of the neocortex (14 mm embryo). Growth is most rapid during the last 6 weeks of fetal life. By 28 weeks' gestation, the adrenal gland may be as large as the fetal kidney, and by term it may be equal to the size of the adult adrenal. The fetal zone accounts for the largest percentage of growth, and after birth the adrenal gland decreases in size due to involution and necrosis of fetal zone cells (Fig. 11-8).

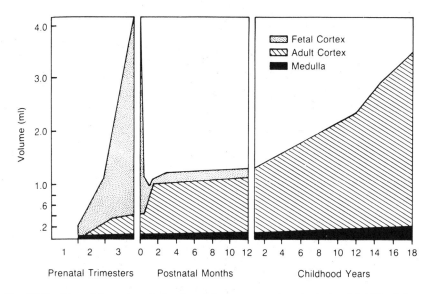

Fig. 11-8 Size of the adrenal gland and its component parts during fetal life, infancy, and childhood. (Adapted from Carr BR and Simpson ER: Endocr Rev 2:306, 1981, with permission.)

Studies of the fetal adrenal gland have attempted to determine what factors stimulate and regulate its growth and steroidogenesis and why the fetal zone atrophies after delivery. Normal adrenal development is dependent on two genes encoding orphan nuclear receptors, *SF-1* (*S*teroidogenic *F*actor-1) and *DAX-1* (*D*osage-sensitive sex reversal, *A*drenal hypoplasia congenita on the *X* chromosome). All investigations have shown that ACTH stimulates steroidogenesis *in vitro*. Furthermore, clinical evidence shows that ACTH is the major trophic hormone of the fetal adrenal gland *in vivo*. In anencephalic fetuses the plasma levels of ACTH are very low and the fetal zone is markedly atrophic. Maternal glucocorticoid therapy effectively suppresses fetal adrenal steroidogenesis by suppressing fetal ACTH secretion. Further evidence that ACTH regulates steroidogenesis early in fetal life is provided by the observation that elevated levels of 17α-hydroxyprogesterone in amniotic fluid are found in fetuses with congenital adrenal hyperplasia due to the absence of 21-hydroxylase (CYP21) activity. Despite these observations, other ACTH-related peptides, POMC derivatives that are formed in the fetal pituitary or placenta, have been proposed as possible trophic hormones for the fetal zone, but the evidence for this proposal is weak. Other hormones or growth factors, including PRL, hCG, GH, hPL, and epidermal and fibroblast growth factors, have no consistently significant effect on steroidogenesis or adenylyl cyclase activity in preparations of fetal zone organ cultures, monolayer cells, or membrane preparations *in vitro*. However, the role of these or other hormones in promoting growth of adrenal cells is unclear.

After birth the adrenal gland shrinks by over 50% owing to regression of fetal zone cells. This suggests that a trophic substance other than ACTH is withdrawn from the maternal or placental compartment or that the secretion rate of some other trophic hormone is altered to initiate regression of the fetal zone.

The medulla of the fetal adrenal gland is formed by 10 weeks' gestation. In contrast to the fetal adrenal cortex, the adrenal medulla is relatively immature at term. The secretion of cortisol by the adrenal cortex that surrounds the medulla stimulates the formation of epinephrine from norepinephrine. However, most of the chromaffin tissue in the human fetus is formed in para-aortic paraganglia rather than in fetal adrenal medullary tissue. Both epinephrine and norepinephrine can be detected in the human fetal medulla by 10–15 weeks' gestation. Except for the effect of cortisol, the regulation of catecholamine secretion in the human fetus has not been fully elucidated. In other species, hypoxia and trauma, as well as advancing gestation and maturation, are related to the release of catecholamines by the adrenal medulla.

Fetal Parathyroid Gland and Calcium Homeostasis

The level of calcium in the fetus is regulated largely by the transfer of calcium from the maternal compartment across the placenta. The maternal compartment undergoes a number of adjustments that ultimately allow for a net transfer of sufficient calcium to the fetus to sustain fetal bone growth.

The changes in the maternal compartment that permit fetal accumulation of calcium include an increase in maternal dietary intake, an increase in circulating maternal 1,25-dihydroxyvitamin D [1,25-(OH)$_2$D] (also known as *calcitriol*), and an increase in circulating parathyroid hormone (PTH). No significant changes are observed in maternal calcitonin levels. The levels of total calcium and phosphorus decline in maternal serum, but ionized calcium levels remain unchanged. The *placental calcium pump* allows for a positive gradient of calcium and phosphorus to the fetus. This is mediated by secretion of parathyroid hormone-related proteins (PTHrP) partly from the amnion and the placenta, which act via receptors on the trophoblast to promote active calcium transport. Circulating fetal calcium and phosphorus levels increase steadily throughout gestation. Fetal levels of total and ionized calcium as well as phosphorus exceed maternal levels at term.

The fetal parathyroid gland contains PTH, and the gland is capable of hormone secretion by 10–12 weeks' gestation. Fetal plasma levels of PTH reportedly are low but increase after delivery. However the fetal parathyroid secretes large amounts of PTHrP during gestation, which may increase placental active calcium transport. The fetal thyroid contains calcitonin, and in contrast to maternal plasma levels, calcitonin levels in the fetus are elevated. Because there is no transfer of PTH or calcitonin across the placenta, the consequences of the observed change in these hormones on fetal calcium are consistent with an adaptation to conserve calcium and stimulate bone growth within the fetus.

Plasma levels of the various forms of vitamin D are lower in the fetus than in the mother. The placenta and decidua are capable of 1α-hydroxylation and of formation of the active metabolite $1,25\text{-}(OH)_2D$ or calcitriol. However, the role, if any, of this hormone in the fetus is unknown, as its major effect is on intestinal absorption of calcium.

After birth, serum calcium and phosphorus levels fall in the neonate. Levels of PTH begin to rise 48 hours after birth, and calcium and phosphorus levels gradually increase over the following several days, depending on dietary intake of milk.

Fetal Endocrine Pancreas

The human fetal pancreas appears during the fourth week of fetal life. The α cells containing glucagon and the δ-cells containing somatostatin develop early, before β-cell differentiation, although insulin can be recognized in the developing pancreas before apparent β-cell differentiation. Total human pancreatic insulin and glucagon content increase with fetal age and are higher than the concentrations in the adult human pancreas.

In contrast to the pancreatic content of insulin, fetal insulin secretion is low and relatively unresponsive to acute changes in glucose in *in vitro* studies of pancreatic cells, in cord blood at delivery, and in blood samples obtained from the scalp of the fetus at term. In contrast, fetal insulin secretion *in vitro* is responsive to amino acids and glucagon as early as 14 weeks' gestation. Although the acute response to glucose is impaired in the fetal pancreas, β cells that are chronically exposed to elevated glucose levels, as may occur in maternal diabetes mellitus, undergo hypertrophy so that the rate of insulin secretion increases.

Glucagon has been detected in human fetal plasma as early as 15 weeks' gestation. Although secretion of glucagon is stimulated in late pregnancy by amino acids and catecholamines, acute changes in glucose appear to have little effect on fetal pancreatic glucagon secretion.

Maternal Compartment

Various maternal adaptations involving the endocrine system occur during pregnancy. Many diseases of the maternal endocrine system, if untreated, are associated with infertility and reduced conception rates. If conception occurs, the more serious the disorder, the more likely it will affect the fetus adversely, as in diabetes mellitus. Hormones or drugs used to treat the endocrine disorders may be transported across the placenta and alter the environment and development of the fetus.

Hypothalamus and Pituitary

Little is known about the endocrine alterations of the maternal hypothalamus during pregnancy. Tumors of the hypothalamus or functional disorders of the hypothalamus commonly result in infertility due to amenorrhea and resulting chronic anovulation. The anterior pituitary undergoes a two- to threefold enlargement during pregnancy due primarily to hyperplasia and hypertrophy of the lactotropes (PRL-secreting cells) thought to result from estrogen stimulation. Thus, PRL plasma levels parallel the increase in pituitary size throughout gestation.

In contrast to lactotropes, the number of somatotropic cells in the pituitary decreases during pregnancy. Maternal levels of GH are low and do not change during pregnancy. Maternal levels of LH and FSH levels are also low during pregnancy. The response of gonadotropins to an infusion of GnRH is severely blunted during pregnancy. The loss of responsiveness to GnRH is thought to be caused by a negative feedback inhibition from the elevated levels of estrogen and progesterone during pregnancy. Levels of TSH are within the normal nonpregnant adult range throughout pregnancy. Furthermore, the response of TSH to a dose of TRH is similar to that in nonpregnant women.

Numerous studies have examined the levels of ACTH- and POMC-related peptides in maternal blood throughout pregnancy. The maternal plasma levels of β-endorphin remain relatively low throughout pregnancy. β-Endorphin levels do increase in maternal blood with advancing labor, but β-endorphin levels in cord blood are similar in infants delivered vaginally and delivered by elective cesarean section from women not in labor. However, fetal hypoxia is associated with significant increases in β-endorphin levels in cord blood. The plasma levels of maternal ACTH have been reported to increase from early to late gestation, but values were either in the normal range or lower than those in nonpregnant women, suggesting that ACTH may be suppressed by estrogen and progesterone. The slight increases in ACTH levels that appear to occur during the course of gestation might be explained by the increased secretion of placental ACTH that is not subject to feedback control. Maternal ACTH rises to very high levels during labor and delivery. The levels of ACTH in umbilical cord plasma parallel those of β-endorphin and, because neither crosses the placenta, offer further evidence that in the fetus, as in the adult, these two peptides are processed from a common precursor.

Corticotropin-releasing hormone increases in maternal serum throughout pregnancy and peaks during labor and delivery. Levels of CRH at term may be 50- to 100-fold higher than those in nonpregnant women. This is due to an increase of CRH synthesis by the placenta. There is also an increase in carrier protein, which binds CRH and may blunt the increase in CRH biological activity. Despite this, maternal CRH levels correlate with rising ACTH and cortisol levels over the course of gestation and labor.

Maternal plasma AVP levels remain low throughout gestation and are not believed to play a role in human parturition. Maternal oxytocin levels are reported to be low and do not vary throughout pregnancy but increase during the later stages of labor.

Thyroid

The thyroid gland increases slightly in size during pregnancy as a result of increased vascularity and mild glandular hyperplasia, but a true goiter is not present. There is a modest increase in oxygen consumption (basal metabolic rate) during pregnancy secondary to fetal requirements.

During pregnancy the mother is in a euthyroid state. Serum total T_4 and T_3 increase markedly but do not indicate a hyperthyroid state, as there is a parallel increase in thyroxine-binding globulin (TBG). Thus the levels of free T_3 and T_4 are not increased in pregnancy (Fig. 11-9). The elevation of total T_4 and T_3 is due to increased TBG from estrogen exposure. A similar finding is observed in women taking oral contraceptives. Reduced T_3-resin uptake is also observed in pregnancy and in women taking oral contraceptives. There is little if any transfer of T_4, T_3, or TSH across the placenta. Thyrotropin-releasing hormone is capable of crossing the placenta, but under normal physical conditions there is little TRH circulating in peripheral maternal plasma. In contrast, in pregnancies complicated by maternal Graves' disease, thyroid-stimulating immunoglobulins (TSI) can cross the placenta and cause fetal hyperthyroidism.

Adrenal

Compared to changes in the fetal adrenal, the maternal adrenal gland does not change morphologically during pregnancy. During pregnancy both glucocorticoids and mineralocorticoids increase with advancing gestation (Fig. 11-9). In contrast, maternal serum DHEA and DHEA-S levels fall as pregnancy progresses due to increased placental utilization as precursors for estrogen synthesis.

The increase in total plasma cortisol is due principally to a concomitant increase in cortisol-binding globulin (CBG), also known as *transcortin*. Placental CRH production may also play a role in increasing maternal ACTH and cortisol. There is a slight increase in free plasma cortisol and urinary-free cortisol, but pregnant women do not exhibit any overt signs of hypercortisolism. Little maternal cortisol crosses the placenta, as it is inactivated to cortisone by the trophoblast (by the enzyme 11β-hydroxysteroid dehydrogenase type 2).

Aldosterone levels increase with advancing gestation, reflecting increased secretion of aldosterone by the zona glomerulosa. The levels of renin and angiotensinogen rise in pregnancy, which leads to elevated angiotensin II levels and markedly elevated levels of aldosterone.

Parathyroid

Calcium and PTH changes during normal pregnancy were discussed in the section Fetal Parathyroid Gland and Calcium Homeostasis.

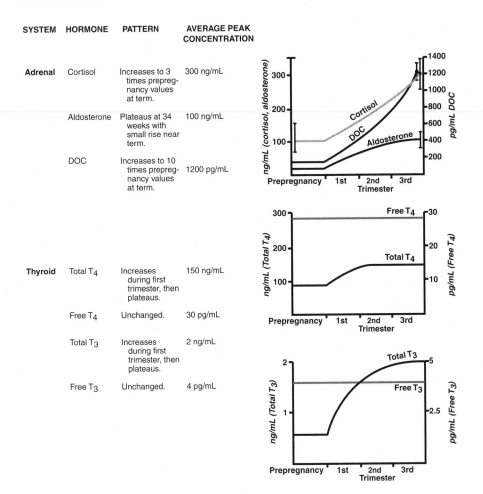

SYSTEM	HORMONE	PATTERN	AVERAGE PEAK CONCENTRATION
Adrenal	Cortisol	Increases to 3 times prepregnancy values at term.	300 ng/mL
	Aldosterone	Plateaus at 34 weeks with small rise near term.	100 ng/mL
	DOC	Increases to 10 times prepregnancy values at term.	1200 pg/mL
Thyroid	Total T$_4$	Increases during first trimester, then plateaus.	150 ng/mL
	Free T$_4$	Unchanged.	30 pg/mL
	Total T$_3$	Increases during first trimester, then plateaus.	2 ng/mL
	Free T$_3$	Unchanged.	4 pg/mL

Fig. 11-9 Maternal serum levels of adrenal and thyroid hormones during pregnancy. DOC, deoxycorticosterone; T$_4$, thyroxine; T$_3$, triiodothyronine. (Adapted from Taylor RN, Lebovic DI, and Martin-Cadieux MC: In: *Basic and Clinical Endocrinology*, 6th ed., FS Greenspan and DG Gardner, eds., McGraw-Hill, New York, p. 578, 2001, with permission.)

Endocrine Pancreas

The metabolic adaptation of pregnancy in which glucose is spared for the fetus is related to an appropriate bihormonal secretion by the maternal endocrine pancreas. In response to a glucose load, there is a greater release of insulin from the β cells and a greater suppression of glucagon release from the α cells compared to the nonpregnant state. In association with the increased release of insulin, the maternal pancreas undergoes β-cell hyperplasia and islet cell hypertrophy accompanied by an increase in blood flow to the endocrine pancreas. During pregnancy, fasting blood glucose levels fall, but rise more in response to a glucose load than in nonpregnant women. The increased release of insulin is related to a relative insulin resistance.

The insulin resistance is due to hormones secreted by the placenta that spare transfer of glucose to the fetus, including hPL. Glucagon levels are suppressed in response to a glucose load, with the greatest suppression occurring near term.

Endocrinology of Parturition

The mechanism by which labor is initiated in women is not completely understood. It is of vital importance that the etiology of the onset of parturition is clarified so as to eventually prevent preterm (or premature) birth. The sequelae of prematurity include not only increased neonatal mortality, but also significant morbidity that can result in severe physical and mental impairment of the newborn. Several theories have been proposed to explain the onset of labor. Initial studies in animal models and humans focused on endocrine changes in the fetal–placental unit. In recent years, molecular biology techniques have greatly increased our understanding of the changes occurring at the myometrial level during initiation and maintenance of labor; however, our overall understanding of the process of human labor, both at term and in preterm labor, remains incomplete. It is likely that multiple pathways operate in a variety of clinical states, such as preterm labor with and without the presence of fetal/placental infection compared with normal labor at full term (defined as 37 weeks or greater).

Fetal Adrenal

The cause of labor in certain mammalian species, most notably the sheep, appears to be regulated by signals first occurring in the fetal pituitary (ACTH), which lead to increased cortisol secretion by the fetal sheep adrenal gland. In turn, increased fetal cortisol levels stimulate 17α-hydroxylase activity (CYP17) in sheep placenta leading to decreased progesterone and increased estrogen production, which triggers the onset of labor. Administration of corticoids or ACTH to the sheep fetus stimulates labor, and the removal of the fetal pituitary or adrenal prolongs labor.

In the human, however, the role of fetal adrenal steroid secretion in the onset of labor is less clear. For example, cortisol or ACTH administration to the mother or fetus does not stimulate parturition. Fetal plasma levels of cortisol do not increase markedly before labor. In contrast, conditions that result in low levels of estrogen in the maternal compartment are often accompanied by prolonged or postdate pregnancy, failure of cervical ripening, or poor cervical dilatation during labor. Such conditions include anencephaly or failure of brain development, congenital absence or hypoplasia of the fetal adrenal, and steroid sulfatase deficiency. In each of these cases, inadequate fetal adrenal hormone precursor is available for placental aromatization to estrogen. In addition, local application of estrogen to the cervix leads to ripening.

It is believed that estrogen derived from fetal adrenal precursors does not directly cause the onset of labor, but instead may modify or fine-tune other events leading to the onset of parturition. One of the effects of estrogen is the stimulation of prostaglandin synthesis in the tissues of the uterus and fetal membranes.

Progesterone Withdrawal

Progesterone inhibits uterine contractions during most of gestation, and in the majority of mammalian species, a decline in maternal levels of progesterone precedes the onset of parturition. In both primates and humans, however, there is no significant decrease in plasma progesterone levels before labor. However, a *functional progesterone withdrawal* has been postulated. This could occur via a change in the ratio of the two progesterone receptor isoforms PR-A and PR-B, and a relative increase in the inhibitory PR-A isoform has recently been reported to occur in term human labor. Other possible mechanisms include a local increase in inactivation or clearance of progesterone within the uterus or a block of progesterone intracellular action within the myometrium.

Oxytocin

Oxytocin has been used in clinical obstetrics for years to induce or augment labor. When sensitive radioimmunoassays became available to detect low levels of oxytocin in maternal and fetal blood, it was determined that oxytocin levels do not rise before the onset of labor. The role of oxytocin is believed to be the regulation of the expulsive phase of labor and contraction of the uterus to reduce blood loss following delivery. However oxytocin may not be essential for labor, as evidenced by normal delivery in some women with diabetes insipidus lacking both AVP and oxytocin.

Relaxin

Relaxin is a two-chain peptide that is synthesized by the corpus luteum, the decidua, and parts of the placenta. Relaxin ripens the cervix in various animal species, involving increased levels of matrix metalloproteinase enzymes. In many mammals, a significant increase in the circulating level of relaxin occurs prior to parturition. In humans, the level of plasma relaxin is highest in the first trimester of pregnancy but declines and thereafter remains constant until delivery. Relaxin has been reported to decrease myometrial contractility *in vitro*. Interest in relaxin has greatly increased with the recent cloning of two relaxin receptors, although its precise role in labor remains to be elucidated. Elevated maternal serum relaxin levels have been found in preterm labor, and its role may be to induce cervical remodeling.

Corticotropin-Releasing Hormone

Levels of CRH in the placenta increase exponentially in late gestation, producing an increasing maternal serum CRH concentration beginning at around 28 weeks. In the last 3 weeks of pregnancy, CRH-binding protein in maternal serum decreases, further increasing free CRH. Placental CRH production may be negatively regulated by progesterone, and both progesterone and nitric oxide decrease placental cell CRH output *in vitro*. However, glucocorticoids increase placental cell CRH output *in vitro* and increase maternal serum CRH levels *in vivo*. It is not known whether cortisol of fetal origin, for example as produced in acute or chronic hypoxic states, acts on the placenta and membranes to increase CRH output. If this mechanism occurs, stimulation of fetal pituitary ACTH by placental CRH could result in a positive feedback loop, further increasing fetal cortisol output.

Receptors of CRH are found in fetal membranes and myometrium, and CRH stimulates prostaglandin production from fetal membranes and maternal decidua, thus promoting myometrial contractility. In addition, CRH may have direct actions on myometrium, in synergy with other mediators that promote contraction. Elevated levels of maternal plasma CRH have been found in women in preterm labor who are destined to deliver within 24–28 hours, compared with those who continue pregnancy despite threatened preterm labor. Thus CRH may be involved in initiation of term or preterm labor.

Prostaglandins

Because of the complexities and discrepancies of parturition in different mammalian species, a paracrine mechanism has been proposed to explain the onset of parturition in humans. This mechanism is related to the close proximity of the fetus, amniotic fluid, fetal membranes (amnion and chorion), and contiguous layer of the uterine decidua and myometrium. Signals not yet identified, originating in the fetus, may by a paracrine mechanism be transmitted to fetal membranes and uterine tissues, leading to increased production of prostaglandins. Accumulating evidence suggests that prostaglandins and prostanoids play a crucial role in human parturition. They are synthesized by the enzyme cyclooxygenase-2 (COX-2), which is induced in both trophoblast and myometrial cells in human labor. The trigger for release of prostaglandins is unknown but is thought to be of fetal origin and is regulated by hormone changes in the fetal–placental–maternal unit.

Prostaglandins, when administered to pregnant women, cause cervical ripening, softening, dilatation, and the onset of uterine contractions resulting in labor. The administration of prostaglandin inhibitors to pregnant women can prevent or delay preterm labor. Moreover, marked increases occur in the levels of prostaglandins in amniotic fluid and in fetal membranes before the onset of labor. Injury to the fetal membranes resulting in increased prostaglandin release results from uterine infections, stripping of the membranes from the cervix, and the instillation of hypertonic saline into the amniotic sac. Thus prostaglandins, along with other procontractile mediators such as endothelin-1 and platelet-activating factor, mediate part of the increase in uterine contractility that is integral to the process of labor. However, they may not necessarily be involved in the initiation of human parturition.

This chapter is dedicated to Yasmin and Layla Rehman.

SUGGESTED READING

Byrd W: Fertilization, embryogenesis, and implantation. In: *Textbook of Reproductive Medicine*, 2nd ed., BR Carr and RE Blackwell, eds., Appleton & Lange, Stamford, CT, pp. 1–20, 1998.

Carr BR: The maternal-fetal-placental unit. In: *Principles and Practice of Endocrinology and Metabolism*, 3rd ed., KL Becker, ed., Lippincott, Philadelphia, pp. 1059–1072, 2001.

Carr BR and Rainey WE: The adrenal. In: *Infertility and Reproductive Medicine Clinics of North America*, Vol. 5, JP Bruner, ed., Saunders, Philadelphia, pp. 749–764, 1994.

Carr BR and Simpson ER: Lipoprotein utilization and cholesterol synthesis by the human fetal adrenal gland. Endocr Rev 2:306–326, 1981.

Casey ML and MacDonald PC. Endocrine changes of pregnancy. In: *Williams Textbook of Endocrinology*, 9th ed., JD Wilson, DW Foster, HM Kronenberg, and PR Larsen, eds., Saunders, Philadelphia, pp. 1259–1271, 1998.

Cunningham FG, Gant NF, Leveno KJ, Gilstrap LC, Hauth JC, and Wenstrom KD: Physiology of Pregnancy. In: *Williams Obstetrics*, 21st ed., McGraw-Hill, New York, pp. 63–200, 2001.

Fisher DA: Endocrinology of fetal development. In: *Williams Textbook of Endocrinology*, 9th ed., JD Wilson, DW Foster, HM Kronenberg, and PR Larsen, eds., Saunders, Philadelphia, pp. 1273–1301, 1998.

Harper MJK: Gamete and zygote transport. In: *The Physiology of Reproduction*, 2nd ed., Vol. 1, E Knobil and JD Neill, eds., Raven Press, New York, pp. 127–188, 1994.

Knobil E and Neill JD. *Encyclopedia of Reproduction*, Vols. 1–4, Academic Press, San Diego, CA, 1998.

Laufer N, Simon A, Hurwitz A, and Glatstein IZ: In vitro fertilization. In: *Infertility*, 2nd ed., MM Seibel, ed., Appleton & Lange, Stamford, CT, pp. 703–749, 1997.

Molitch ME: Endocrine disease in pregnancy. In: *Principles and Practice of Endocrinology and Metabolism*, 3rd ed., KL Becker, ed., Lippincott, Philadelphia, pp. 1077–1091, 2001.

Parker CR Jr: The endocrinology of pregnancy. In: *Textbook of Reproductive Medicine*, 2nd ed., BR Carr and RE Blackwell, eds., Appleton & Lange, Stamford, CT, pp. 19–44, 1998.

Pederson RA and Burdsal CA: Mammalian embryogenesis. In: *The Physiology of Reproduction*, 2nd ed., Vol. 1, E Knobil and JD Neill, eds., Raven Press, New York, pp. 319–390, 1994.

Society for Assisted Reproductive Technology: Assisted reproductive technology in the United States: 1999 results generated from the American Society for Reproductive Medicine/Society for Assisted Reproductive Technology registry. Fertil Steril 78(5):918–931, 2002.

Steinkampf MP, Davis OK, and Rosenwaks Z: Assisted reproductive technology. In: *Textbook of Reproductive Medicine*, 2nd ed., BR Carr and RE Blackwell, eds., Appleton & Lange, Stamford, CT, pp. 665–678, 1998.

Tulchinsky D and Little AB, eds: *Maternal-Fetal Endocrinology*, Saunders, Philadelphia, 1994.

Veech LI: *Atlas of the Human Oocyte and Early Conceptus*, Williams & Wilkins, Baltimore, 1986.

Wassarman PM: Fertilization in mammals. Sci Am 259:78–84, 1988.

Weitauf HM: Biology of implantation. In: *The Physiology of Reproduction*, 2nd ed., Vol. 1, E Knobil and JD Neill, eds., Raven Press, New York, pp. 391–440, 1994.

Word RA: Parturition. In: *Textbook of Reproductive Medicine*, 2nd ed., BR Carr and RE Blackwell, eds., Appleton & Lange, Stamford, CT, pp. 45–56, 1998.

Yanagimachi R: Mammalian fertilization. In: *The Physiology of Reproduction*, 2nd ed., Vol. 1, E Knobil and JD Neill, eds., Raven Press, New York, pp. 189–318, 1994.

12

Growth Regulation

PINCHAS COHEN
RON G. ROSENFELD

ENDOCRINE REGULATION OF GROWTH

Growth Hormone Secretion and Action

While multiple hormones influence somatic growth, the main regulator of postnatal growth is growth hormone (GH). Growth hormone is secreted in a pulsatile manner from the anterior pituitary primarily as a 22 kD molecule (although other forms may be found). The development of the pituitary gland, as well as GH gene expression, is regulated by the multiple pituitary transcription factors listed in Table 12-1. *Pit-1* and *Prop-1* are genes (which thus encode proteins) that are often mutated or deleted in cases of congenital hypopituitarism.

Under normal waking conditions, GH levels are often low or undetectable, but several times during the day, and particularly at night during phase 3 of sleep, surges of GH secretion occur. Secretion of GH is mainly under hypothalamic control, and this, in turn, is regulated by catecholaminergic neurotransmitters from higher cortical centers (see Chapter 6). The hypothalamic hormones growth hormone-releasing hormone (GHRH) and somatostatin respectively stimulate and inhibit GH secretion. Recently, a new hormone named *ghrelin* has been discovered that is secreted from the stomach and acts to increase GH secretion through a specific receptor as well as to enhance appetite (see also Chapters 6 and 16). Many other factors influence GH secretion, notably, glucose that inhibits and certain amino acids that stimulate GH secretion. Exogenous physiological and pharmacological factors are known to stimulate GH secretion. Indeed, some of these agents, including the drugs clonidine and L-dopa, as well as exercise, are used in GH stimulation tests. In plasma, most GH is bound to a carrier protein called *GH-binding protein*, a cleavage product of the extracellular domain of the GH receptor.

The Insulin-like Growth Factors

In the liver and other target cells, such as bone and fat, GH induces the production of somatomedins, or insulin-like growth factors (IGF-I and IGF-II), through interaction with its receptor. Growth hormone receptor signal transduction involves the

Table 12-1   Homeodomain Transcription Factors Involved in Human Pituitary
Development and Differentiation

HESX1 (homeobox gene expression in embryonic stem cells)
PROP1 (prophet of Pit1)
POU1F1 (POU domain/Pit1)
RIEG (Rieger's syndrome gene)
LHX3 (LIM homeodomain protein)

activation of a complex Janus kinase/signal transducer and activator of transcription (JAK-STAT) pathway (see Chapter 3) that activates rapid metabolic effects as well as transcriptional signaling for IGF-I and related genes. The IGFs are found in plasma bound to a family of proteins called *IGF-binding proteins* (IGFBPs), which are also GH dependent. Most IGFs are bound to IGFBP-3 and to a third protein known as the *acid labile subunit* (ALS). The somatomedins, particularly IGF-I (previously known as *somatomedin C*), interact with target organs such as growing cartilage to induce growth and feedback on the pituitary to inhibit GH secretion. Both IGFs and their main serum-binding proteins (IGFBP-3 and ALS) are reduced in GH deficiency and elevated in conditions of GH excess. This cascade of growth control, known as the *somatomedin hypothesis*, is summarized in Figure 12-1.

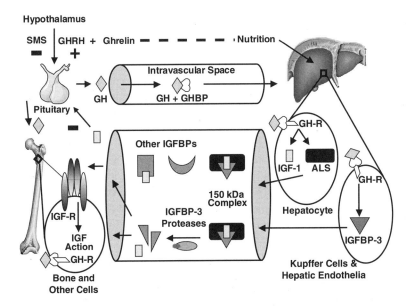

Fig. 12-1   Diagram showing regulation of growth. Growth hormone (GH) secretion is regulated by growth hormone-releasing hormone (GHRH), ghrelin, and somatostatin (SMS). In plasma, GH is bound to the GH-binding protein (GHBP). In the liver, GH mediates secretion of insulin-like growth factor (IGF)-I, IGF-binding protein (IGFBP)-3, and the acid-labile subunit (ALS) by binding to the GH receptor (GH-R). The IGFs mediate growth by binding to the IGF receptor (IGF-R).

Additional Growth Regulators

Other endocrine factors that are involved in the regulation of growth include thyroid hormone, which is essential for normal linear skeletal growth, and glucocorticoids, which can stunt growth when present in excess. Sex steroids, through several direct and indirect mechanisms, can accelerate growth and normally facilitate the pubertal growth spurt. When they are present in excess at an earlier age, the resulting acceleration of growth is associated with premature closure of the epiphysis and reduced adult height. Parathyroid hormone and vitamin D are essential for normal skeletal ossification, and the absence of or resistance to these agents is associated with abnormal growth patterns. Table 12-2 lists various endocrine factors involved in growth. Nonendocrine factors affecting growth are many and incompletely understood; by far the most important are genetic factors that determine the growth rate, the age of puberty, and the adult height. Psychological and social influences can prevent the genetic potential for growth from being fully expressed.

Malnutrition, either through dietary deficiencies, malabsorption, or as a manifestation of chronic illness, can interrupt normal growth. Interestingly, GH levels are often elevated in these conditions, but IGF-I levels are depressed.

Growth Patterns and Growth Curves

One critical growth period is the pubertal growth spurt, which is regulated by changes in GH secretion and by modulation of GH action, both related to the effects of sex steroids (for additional details see Chapter 6). Puberty is associated with an increase in the number and amplitude of nightly GH surges and a rise in serum IGF-I, both of which parallel the increase in the growth velocity of puberty. This peak height velocity occurs earlier in girls than in boys. Similarly, growth arrest due to epiphyseal fusion occurs earlier in girls. This earlier growth spurt, and the fact that puberty begins about a year earlier in girls, accounts for much of the difference in adult height between men and women. It is interesting that peak height velocity does not parallel the levels of estrogen (which rise later in girls) or testosterone (which rise earlier in boys).

The growth of an individual is a dynamic function of height increment over time. Accordingly, to evaluate growth accurately, one must obtain accurate serial measurements of a child's height and plot them on a growth curve. The data thus obtained should be analyzed after a sufficiently long period of time has elapsed between measurements (a minimum of 6 months to 1 year). Growth curves are based

Table 12-2 Hormones and Growth Factors Involved in Growth

Thyroid Hormones and Their Receptors
Fibroblast growth factors (FGFs) and their receptors
Epidermal growth factors (EGF)
Glucocorticoids and their receptors
Parathyroid hormone
Vitamin D and its receptor
Androgens and estrogens
Glypicans

on normative population data, and the ones commonly available reflect the North American means compiled by the National Center of Health statistics of the U.S. Public Health Service. An example of such a chart is given in Figure 12-2. It is preferable to use those growth curves that show the standard deviations from the mean or Z score. These types of curves allow a more precise estimation of the degree of short stature when it exists. However, it must be emphasized that growth

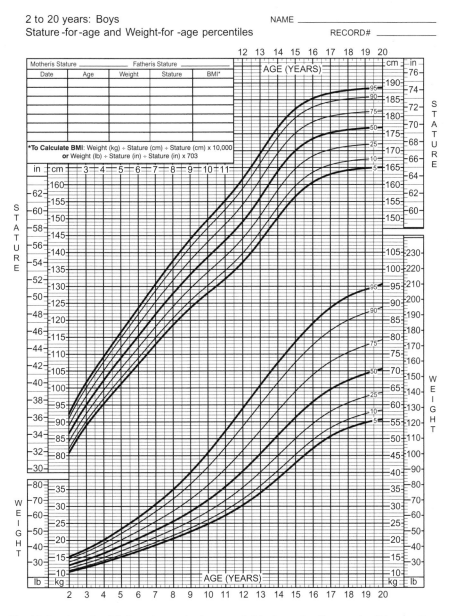

Fig. 12-2 A male childhood growth chart available from the Centers for Disease Control demonstrating normative ranges for height.

curves are cross-sectional, rather than longitudinal, and are particularly nonrepresentative during adolescence, when growth acceleration may normally occur at widely divergent ages. Consequently, it is preferable to perform consecutive measurements of height, which are then used to calculate growth velocity and are plotted on a growth velocity chart. Such charts are available at the website of the Centers for Disease Control (CDC.gov).

THE INSULIN-LIKE GROWTH FACTOR AXIS

Insulin-like Growth Factors

Insulin-like growth factors I and II are two closely related peptide hormones of approximately 7 kD in size. The IGFs were first identified in 1956 and were originally named *sulfation factors* or *somatomedins*. They belong to a family of peptide hormones that include relaxin and insulin, and share a high degree of structural similarity with proinsulin. Like proinsulin they are composed of A, B, and C domains, but also include a D domain that together form the mature IGF peptide. Both IGF-I and IGF-II are synthesized with an additional extension peptide known as the *E peptide*. In the liver and most other sites of IGF production this peptide is removed as part of the posttranslational processing of IGF-I and IGF-II. In some cases, however, larger forms of IGFs (particularly IGF-II) containing the E peptide are secreted. These larger molecular weight forms are also subject to glycosylation and may range in size from 10 kD to over 20 kD.

Both IGF-I and IGF-II have a complex gene structure, with the IGF-I gene spanning 95 kb (containing six exons) at the long arm of chromosome 12 and the IGF-II gene consisting of nine exons and having a total genomic size of 35 kb. Both genes are subject to multiple splicing, and their mRNA species exist in several different sizes. The IGF-II gene is located on the short arm of chromosome 11 (near the insulin gene) in an area that appears to be paternally imprinted. This phenomenon may be related to the fact that IGF-II is a major fetal growth factor, although the postnatal roles of IGF-II are not well defined.

The IGFs are important metabolic and mitogenic factors involved in cell growth and metabolism. They are produced in the liver, in bone cells, and in other tissues, at least partially under GH control. Circulating IGFs have direct (endocrine) effects on somatic growth and on the proliferation of many tissues and cell types, both *in vivo* and *in vitro*. However, the IGFs are also thought to be significant autocrine–paracrine factors involved in cellular proliferation. Locally produced IGFs have been demonstrated in bone, brain, prostate, muscle, mammary tissue, and other sites, where they are considered to be responsible for tissue growth and differentiation.

Insulin-Like Growth Factor Receptors

The IGFs interact with specific receptors, designated *type I* and *type II* IGF receptors, as well as with the insulin receptor. The type I IGF receptors binds IGF-I with high affinity, IGF-II with slightly lower affinity, and insulin with low affinity. The insulin receptor can bind IGF-I and IGF-II, but with much lower affinity than insulin. The type II IGF receptor binds only IGF-II with high affinity.

The mitogenic effects of IGFs are thought to be mediated primarily through the type I IGF receptor. The metabolic effects of IGFs are probably mediated through the interactions of IGFs with the insulin receptor but may involve interaction with the type I IGF receptor and/or the insulin-IGF hybrid receptors. It is unclear what function the type II IGF receptor plays in mediating IGF action.

The type I IGF receptor and the closely related insulin receptor are heterotetramers composed of a pair of α- and β-subunits, which result from posttranslational processing of a single gene product that encodes for the entire receptor. The two α-subunits are linked by disulfide bonds and are primarily extracellular; they are involved in ligand binding. The β-subunits are connected to the α-subunit by disulfide bonds and function as intracellular tyrosine kinases. They undergo autophosphorylation after the interaction of the receptors with their ligands, followed by a conformational change. Subsequently, these kinases appear to phosphorylate a cytoplasmic molecule known as the *insulin-responsive substrates* (IRS), which activate both the protein kinase B (also called Akt) and mitogen-activated protein kinase (MAPK) pathways and are involved in mediating many of the effects of insulin and IGFs.

Recently, evidence has been emerging of the existence of a class of receptors for the IGF family, which has biological properties intermediate between the insulin and the type I IGF receptor. Analysis of tissues where these receptors appear to be common (such as placenta), as well as transfection experiments, revealed that these receptors are composed of one insulin receptor a-β dimer and one type I IGF receptor a-β dimer. This receptor has been labeled the *hybrid receptor* and appears to have high affinity for insulin, as well as for IGFs. The physiological role of the hybrid receptor remains elusive, but it may explain the potent insulin-like effects seen with intravenous administration of IGF-I to humans. While IGF-I binds to the insulin receptor with only 1%–2% of the affinity of insulin, it mediates hypoglycemia *in vivo* with 7%–10% the effectivity of insulin.

The cDNA for a newly described member of this family of receptors has recently been cloned and, due to its high homology with the insulin receptor, has been designated the *insulin receptor-related receptor* (IRR). There are no known ligands for the IRR, and both IGFs and insulin bind to it very poorly. It appears, however, to be expressed in a specific manner in renal and neural tissues and may have a role in fetal development. In chimeric transfection experiments it has been documented to be a very potent mediator of cellular proliferation.

The type II IGF receptor is structurally distinct, binds primarily IGF-II, but also serves as a receptor for mannose-6-phosphate–containing ligands. It is not a member of the insulin receptor family, but rather displays homology to certain cytokine receptors. The receptor is 270 kD in size and has 15 repeat extracellular domains. The type II IGF receptor has a very short intracellular domain and an unknown mechanism of signal transduction. It has been associated with changes in calcium influx and has been reported to mediate cell motility. Recently, it has been suggested that the type II IGF receptor serves as a targeting mechanism to mediate lysosomal destruction of excess IGF-II during fetal life. Furthermore, it has been shown in mice that this receptor is maternally imprinted and negatively controls the size of the fetus, further strengthening this hypothesis. The IGFs and their cell surface receptors are depicted schematically in Figure 12-3.

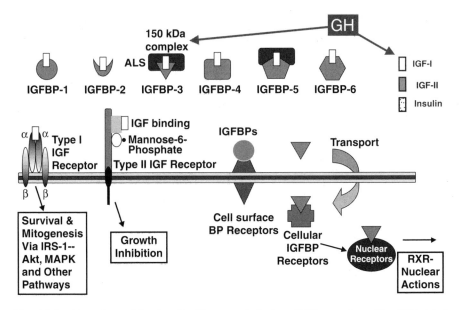

Fig. 12-3 Overview of the insulin-like growth factors (IGF) receptors. The IGFs bind to the Type I IGF receptor as well as to the Type 2 IGF receptor and six insulin-like growth factor binding proteins (IGFBPs), all of which have regulatory effects on cell function. Akt, protein kinase B; IRS-1, insulin-responsive substrate-1; MAPK, mitogen-activated protein kinase; RXR, retinoid-X receptor.

The roles of the components of the IGF system in growth can be appreciated by the phenotypes of knockout mice for various axis components described in Table 12-3.

Insulin-like Growth Factor Binding Proteins

A class of proteins with high affinity for the IGFs, the IGFBPs, have been shown to be involved in the modulation of the proliferative and mitogenic effects of IGFs on cells. The molecular mechanisms involved in the interaction of the IGFBPs with the IGFs and their receptors remain unclear, but these molecules appear to regulate the availability of free IGFs for interaction with the IGF receptor. The human IGFBP family consists of at least six proteins. IGFBP-1 is a 25 kD protein found in high concentrations in amniotic fluid and is also secreted by hepatocytes. IGFBP-2 has a molecular weight of 31 kD, is found in serum, cerebrospinal fluid (CSF), and seminal plasma, is secreted by many cell types, and is expressed in many fetal and adult tissues. IGFBP-3 is the major binding protein in postnatal serum and is synthesized by hepatocytes and other cells. In plasma, IGFBP-3 is found as part of a 150 kD complex that also includes an acid-labile subunit and an IGF molecule. IGFBP-4 is a 24 kD protein that has been identified in serum and in seminal plasma, as well as in numerous cell types. IGFBP-5 is found in CSF and, in smaller amounts, in serum; it is also observed in rapidly growing fetal tissues. IGFBP-6 is found in CSF and is

Table 12-3 Physical and Biochemical Features of the Various GH/IGF-I Knockout Mouse Models

Knockout	Birth weight (% of WT birth weight)	Other features	Postnatal course
IGF-I	60%	Normal placenta	Slow growth; die before adulthood
IGF-II	60%	Small placenta	Normal growth rate
IGF-I + IGF-II	30%	Small placenta; no respirations	Immediate postnatal death
IGF-I receptor	45%	No respirations	Immediate postnatal death
IGF-II receptor	130%	Edema	Death *in utero*
IGF-I receptor + IGF-II receptor	100%		Normal growth rate
IGF-I and GH receptor	17%		Postnatal growth retardation
IRS-1	50%–70%	Carbohydrate intolerance	Survive with normal growth rate
Insulin genes (Ins1 + Ins 2)	80%–85%	Diabetes	Early death from diabetes
Insulin receptor	90%	Diabetes; hypotrophy of subcutaneous fat	Early death from diabetes
PAPP-A	60%	IGFBP-4 proteolysis lost	Slow postnatal growth

GH, growth hormone; IGF-I, insulin-like growth factor I; IGFBP-4, insulin-like growth factor-binding protein; IRS-1, insulin-responsive substrate-1; PAPP-A, pregnancy-associated plasma protein-A; WT, wild type.

produced by transformed fibroblasts; IGFBP-6 has relative specificity for IGF-II over IGF-I. A high degree of structural homology among the six cloned complementary DNAs (cDNAs) for the binding proteins and remarkable sequence conservation across species have been demonstrated. The IGFBPs are tightly regulated by various endocrine factors and are uniquely expressed during ontogeny. They are depicted schematically in Figure 12-3.

Insulin-Like Growth Factor-Binding Protein Proteases
Recently recognized as potential modulators of IGF action is a group of enzymes capable of cleaving IGFBPs. First identified in pregnancy serum, IGFBP-3 proteolytic activity is responsible for the disappearance of intact IGFBP-3 from the serum of pregnant individuals, with no change in IGFBP-3 immunoreactivity. The IGFBP proteases have also been reported in the serum of severely ill patients in states of cachexia, in patients with GH receptor deficiency, and in prostate cancer patients. Seminal plasma contains an IGFBP-3 protease that has been identified as prostate specific antigen (PSA). This IGFBP protease belongs to the kallikrein family. It has been speculated that the IGFBP proteases are important modulators of IGF bioavailability and bioactivity through their modification of the IGF carrier proteins. The proteolytic activity may play a role in regulating IGF availability at the tissue level by altering the affinity of the binding proteins for the growth factors, releasing free IGFs and allowing increased receptor binding. One of the proteases found in pregnancy serum, pregnancy-associated plasma protein-A (PAPP-A), is responsible for

cleavage of IGFBP-4. Recent evidence demonstrates that PAPP-A null mice are small, suggesting that excess IGFBPs due to a lack of a protease leads to a functional deficiency of IGFs and poor growth (Table 12-3).

Action of Insulin-Like Growth Factor-Binding Proteins

The molecular mechanisms involved in the interaction of the IGFBPs with the IGFs and their receptors are being elucidated, and three possible models for their actions have been suggested. The first mechanism is that these molecules regulate the availability of free IGFs for interaction with the IGF receptors. Indeed, the addition of IGFBPs to many *in vitro* cell culture systems results in the inhibition of IGF actions within these experimental systems. Additionally, several trophic hormones have been shown to suppress IGFBP production by their target cells. These include thyroid-stimulating hormone (TSH) inhibiting IGFBP-2 in thyroid cells, follicle-stimulating hormone (FSH) inhibiting IGFBP-3 in Sertoli cells, and FSH inhibiting the production of an IGFBP produced by granulosa cells. On the other hand, transforming growth factor (TGF) and 1,25-$(OH)_2$ vitamin D, which are inhibitory for cells, stimulate the production of IGFBP-3 and -4. In these models, it has been assumed that the suppression or stimulation of an inhibitory IGFBP stimulates or inhibits cell growth, respectively.

In other systems, however, IGFBPs have been demonstrated to enhance IGF action, under circumstances that may involve cellular processing of the IGFBPs. These IGF-enhancing actions of IGFBPs have been demonstrated for IGFBP-1 through -5. It appears that a processing step, such as an affinity change involving proteolysis or phosphorylation, may be required for the activation of this function. Finally, as recently shown in several *in vitro* systems, including a cell transfection model, IGFBPs have an IGF-independent mechanism of cell inhibition.

The mechanism by which IGFBPs interact independently with cells has not yet been fully elucidated. IGFBP-1 and IGFBP-2 contain an arginine-glycine-aspartate (RGD) amino acid sequence that may allow them to interact with integrin receptors. IGFBP-3 does not contain such a sequence, but has recently been shown to bind to specific binding sites on the cell membrane and to be present inside the nucleus, where it binds nuclear receptors and regulated transcriptional as well as signaling events.

ADDITIONAL GROWTH-REGULATING PEPTIDES

The Fibroblast Growth Factor Family of Peptides and Receptors

Fibroblast growth factors (FGFs) constitute an important and rapidly expanding family of peptide cytokines that are important in the regulation of many tissues. Initially it was suggested that these factors may be specific for cells of stromal lineage, but it appears that many other cells respond to FGFs as well. At least seven different FGFs (FGF-1 through -7) have been identified, including the best-characterized acidic FGF (aFGF or FGF-1), basic FGF (bFGF or FGF-2), and keratinocyte growth factor (KGF or FGF-7). The FGFs mediate their actions by binding to at least three receptors—FGFR1, FGFR2, and FGFR3—that have distinct tissue distributions. For the most part, FGFs appear to be autocrine–paracrine growth factors that participate in organ growth and differentiation as well as in carcinogenesis but not in somatic growth. An exception to this rule is the observation that the genetic form of dwarfism known as *achondroplasia* is caused by a mutation in the *FGFR3* gene, suggesting that normal FGFR3 signaling is essential for the normal growth of long bones. A human mutation in the *FGFR2* gene causes craniosynostosis, a disease characterized by abnormal closure of the bones in the skull but normal long bone growth. So far, targeted disruptions of murine FGF-2 and FGF-5 have been reported, and the phenotypes associated with them do not include growth abnormalities. Future studies will further define the role different components of the FGF systems play in somatic and tissue growth.

The Epidermal Growth Factor System

Epidermal growth factors (EGFs) and their receptors are ubiquitous in many tissues and participate in developmental processes such as precocious eyelid opening and tooth eruption. The mitogenic actions of EGF have been extensively explored in cell culture systems, and the receptor for EGF was characterized as a prototype model for signal transduction involving tyrosine kinases, and the now extensive *in vitro* data indicate multiple cellular functions of EGF. Epidermal growth factor has been identified in most body fluids of several mammalian species; however, neither EGF antibody administration to newborn animals nor gene targeting of EGF has caused major deleterious effects, as might be expected from the *in vitro* studies. The EGF family of growth factors does appear to be important in mammalian development and function, although the precise roles and significance are not yet clear. Members of the EGF family may have a role in embryogenesis and fetal growth since receptors have been identified in fetal tissues. It has been proposed that abnormal EGF–EGF receptor interactions may be instrumental in the development of cancer, but it appears that they are not involved in somatic growth.

Other Growth-Promoting Peptides

An ever-increasing number of growth factors is being recognized, and multiple hormones and peptides are being characterized as having growth-promoting activities in certain cell types. In general, these molecules appear to lack somatic growth-promoting effects, but play important autocrine–paracrine as well as endocrine roles. Notable among these are groups of growth factors that have tissue-specific effects. Endothelin, platelet-derived growth factor (PDGF), and vascular-epithelial growth factor (VEGF) regulate angiogenesis and other vascular processes in addition to modulating the function of numerous cultured cells. A variety of hematopoetic growth factors such as granulocyte colony-stimulating factor (GCSF), macrophage colony-stimulating factor (MCSF), erythropoetin, and thrombopoeitin promote the growth of the different lineages of the hematopoetic cells. The growth of various cell of the immune system is stimulated by an array of cytokines including interleukins and interferons. The complex array of cells that comprise the nervous system is under the regulatory influence of specific growth factors. Other growth factors that have been attributed to specific tissues (such as hepatocyte growth factor

[HGF]) are being recognized as having general growth-promoting effects in numerous tissues. Additional organ-specific growth-regulatory processes are being described in the gastrointestinal tract, kidneys, and other organs.

Growth Inhibitory Peptides

Of particular interest is a class of cytokines that can negatively modulate cellular growth. Transforming growth factor-beta (TGF-β) can act both as an agent that mediates cellular growth and malignant transformation and as a growth inhibitory substance that has the potential to arrest the growth of normal and neoplastic cells. Tumor necrosis factors (TNF) and other compounds have been described as having similar effects. These molecules may regulate the entry of cells into programmed cell death (apoptosis). The growth inhibitory processes of TGF-β and other cytokines may prove to be of great importance in the development of cancer treatments.

DISORDERS OF GROWTH

Short Stature

Definition and Epidemiology of Short Stature

Since height is a normally distributed function, it is simple to provide a statistical definition of *normal height* as that falling between 2.0 standard deviations (SD) (Z scores) above and below the mean for each age group. This will include those individuals between the 2nd and 98th percentiles but will exclude approximately 4% of the population, many of whom represent variants of the normal state. Additionally, applying the standards of the North American population to other ethnic groups, particularly Asian and Hispanic immigrants, may prove to be an inappropriate screening method for pathological short stature. The use of population- or disease-specific growth curves (e.g., Turner's syndrome) may overcome this problem. On the other hand, it is important to consider all individuals in the context of the society in which they live and to attempt to avoid using treatment criteria based exclusively on ethnic background.

Since short stature is a significant problem at any age, even when it is a transient phenomenon, some emphasis should also be placed on predicting the adult height of an individual. Factors influencing adult height include mean parental height, current height and sexual maturation rating, chronological age, and bone age. Many methods have been developed for calculating estimated adult height. The initial step and the most easy-to-use method of predicting adult height is to determine the mean parental height (preferably obtained by direct measurements) and add or subtract (for males and females, respectively) 6.5 cm or 2.5 in. In the absence of chronic illness or endocrine disease, this often provides a fair estimation of the genetic potential. Another simple method is the *chart method*, which consists of determining the height percentile (or Z score) of the patient and extrapolating it to the adult height at the same percentile. While the above methods can provide a low-cost and immediate estimate of predicted adult height, when evaluating a child with short stature the use of a bone age radiograph allows for a much more accurate prediction.

Differential Diagnosis of Short Stature

A height greater than 2.0 SD below the mean for age during childhood can have many causes, including, as shown in Table 12-4, multiple endocrine and systemic disorders. Of these, the normal variants are by far the most common. When normal variant short stature is associated with delayed puberty, skeletal maturation, and growth, it is termed *normal variant constitutional delay* (NVCD). When it is found in individuals with normal progression through puberty and normal skeletal maturation, it is termed *normal variant short stature* (NVSS). The latter is a growth pattern representing the genetic potential for growth of that individual and is not associated with any endocrine or systemic pathology of any kind.

Normal variant short stature is often, but not always, associated with a history of short stature in at least one parent. These patients commonly have normal birth weights, and in the first few years of life their growth pattern usually settles at or just below the third percentile and then follows this percentile with a pubertal growth spurt at a normal age. The adult height achieved by these patients is typically below the third percentile (64 in. or 162 cm for males and 59 in. or 150 cm for females) and is predictable by bone age measurements. Criteria for the diagnosis of NVSS include the exclusion of organic or emotional pathology by history, physical exam, and simple laboratory tests outlined later.

Normal variant constitutional delay occurs in both sexes, although males are more likely to have this condition. A history of delayed maturation is usually present in at least one parent. The growth pattern typically observed in this condition consists of growth at or slightly below the fifth percentile throughout childhood, with further deviation from the normal growth curve at the time puberty should normally occur. Puberty develops late in these patients, but when it does, it is associated with a near-normal growth spurt and the adult height achieved is entirely normal. The diagnosis of NVCD is made by exclusion. Systemic and endocrine causes must be ruled out by the appropriate tests before NVCD is diagnosed.

Other Causes of Short Stature

Other causes of growth failure may be the result of chromosomal disorders; among these, the most common is Turner's syndrome. This condition is classically caused by a monosomic 45,X state, but other abnormalities of the X chromosomes, including partial deletions and mosaic states, may manifest the same clinical findings (see Chapter 8). Short stature is the most common finding in Turner's syndrome, with primary ovarian failure being the other important feature. Prader-Willi syndrome is a condition that is usually associated with abnormalities of chromosome 15; it includes short stature, hypogonadism, and obesity.

Children born small for gestational age (SGA) are at risk for developmental, metabolic, and growth problems later in life. About 10% of SGA children fail to catch up by midchildhood. This group of children has been shown to respond well to GH therapy in terms of improved growth and final height.

Growth failure associated with systemic disease and malnutrition is usually characterized by normal or elevated GH, but depressed somatomedin levels. During adolescence, these conditions are often associated with delayed puberty as well as delayed bone age and must be differentiated from NVCD. In underdeveloped countries, overt protein-calorie malnutrition is the most common form of malnutrition, but in developed countries, self-inflicted malnutrition (anorexia nervosa and bulimia) or malnutrition associated with chronic disease is also common.

Gastrointestinal disease may also cause growth retardation, often with few or no appreciable symptoms, usually as a result of malabsorption. Many systemic diseases treated with steroids are associated with growth retardation secondary to the effects of these agents on epiphyseal growth. Of these, asthma, inflammatory bowel disease, and rheumatoid arthritis are the conditions most commonly encountered. Insulin-dependent diabetes mellitus, when not adequately controlled, is associated with depressed somatomedin levels and poor growth.

Endocrine Causes of Short Stature

It is helpful to bear in mind that chronic illness frequently tends to retard weight to a greater degree than height, whereas endocrinopathies tend to do the opposite. Endocrine abnormalities account for only a fraction of the cases of short stature; it is, however, imperative to diagnose these children promptly, since adequate therapy can normalize the growth and eliminate the other abnormalities associated with these disorders.

Hypothyroidism in childhood is generally associated with poor linear growth. Indeed, poor growth and/or delayed puberty may be the presenting signs of chronic hypothyroidism. Congenital hypothyroidism usually results from anatomically abnormal or absent glands or from enzymatic defects in thyroid hormone metabolism. Acquired hypothyroidism is usually caused by autoimmune thyroiditis. It is important to note that hypothyroidism may coexist with GH deficiency and that it may also cause false negative results on provocative GH testing. It is therefore imperative to consider hypothyroidism as the first step in short stature evaluation.

Glucocorticoid excess, either iatrogenic or due to Cushing disease or primary adrenal hypercortisolism, is associated with attenuation of the growth rate. This finding is associated with truncal obesity and the other findings of Cushing syndrome. Congenital abnormalities of bone mineral metabolism, such as vitamin D–resistant rickets and pseudohypoparathyroidism, display classic findings that are generally noticeable prior to adolescence.

Growth Hormone Deficiency

Familial GH deficiency displays a variety of hereditary patterns, depending on the type of the GH gene mutation involved. Congenital GH deficiency may also be caused by a deficiency of the *Pit1* or related genes and may be associated with additional pituitary hormone deficiencies. Congenital GH deficiency as part of panhypopituitarism can also include abnormal secretion of corticotropin, thyrotropin, vasopressin, or gonadotropins. Congenital GH deficiency is usually recognized early in life, with the constellation of hypoglycemia, small phallus, relative adiposity, and subnormal length. Sporadic GH deficiency can be either idiopathic (most common) or secondary to pathological processes at the level of the pituitary or hypothalamus.

Patients with such disorders are more likely to present at adolescence and represent a critical group of patients that must be differentiated from the normal variants of short stature. Space-occupying lesions of the brain are the second most frequent cause of GH deficiency. Midline brain tumors, in particular craniopharyngioma are the most common, although many different types of neoplasia can involve the hypothalamic–pituitary area. Craniopharyngiomas are slowly growing, benign suprasellar tumors that infringe mainly on the pituitary and the optic chiasm. The most common symptoms of this tumor are growth failure, headache, and visual disturbances. Partial or complete hypopituitarism may develop, and the growth failure may be associated with pubertal delay, further complicating the diagnostic picture. Surgery is the treatment of choice for these tumors but subsequently is often associated with varying degrees of hypopituitarism. Other types of brain tumors, infiltrative processes such as sarcoidosis, histiocytosis X, and posttraumatic and postinflammatory conditions, can all cause GH deficiency and growth failure.

A growing number of children presenting with GH deficiency and growth failure in adolescence are survivors of malignancies who received CNS irradiation and chemotherapy. Children cured of common acute lymphoblastic leukemia represent the majority of this group since they have often undergone prophylactic radiotherapy with greater then 2000 rads and have received intrathecal cytotoxic agents, which may result in clinical symptoms of hypopituitarism years after the primary disease has been treated. Even though the diagnosis of GH deficiency may seem obvious in some of these cases, it is important to perform the full diagnostic workup on these children so that other pituitary deficiencies may be diagnosed as well.

While some extremely short children may pass provocative GH tests, they may nevertheless respond to GH therapy. This group of children, characterized as having *non-GH-deficient short stature*, has recently been approved for GH therapy in this country by the Food and Drug Administration.

Insulin-Like Growth Factor Deficiency

Recently, it has been recognized that many short children who pass GH stimulation tests have low levels of IGF-I, which appears to be the cause of their short stature. The most severe IGF deficiency is Laron-type dwarfism (or growth hormone receptor deficiency, GHRD), which is caused by mutations or deletions of the GH receptor gene and is associated with elevated GH levels and with depressed IGF and IGFBP-3 levels. However, a larger group of patients with genetically unexplained IGF deficiency exists and may benefit from either IGF-I therapy (which is under development) or from GH therapy.

Table 12-4 lists several of the aforementioned causes of short stature.

Evaluation of Short Stature

Historical features that aid in the diagnosis of short stature include the pregnancy and perinatal history, the growth pattern, the general medical history, and any symptoms of systemic disease. The family history should be probed for parental heights and growth and maturation patterns.

In the child with clinically significant short stature, when a systemic disease is not the obvious cause of the growth problem, laboratory evaluation is frequently necessary. The presence of occult chronic disease causing short stature can be usu-

Table 12-4   Causes of Short Stature

Normal Variants

Normal variant short stature (NVSS)
   Familial
   Sporadic
Normal variant constitutional delay (NVCD)

Abnormal Variants

Chromosomal disorders
   Turner's syndrome
   Down's syndrome (trisomy 21)
   Other chromosomal conditions
Dysmorphic syndromes
Skeletal dysplasias (primary and secondary)
   Achondroplasia (fibroblast growth factor receptor-3 [FGFR3] deficiency)
Systemic disease
   Malnutrition
   Eating disorders
   Malabsorption
   Other occult chronic diseases
Psychosocial dwarfism
Endocrine disorders
   Growth hormone deficiency
   Insulin-like growth factor (IGF) deficiency
   Hypothyroidism
   Glucocorticoid excess
Congenital abnormalities of bone metabolism

ally ruled out with a complete blood count, a urinalysis, and a blood chemistry panel. Thyroid function can be evaluated with a TSH and free thyroxine test. In girls a karyotype is obligatory in order to rule out Turner's syndrome, even if no other stigmata exist. A bone age is essential for the diagnostic evaluation and prognosis of all short adolescents, and IGF-I and IGFBP-3 levels can provide important insight into the etiology of the short stature. The overwhelming majority of children with GH deficiency will have low immunoassayable IGF-I levels. Finally, in the adolescent male suspected to have NVCD and considered for therapy, a serum testosterone level is often helpful.

If the child being evaluated is shorter than 2.0 SD below the mean for age and has a low growth velocity and a low IGF-I level, GH testing should be performed. In normal children, random, unstimulated GH levels are typically under 5 ng/ml; therefore, if GH deficiency is suspected, GH should be measured after appropriate pituitary stimulation. The GH stimulation tests commonly employed include GH levels 30, 60 and 90 minutes assayed after clonidine or arginine administration. It is recommended that cortisol levels also be assayed as part of a pituitary evaluation to rule out pituitary–adrenal axis dysfunction. Magnetic resonance imaging of the head is recommended in patients with documented GH deficiency to evaluate possible local pathology.

Management of Short Stature

Normal variant constitutional delay is associated with normal predicted adult height and, in the case of the socially well adjusted adolescent, reassurance is the most important aspect of therapy, since these patients will all enter puberty eventually and will experience a growth spurt at that time. Counseling of the patient and the family should center on the expected growth that follows puberty. If, however, the patient feels that he or she has become so stigmatized by the combination of short stature and sexual immaturity that reassurance alone is insufficient, testosterone therapy should be considered. The therapy most commonly recommended is testosterone enanthate, 200 mg intramuscularly every 3–4 weeks with three to four injections. The great majority of patients so treated are satisfied with this therapy, and their adult height is not compromised.

Turner's syndrome patients have been shown to benefit from growth-enhancing therapy, and the currently recommended regimen for their management involves initiation of GH regardless of the response to provocative testing. This should be done as soon as they fall below the third percentile and should be continued until the completion of growth. Disease-specific growth curves for Turner's syndrome allow the physician to monitor the response to therapy by documenting the patient's growth relative to expected growth in patients with Turner's syndrome. Other chromosomal and genetic syndromes do not respond to therapy quite as well and have not yet been adequately studied with regard to GH treatment.

Growth hormone deficiency of any type requires GH therapy, and with the unlimited availability of recombinant GH, therapy can be provided to all these patients. If the diagnosis of classic GH deficiency is made, GH therapy should be started immediately. Growth hormone is best given daily, at bedtime, as a subcutaneous injection at a dose ranging from 25 to 50 μg/kg/day (up to 100 μg/kg/day during puberty).

Complications of Therapy

Antibodies to GH can occur in response to some forms of recombinant GH, but they have clinical significance only in GH gene deletions. Slipped capital femoral epiphysis is more common in GH-deficient children and may have an increased incidence with GH therapy. Breast enlargement can occur in GH-treated boys. Concerns about leukemia, diabetes, and tumor recurrence have not been substantiated. Monitoring of serum IGF-I during therapy and maintaining it in the normal range may minimize these theoretical risks. Additional considerations include the local side effects that can be associated with any injectable drug and the possible effects of GH on carbohydrate and lipid metabolism. Finally, GH therapy may be a significant burden on the average family budget, with current costs ranging between $10,000 and $50,000 a year. All of the above considerations should be weighed and discussed before embarking on therapy.

Tall Stature

As with short stature, the normal distribution of height predicts that 2.5% of the population will be taller than 2.0 SD above the mean. However, the social acceptability and even desirability of tallness (heightism) makes tall stature a much less frequent complaint among adolescents. In North America, it is extremely unusual for males to seek help regarding excessive height, although in Europe it is somewhat more common. Even in females, tall stature has become more socially acceptable, although tall girls may still approach their physician with a desire to curb their growth rate.

By far the most common cause of tall stature (as with short stature) is normal variant familial or constitutional tall stature. Almost invariably, a family history of tallness can be elicited and no organic pathology is present. The child is often tall throughout childhood and enjoys excellent health. The parent of the constitutionally tall adolescent may reflect unhappily on his or her own adolescence as a tall teenager. There are no abnormalities in the physical exam, and the laboratory studies, if obtained, are always negative.

Pituitary gigantism is an extremely rare cause of tall stature, representing the pediatric equivalent of acromegaly (see Chapter 6). It is caused by a GH-secreting pituitary tumor and is associated with elevated and nonsuppressible GH levels accompanied by an increase in IGF-I. Typical features include disproportionate enlargement of the jaw, hands, and feet. Visual field defects and neurological abnormalities are common. Klinefelter syndrome (XXY syndrome) is a relatively common (1 in 500–1000 live male births) abnormality associated with tall stature, mild mental retardation, gynecomastia, and a decreased upper to lower body segment ratio (see also Chapter 8). The testes are invariably small, although androgen production by Leydig cells is often in the low normal range. Spermatogenesis and Sertoli cell function are defective, and infertility results. XYY syndrome is associated with tall stature and possible behavioral and mental problems. Marfan syndrome is an autosomal dominant connective tissue disorder consisting of tall stature, increased arm span, and decreased upper to lower body segment ratio.

The Insulin-Like Growth Factor Axis in Disease States

The serum levels of IGFs and IGFBPs are regulated ontogenically. Levels of IGF-I, IGF-II, and IGFBP-3 rise slowly throughout childhood and increase further during puberty. Serum IGF and IGFBP-3 levels remain stable during most of adult life and fall slowly during aging. Levels of IGFBP-2 and IGFBP-4, on the other hand, appear to rise in aging people. Levels of IGFBP-1 are highest after birth and gradually decline afterward.

Insulin-Like Growth Factor-Binding Protein in Growth Disorders

Serum concentrations of several IGF axis parameters are sensitive to the GH secretory status. Serum IGF-I, IGF-II, and IGFBP-3 levels are reduced in GH deficiency and are dramatically low in GH receptor deficiency (GHRD). Levels of IGF-I and IGFBP-3 are elevated in acromegaly. Furthermore, serum IGF-I and IGFBP-3 rise in response to GH therapy in GH-deficient patients. Nutrition plays a minor role in the regulation of serum IGFBP-3, although serum IGF levels are reduced in starvation and in poorly controlled diabetes. In all of these situations, the serum IGF-I and IGFBP-3 levels appear to correlate positively with GH and growth. However, IGF-II does not always maintain a direct relationship with these parameters and may not be directly regulated by GH.

While GH treatment consistently increases serum IGFBP-3, conflicting results have been reported regarding the effects of IGF-I therapy. In animal models, IGF-I appears to induce the production of IGFBP-3 and IGFBP-2. However, in preliminary reports on the use of IGF-I in human patients with GHRD, IGF-I appears to stimulate growth without inducing the production of IGFBP-3.

Serum IGFBP-2 levels appear to be inversely related to the GH secretory status. Concentrations of IGFBP-2 are increased in GH deficiency and GHRD and reduced in acromegaly. Furthermore, IGF-I treatment or elevated IGF-II levels (in certain tumors) are associated with suppression of GH secretion and increases in IGFBP-2. Other IGFBPs do not seem to be directly related to GH status.

The Insulin-Like Growth Factor Axis in Diabetes

In addition to their growth-promoting actions, IGFs have potent metabolic activities. Both IGF-I and IGF-II have been shown to be important regulators of glucose homeostasis *in vivo* as well as *in vitro*.

One of the postulated roles of IGFBPs is the prevention of the potential hypoglycemia that could arise from high plasma levels of free IGFs. It is thought that IGFBP-1 is the primary binding protein involved in modulating acute regulation of serum glucose levels by IGF peptides. Levels of serum IGFBP-1 measured by radioimmunoassay are strongly correlated with metabolic state. *In vivo* in humans, insulin appears to be the primary regulator of IGFBP-1; IGFBP-1 levels are inversely correlated with plasma insulin in essentially all conditions tested. Elevations of serum IGFBP-1 are seen in the hypoinsulinemia associated with fasting, Type 1 diabetes mellitus, and exercise. Reduced IGFBP-1 levels are seen in patients with insulinoma, after a meal or a glucose challenge, or during euglycemic-hyperinsulinemic clamps. The apparently inverse correlation observed between serum IGFBP-1 and GH levels in GH deficiency and in acromegaly may also be related to the changes in insulin levels that are well described in these conditions. The relationship between serum IGFBP-1 and insulin is maintained with increasing age, in relation to nutritional state, and during the circadian rhythm.

Uncontrolled insulin-dependent diabetes mellitus is often associated with growth retardation. Abnormalities of IGFs and IGFBPs are frequently reported in this condition. Total plasma IGF levels are reduced, and serum IGFBP-3 levels have also reported to be low. Both of these observations may represent a state of partial GH resistance in the poorly controlled diabetic patient. Additionally, elevated IGFBP-1 levels have been suggested to have an inhibitory role in cartilage growth in insulin-dependent diabetes. Acute administration of insulin to diabetic patients results in both metabolic normalization and a fall of IGFBP-1 levels to normal. Improved long-term control of diabetes is associated with normalization of both growth and IGFBP-1 levels. Although a cause-and-effect relationship has not been firmly established, IGFBP-1 may function as a growth-inhibiting IGF antagonist in both uremic and diabetic serum.

The Insulin-Like Growth Factor Axis in Proliferative Disorders

Several neoplastic conditions are characterized by altered expression of IGFs and related molecules. Insulin-like growth factor-I mRNA has been detected in tumors of neuroectodermal origin and in breast, bone, and liver tumors. Insulin-like growth factor-II has been reported to be expressed in excess in several benign and malignant conditions. High molecular weight IGF-II has been associated with stromal tumors causing hypoglycemia. Insulin-like growth factor-II mRNA has been reported in colon, breast, liver, and kidney tumors. Of note is that some cases of Wilms' tumor are associated with duplication in the short arm of chromosome 11, which includes the site of the IGF-II gene. Consequently, IGF-II is overexpressed in the tumor and may stimulate tumor growth.

The IGFBPs have recently been suggested to be abnormally expressed in some tumors. However, few of the reports demonstrating IGFBP expression in tumor cells used a comparable control tissue in a manner that convincingly demonstrated altered expression. Thus, although it is clear that most tumors secrete IGFBPs, no definitive examples of abnormalities in IGFBP expression are available. Serum IGFBP-2 levels have been reported to be increased in several malignancies, including leukemia and prostate cancer. Whether this elevation in serum IGFBP-2 levels represents an early tumor marker, a paraneoplastic phenomenon, or a tumor secretory product is not yet known.

The IGF axis is clearly involved in many cases of neoplastic transformation. It has been proposed that altered IGF–IGFBP–IGF-R balance in the autocrine–paracrine environment of the developing neoplasia may influence or promote tumor growth.

CONCLUSION

Over the past few years, the medical and scientific literature has witnessed an explosion of information regarding the physiology of growth and growth factors in general and the various components of the IGF axis in particular. Undoubtedly, the coming years will bring even more new information on the physiology and pathology of these key cellular regulators. Furthermore, these discoveries are likely to lead to the increasing use of diagnostic tests, as well as to therapeutic applications of these agents.

SUGGESTED READING

Ferry RJ Jr, Katz LE, Grimberg A, Cohen P, and Weinzimer SA: Cellular actions of insulin-like growth factor binding proteins. Horm Metab Res 31:192–202, 1999.

Firth SM and Baxter RC: Cellular actions of the insulin-like growth factor binding proteins. Endocr Rev 23:824–840, 2000.

Giustina A and Veldhuis JD: Pathophysiology of the neuroregulation of growth hormone secretion in experimental animals and the human. Endocr Rev 19:717–797, 1998.

Grimberg A and Cohen P: Role of IGFs in growth control and carcinogenesis. J Cell Physiol 183:1–9, 2000.

Le Roith D: Seminars in medicine of the Beth Israel Deaconess Medical Center. Insulin-like growth factors. N Engl J Med 336:633–640, 1997.

Lee KW and Cohen P: Nuclear effects: unexpected intracellular actions of insulin-like growth factor binding protein-3. J Endocrinol 175:33–40, 2002.

Longo VD and Finch CE: Evolutionary medicine: from dwarf model systems to healthy centenarians? Science 299:1342–1346, 2003.

Monzani R and Cohen P: IGFs and IGFBPs: role in health and disease. Best Prac Res Clin Endocrinol Metab 16:433–447, 2002.

Scully KM and Rosenfeld MG: Pituitary development: regulatory codes in mammalian organogenesis. Science 295:2231–2235, 2002.

Stock J: Signaling across membranes: a one and a two and a . . . Science 274:370–371, 1996.

Vance ML and Mauras N: Growth hormone therapy in adults and children. N Engl J Med 341:1206–1216, 1999.

13

The Thyroid

JAMES E. GRIFFIN

Thyroid hormones are important for the normal growth and development of the maturing human. In the adult, thyroid hormones maintain metabolic stability by regulating oxygen requirements, body weight, and intermediary metabolism. Thyroid function is under hypothalamic–pituitary control, and thus, like the gonads and adrenal cortex, it serves as a classical model of endocrine physiology. In addition, the physiological effects of thyroid hormones are regulated by complex extrathyroidal mechanisms resulting from the peripheral metabolism of the hormones. These mechanisms are not under hypothalamic–pituitary regulation.

SYNTHESIS AND SECRETION OF THYROID HORMONES

Iodide Kinetics

Adequate iodide intake is necessary for normal thyroid hormone synthesis, as thyroid hormones are the only substances in the body that have iodine in their structure. The major sources of dietary iodide are iodated bread, iodized salt, and dairy products. Individuals may also be exposed to iodide in medications, disinfectants, and radiographic contrast agents. The minimum dietary requirement of iodide is about 75 μg/day. This amount, or half of the recommended daily allowance of iodide (150 μg/day), could be obtained from 10 g of salt alone if iodized at the recommended World Health Organization rate of 1 part potassium iodide (KI) in 100,000 parts sodium chloride (NaCl). In the United States, iodized salt contains 1 part KI in 10,000 parts NaCl.

Dietary iodine intake in the United States recently ranges from 150 to 300 μg/day (down from as high as 500 μg/day in the 1970s due to decreased salt intake). The higher number is used in Figure 13-1 to depict normal iodine metabolism. Iodine is ingested in both inorganic and organically bound forms, and the organically bound form is converted to inorganic iodide. Iodide itself is efficiently absorbed; little is lost in the stool. Absorbed iodide is largely confined to the extracellular fluid. Its concentration there is normally about 1 μg/dl, and the total extracellular fluid pool is about 250 μg. The major sites of removal of iodide from the extracellular fluid are the thyroid and the kidneys. Iodide clearance in humans appears to

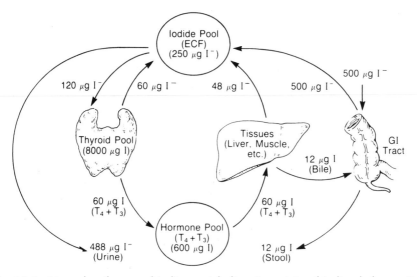

Fig. 13-1 Normal pathways of iodine metabolism in a state of iodine balance. T_3, 3,5,3'-triiodothyronine; T_4, thyroxine; ECF, extracellular fluid; GI, gastrointestinal. Arrows indicate daily flux from one compartment to another. Numbers in parentheses indicate pool sizes. (Redrawn from Larsen PR and Ingbar SH: In: *Williams Textbook of Endocrinology*, 8th ed., JD Wilson and DW Foster, eds., Saunders, Philadelphia, p. 361, 1992.)

be largely independent of serum iodide concentration. Total renal iodide excretion approximates intake. Iodide removed from the serum by the thyroid is returned to the circulation as iodothyronines (thyroid hormones), whose iodine is largely returned to the extracellular fluid after peripheral deiodination. The hormone pool of iodide includes that in the circulation as well as thyroid hormones in the tissues. The largest pool of iodine is in the thyroid, which contains about 8000 μg, virtually all in iodinated amino acids (Fig. 13-1). The thyroid iodine pool has a slow turnover of about 1% daily.

Iodide Transport and Organification

An overall scheme of thyroid hormone biosynthesis, secretion, and metabolism is depicted in Figure 13-2. The thyroid concentrates inorganic iodide from the extracellular fluid by an active, saturable, energy-dependent process. This iodide carrier is a 643-amino acid transport protein termed the *sodium iodide symporter* (NIS). It is located on the basolateral membrane of the acinar cell. It is a 643-amino acid intrinsic membrane protein with 13 transmembrane domains. Under normal conditions, the rate of inward clearance of iodide by the thyroid exceeds the rate of incorporation of iodide into amino acids (organification) and back-diffusion so that the thyroid-to-plasma (T:P) ratios of iodide are greater than unity, usually about 20 to 40. Both thyroid-stimulating hormone (TSH) and an internal autoregulatory system influence this sodium iodide symporter. Thyroid-stimulating hormone stimulates iodide transport; in general, an increasing glandular content of organic iodine di-

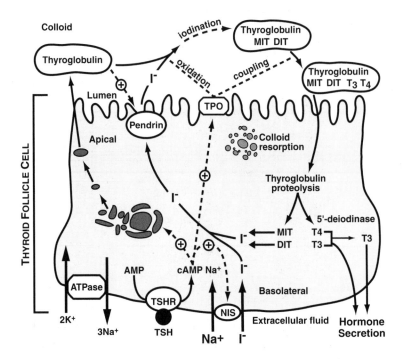

Fig. 13-2   Diagram of the steps of thyroid hormone biosynthesis and release. T_3, 3,5,3′-triiodothyronine; T_4, thyroxine; DIT, diiodotyrosine; MIT, monoiodotyrosine; NIS, sodium iodide symporter; TPO, thyroid peroxidase; TSH, thyroid-stimulating hormone; TSHR, TSH receptor. (Adapted from Spitzweg et al, 2000, p. 323.)

minishes iodide transport and its response to TSH. Iodide transport by the NIS is inhibited by certain anions, notably perchlorate and thiocyanate. Other tissues such as the salivary glands and gastric mucosa are known to be able to concentrate iodide via the NIS, and the human NIS has been identified in the breast, colon, and ovary.

There is an additional thyroid cell protein involved in iodide transport, a product of the *PDS* gene termed pendrin (Fig. 13-2). Pendrin was discovered as a result of mapping of a rare autosomal recessive condition of impaired thyroid hormone synthesis associated with congenital sensorineural hearing loss termed the *Pendred syndrome* (PDS). Pendrin is a highly hydrophobic 780-amino acid protein with 11 putative transmembrane-spanning regions initially thought to be a member of a sulfate transport protein family. It is now recognized to transport chloride, iodide, and bicarbonate. Pendrin is expressed in the apical membrane of the thyroid follicular cell as well as in the inner ear and the kidney. Mutations in pendrin cause an inner ear malformation leading to deafness. In contrast to the sodium-dependent NIS, it does not require the presence of sodium. Pendrin is thought to be needed for iodide transport across the apical membrane of the follicular cell into the follicular lumen, where it can be incorporated into thyroglobulin. Pendrin appears to be positively regulated by the autocrine action of follicular thyroglobulin (Fig. 13-2).

The two principal thyroid hormones are thyroxine (3,5,3′,5′-tetraiodo-L-thyronine), or T_4, and 3,5,3′-triiodo-L-thyronine, or T_3 (see Fig. 13-3 for the chem-

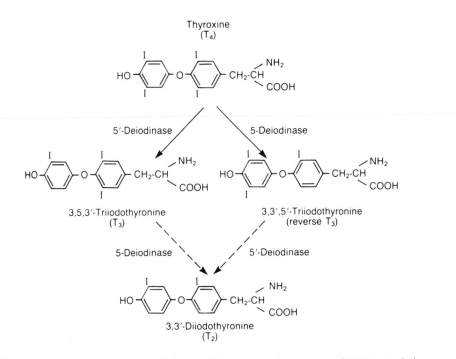

Fig. 13-3 Structures of the principal thyroid hormones, thyroxine, and 3,5,3'-triiodothyronine and part of the pathway of metabolism by deiodination. (From Griffin JE: *Manual of Clinical Endocrinology and Metabolism*, McGraw-Hill, New York, p. 50, 1982.)

ical structures). These hormones are produced from the precursor amino acids diiodotyrosine and monoiodotyrosine. These iodoamino acids are formed by the iodination of tyrosine residues within the matrix of thyroglobulin (Fig. 13-2), a large protein molecule unique to the thyroid. The iodination is catalyzed by thyroid peroxidase, a membrane-bound heme-protein enzyme. The source of the hydrogen peroxide is not known. The active iodinating agent is probably I^+ or hypoiodous acid (HOI) formed by peroxidase-catalyzed oxidation of I^-.

The thyroid has a limited capacity to utilize excess iodides in hormonogenesis. Progressive increases in the concentration of iodide in extracellular fluid are associated with progressively decreasing values of the T:P ratio, while the amount of iodide actively transported into the gland and organified rises progressively until it reaches a maximum followed by a sudden decrease, termed the acute *Wolff-Chaikoff effect*. The increasing iodination occurs despite a falling percentage uptake of circulating iodide. The serum iodide level beyond which iodination decreases is 15–20 μg/dl. The inhibitory effect of excess iodide on iodination in thyroid glands requires iodide organification. Inhibition is of brief duration, and escape from or adaptation to iodide inhibition occurs after a few days in the normal thyroid gland. This is thought to occur by down-regulation of NIS activity lowering the intrathyroidal iodide below the minimal threshold required for the Wolff-Chaikoff effect.

Both T_4 and T_3 form within thyroglobulin (Fig. 13-2) by a coupling reaction involving two diiodotyrosyl residues or a monoiodotyrosyl and a diiodotyrosyl residue, respectively. This coupling reaction occurs separately from iodination and also is catalyzed by thyroid peroxidase. The specific tertiary structure of thyroglobulin is thought to be important for efficient coupling, since disruption of its native structure or substitution of other proteins for thyroglobulin results in very low levels of T_4 formation. Thyroglobulin is a large molecule with a molecular weight of 660,000. Almost all of the thyroglobulin in the normal thyroid gland is present as a soluble protein in the lumen of the thyroid follicle. Only three or four molecules of T_4 are formed in each molecule of thyroglobulin, and certain tyrosines are favored for T_4 formation. The thyroid normally makes much more T_4 than T_3 if iodine intake is adequate, and the T_4 to T_3 ratio of normal thyroglobulin is 15:1.

Storage and Release of Thyroid Hormones

In contrast to most endocrine glands, which do not store appreciable amounts of hormone, the thyroid contains several weeks' supply of thyroid hormones in the thyroglobulin pool. Thyroglobulin must be hydrolyzed to release T_4 and T_3. This cleavage of iodothyronines from thyroglobulin is accomplished by lysosomal proteases within the follicular cell (Fig. 13-2). In response to TSH stimulation, colloid droplets are formed at the apical surface of the follicular cells by endocytosis of adjacent luminal colloid. Lysosomes migrate from the basal end of the follicular cell to fuse with the colloid droplets and release their hydrolytic enzymes. Digestion of thyroglobulin apparently releases all iodinated amino acids in the free form. Iodotyrosines are largely prevented from being released into the circulation by the action of an intracellular deiodinase (Fig. 13-2). The iodide released from monoiodotyrosine and diiodotyrosine is then available for reutilization in the thyroid gland. The free T_4 and T_3 diffuse from the cell into the circulation.

Although the thyroid is capable of deiodinating T_4 to T_3, the contribution of this pathway of T_3 formation to overall T_3 production is considered small (see below).

Thyroglobulin itself is not normally released into the circulation in significant quantities. Some small quantities of thyroglobulin can be measured by sensitive immunoassays in the peripheral blood of most normal subjects. It appears that this thyroglobulin reaches the blood via lymphatics. When the thyroid gland is damaged by disease processes, such as the inflammation associated with thyroiditis, significant quantities of thyroglobulin may leak into the circulation.

Release of thyroid hormones is inhibited by excess iodide. This effect of iodide is used in the treatment of severe hyperthyroidism. It may involve inhibition of adenylyl cyclase activity that increases as part of the normal response to thyroid stimulators.

TRANSPORT OF THYROID HORMONES AND TISSUE DELIVERY

Iodothyronines in the circulation are largely bound to thyroid hormone-binding globulin (TBG), transthyretin, and albumin. Under normal conditions at equilibrium, about 70% of T_4 and 80% of T_3 is bound to TBG. About 10% of T_4 and T_3 is bound to transthyretin. Albumin binds 20% of T_4 and about 10% of T_3. Lipoproteins carry a minor fraction of thyroid hormones. Only about 0.03% of T_4 and 0.3% of T_3 is *free* or dialyzable in *in vitro* studies. Thyroxine binds more tightly to serum-binding proteins than T_3, resulting in a lower metabolic clearance rate and a longer serum half-life. The serum half-life of T_4 is about 7 days, whereas that of T_3 is less than 1 day.

As discussed in Chapter 5, we recognize that the capillary exchangeable or bioavailable thyroid hormone, as assessed by *in vivo* studies, is greater than the free fraction as assessed by *in vitro* analysis. Measured bioavailable T_3 in brain tissue (as an example of peripheral nonhepatic tissues) was found to equal 10% of the albumin-bound T_3, whereas bioavailable T_3 in liver tissue was equal to all of the albumin-bound fraction and more than half of the TBG-bound fraction. The bioavailable T_4 in brain is similar to that of T_3, whereas bioavailable T_4 in liver is primarily the albumin-bound fraction. Thus, like steroid hormones, the capillary exchangeable fraction of thyroid hormones more closely approximates the sum of the free plus the albumin-bound fraction than it does the free fraction.

There is now strong evidence for the presence of plasma membrane carriers for both T_4 and T_3 to enter cells. The process is energy dependent, saturable and requires adenosine triphosphate (ATP). The identified carriers for thyroid hormone transport to intracellular sites of metabolism include the sodium/taurocholate co-transporting polypeptide, various organic anion transporters, and the L-amino acid transporters. Studies of thyroid hormone transport in fasting or ill individuals suggest that impaired transport of thyroid hormones to the intracellular sites of metabolism may be sufficient to account for the changes in thyroid hormone levels seen in these conditions (see below).

THYROID HORMONE METABOLISM

Kinetics of Thyroid Hormone Production and Turnover

As mentioned above, the primary iodothyronine secreted by the thyroid gland is T_4. Most circulating T_3 is produced by monodeiodination of T_4 in peripheral tissues. About 80% of T_4 is monodiodinated either in the 5' or 5 position to form either T_3 or reverse T_3 (Fig. 13-3). About 40% of the 80 mg of T_4 secreted each day is peripherally metabolized via 5'-deiodination to produce about 80% of the 30 mg of T_3 produced each day (Fig. 13-4). Most of this conversion occurs in liver and kidney, and the T_3 that is formed is released into serum. The remaining 20% of T_3 production comes from direct secretion by the thyroid gland. In most systems, T_3 has about 10 times the potency of T_4 (see below). Because under physiological conditions most of the activity of T_4 can be accounted for by the T_3 formed from it, T_4 can be considered a prohormone.

The alternate monodeiodination product of T_4, formed by removal of an inner ring iodine, is 3,3',5'-triiodo-L-thyronine or reverse T_3 (rT_3) (Fig. 13-3). Nearly all rT_3 is produced extrathyroidally, and a little more than a third of secreted T_4 is converted to this metabolite (Fig. 13-4). Serum rT_3 concentrations are lower than T_3 concentrations because of their more rapid metabolic clearance. Reverse T_3 has little or no thyroid hormone biological activity. Both T_3 and rT_3 are further deiodinated to 3,3'-diiodothyronine (Fig. 13-3) as well as to other diiodothyronines and monoiodothyronines that are biologically inactive. Both T_4 and T_3 also form glucuronide conjugates that are excreted via the bile into the feces.

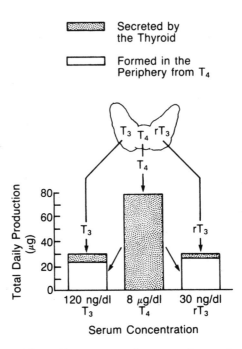

Fig. 13-4 Dynamics of thyroid hormone production and mean serum concentrations. The total daily production and distribution into the components of directed secretion by the thyroid and peripheral conversation of secreted thyroxine are shown. T_4, thyroxine; T_3, 3,5,3'-triiodothyronine; rT_3, reverse triiodothryonine or 3,3',5'-triiodothyronine. (Adapted from Schimmel M and Utiger RD: Ann Intern Med 87:760, 1977, with permission.)

DEIODINASE ENZYMES INVOLVED IN THYROID HORMONE ACTIVATION AND INACTIVATION

There are three distinct iodothyronine deiodinases (Table 13-1). They all have the uncommon amino acid selenocysteine in their active site and make use of the structure formed as a result of a selenocysteine insertion sequence to insert selenocysteine at codon UAG, which is normally a stop codon.

Type 1 deiodinase (D1) has both outer ring (5') and inner ring (5) actively. It is thought to be the primary deiodinase providing T_3 to the circulation with locations in the liver, kidney, thyroid, and brain. It converts T_4 to T_3 and rT_3 to 3,3'-diodothyronine. It has a relatively low affinity for T_4 (Table 13-1) and thus would not be saturated at normal or elevated T_4 concentrations. It is sensitive to inhibition by propylthiouracil, a drug that competes with the thiol cofactor involved with regeneration of the enzyme. Reverse T_3 is actually the preferred substrate for 5' deiodination, and inner ring deiodination of T_4 and T_3 (or preferably their sulfates) is also accomplished by this same enzyme. Fasting may be associated with lowered D1 activity by depletion of cofactors and effects of tumor necrosis factor-α (TNF-α) and interleukin-1. Thyroid hormone excess enhances and thyroid hormone deficiency decreases D1 activity.

Table 13-1   Characteristics of the Human Iodothyronine Deiodinases

	Type 1	Type 2	Type 3
Deiodination site	5′ and 5	5′	5
Physiological roles	Provide T_3 for the circulation	Provide intracellular T_3 in pituitary, brain, and brown adipose tissue; provide T_3 for the circulation	Inactivate T_4 and T_3
	Inactivate T_4 and T_3		
	Degrade rT_3		
Tissue location	Liver, kidney, thyroid, brain	Pituitary, brain, brown adipose tissue, placenta, thyroid, skeletal and cardiac muscle	Brain, placenta, skin
Substrate preference	$rT_3 >> T_4 > T_3$	$T_4 \gtrsim T_3$	$T_3 > T_4$
K_m	$\sim 10^{-7}\ M\ (rT_3)$	$\sim 10^{-9}\ M\ (T_4)$	$\sim 10^{-9}\ M\ (T_3)$
	$\sim 10^{-6}\ M\ (T_4)$	$\sim 10^{-8}\ M\ (rT_3)$	$\sim 10^{-8}\ M\ (T_4)$
Inhibition by propylthiouracil	Sensitive	Resistant	Resistant
Response to thyroid hormone excess	Increase	Decrease	Increase

T_3, triiodothyronine; T_4, thyroxine; rT_3, reverse T_3.
Source: Adapted from Larsen PR: Biochem Soc Trans 25:589, 1997.

Type 2 deiodinase (D2) has outer ring activity and is thought to be an important source of intracellular T_3 in certain tissues as well as a source of circulatory T_3. In humans it is found in the pituitary, brain, brown adipose tissue, thyroid, placenta, and both skeletal and cardiac muscle. It has a much higher affinity for T_4 and rT_3 than does D1 and prefers T_4. The regulation of D2 activity by thyroid status is opposite to that of D1; thyroid hormone deficiency enhances and thyroid hormone excess decreases D2 activity. Fasting and TNF-α decrease D2 activity in muscle. The T_3 formed by intracellular conversion of T_4 by D2 is important for providing more than half of the T_3 occupying the nuclear receptors in the pituitary, brain, and brown adipose tissue. The T_3 formed in the anterior pituitary is necessary for physiological feedback inhibition of T_4 on TSH secretion. In contrast, the majority of nuclear T_3 in the liver and kidney is derived from circulating T_3. Type 2 deiodinase is not sensitive to inhibition by propylthiouracil, perhaps because of slower turnover of D2 compared with D1.

Type 3 deiodinase (D3) has an inner ring (5-deiodinase) activity and is thought to be important for inactivation of T_4 and T_3. It is present in the brain, placenta, and skin. It has higher affinity for T_3 than for T_4 and may serve to protect the fetus from maternal thyroid hormones. It is not sensitive to propylthiouracil. The D3 is enhanced in the brain by thyroid hormone excess and decreased by thyroid hormone deficiency. The opposite regulation of D2 and D3 activities in the brain may work to keep brain T_3 levels constant in conditions of thyroid hormone excess or deficiency.

Effects of Illness and Drugs on Thyroid Hormone Metabolism

The majority of patients hospitalized with nonthyroidal illness have serum T_3 levels below the normal range. These low values are not usually appreciated because serum T_3 levels are not measured. The routine screening tests (free T_4 estimates;

see below) are within the normal range in these patients. Both TSH levels and the TSH response to thyrotropin-releasing hormone (TRH; see below) are also usually normal. However, serum rT_3 levels are elevated, and the depressed T_3 and elevated rT_3 levels return to normal on recovery from illness. These changes are due to a temporary decrease in 5′-deiodinase activity (D1). A decrease in 5′-deiodinase would not only impair T_4 to T_3 conversion but would also impair further deiodination of rT_3, in effect decreasing its clearance. A model for the low T_3 levels of illness is starvation. Total caloric deprivation results in a greater than 50% decrease in serum T_3 levels without major changes in T_4 or TSH. As in nonthyroidal illness, serum rT_3 levels increase about 50% with starvation. An explanation for the decreased 5′-deiodination may be the impaired transport of the iodothyronine substrates for deiodination into the cellular sites of the enzyme. Starvation depletes ATP and thus diminishes cellular uptake.

A major question about the low T_3 state is whether patients with significantly reduced T_3 levels have thyroid hormone deficiency at the tissue level. Although the fact that TSH values are not usually increased would seem to argue against it, it could be postulated that impaired hypothalamic TRH secretion might mask actual thyroid hormone deficiency. When fasted subjects with decreased serum T_3 levels are given exogenous T_3 replacement, muscle protein catabolism is enhanced, as evidenced by increased urinary urea, ammonia, and 3-methylhistidine excretion. This has been taken as evidence of a protein-sparing effect of the low T_3 levels in starvation. In clinical observations of patients with low T_3 levels associated with illness, the basal metabolic rate and the cardiac measurement of thyroid status—pulse wave arrival time—are normal, again suggesting adequate thyroid effects at the tissue level. Dynamic tests of feedback at the hypothalamic–pituitary level, though normal in fasted subjects, may be subtly abnormal in some patients with illness and low T_3 levels. In general, however, there is little evidence for significant thyroid hormone deficiency at the tissue level, and the impaired T_4 to T_3 conversion is probably beneficial in sparing protein catabolism.

Two iodine-containing drugs given to patients with nonthyroidal illness inhibit 5′-deiodinases in all tissues and result in elevated T_4 levels (Fig. 13-5). They are iopanoic acid, a drug used for radiographic visualization of the gallbladder, and amiodarone, a drug used to treat cardiac arrhythmias. These compounds appear to mimic the structure of T_4 in the iodine substitutions on the benzene ring and the presence of an aliphatic side chain (Fig. 13-5). The evidence for inhibition of D2 is that these drugs result in an elevation of TSH levels. On discontinuation of the amiodarone or while waiting for the elimination of iopanoic acid, the alterations in thyroid function tests return to normal.

REGULATION OF THYROID FUNCTION

The Hypothalamic–Pituitary–Thyroid Axis

The function of the thyroid gland is regulated mainly by TSH, an anterior pituitary glycoprotein hormone with an α- and β-subunit and a molecular weight of about 28,000 (see Chapter 5). The α-subunit of TSH is identical to the α-subunit of go-

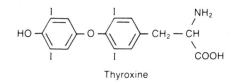

Thyroxine

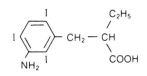

Iopanoic Acid

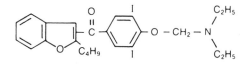

Amiodarone

Fig. 13-5 Structures of thyroxine, the oral cholecystographic agent iopanoic acid, and the antiarrhythmic agent amiodarone. The similarities of iodine substitutions on the benzene rings and aliphatic side chains are shown. (From Griffin JE: Am J Med Sci 289:86, 1985, with permission.)

nadotropins, whereas the β-subunit is distinct and confers on the intact TSH molecule its biological activity. The TSH stimulates the thyroid by interacting with specific cell surface, G protein–linked receptors on thyroid follicular cells to enhance the activity of adenylyl cyclase and thus stimulate the generation of cyclic adenosine monophosphate (AMP) as a second messenger inside the cell. All of the intracellular effects of TSH stimulation can be mimicked by cyclic AMP in the absence of TSH.

The regulation of TSH secretion by the pituitary is primarily under the dual control of the hypothalamic tripeptide TRH and thyroid hormones (Fig. 13-6). Thyrotropin-releasing hormone is derived from a pro-TRH peptide. Like other hypothalamic-releasing hormones, TRH reaches the anterior pituitary via the hypothalamic–pituitary portal circulation (see Chapter 6). It interacts with specific receptors on pituitary thyrotrophs to release TSH and on mammotrophs to release prolactin. Thyrotropin-releasing hormone belongs to the category of stimulating factors whose action starts with the hydrolysis of phosphatidylinositol 4,5-bisphosphate (PIP_2) (see Chapter 3). The hydrolysis of PIP_2 in the cell surface membrane generates two second messengers, inositol trisphosphate (IP_3) and 1,2-diacylglycerol. This hydrolysis is catalyzed by the membrane-bound enzyme phospholipase C and is associated with the rapid elevation of the concentration of free ionized calcium in the cell cytoplasm. The released calcium is thought to stimulate exocytosis. Together with these effects of IP_3, there is a parallel activation of protein kinase C by dia-

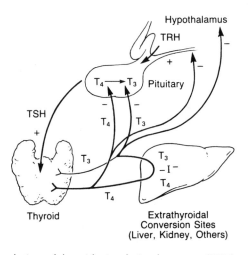

Fig. 13-6 The regulation of thyroid-stimulating hormone (TSH) secretion by the anterior pituitary. Positive effects of thyrotropin-releasing hormone (TRH) from the hypothalamus and negative effects of circulating 3,5,3'-triiodothyronine (T_3) and T_3 from intrapituitary and hypothalamic conversion of thyroxine (T_4).

cylglycerol that leads to phosphorylation of proteins involved in exocytosis and mediates the sustained phase of secretion.

The release of TRH is controlled by central nervous system mechanisms (see Chapter 6). Thyrotropin-releasing hormone is probably released in a pulsatile fashion, as pulsatile TSH secretion has been identified. The release of TSH is not absolutely dependent on TRH because low residual secretion of TSH persists even after the secretion of TRH has been stopped. Thus, the decrease in thyroid activity is more severe following hypophysectomy, which eliminates the source of TSH, than following hypothalamic lesions.

The ability of the thyrotroph to respond to TRH with increased TSH release is controlled by the feedback inhibition of thyroid hormones (Fig. 13-6). Either T_4 or T_3 is capable of inhibiting TSH secretion; however, as previously discussed, T_3 formed in the pituitary by 5'-deiodination (D2) of circulating T_4 appears to be a more important source of thyroid hormone to occupy nuclear receptors and mediate this feedback inhibition than is circulating T_3. Negative feedback by T_3, formed by D2, occurs at both the pituitary and the paraventricular nucleus of the hypothalamus. Negative feedback involves decreased transcription of TSH-α and -β genes and also the pro-TRH gene. It is not known whether thyroid hormones also inhibit TRH release. Studies in which exogenous TRH was administered to normal subjects and patients with thyroid hormone deficiency or thyroid hormone excess indicate that feedback at the level of the pituitary is sufficient to explain the regulation of TSH secretion. The TSH response to administered TRH is enhanced in patients with thyroid hormone deficiency compared to normal subjects. In contrast, thyroid hormone excess diminishes or abolishes the TSH response to TRH. Also, TRH receptors on thyrotrophs are increased in hypothyroidism and decreased in hyperthyroidism.

In addition to TRH and thyroid hormone, other substances of hypothalamic origin play some role in regulating TSH secretion. Somatostatin, another hypothalamic hormone (see Chapter 6), can inhibit TSH secretion. Because injection of antisomatostatin antiserum into normal animals increases TSH levels, somatostatin may be a tonic inhibitor of TSH secretion. The neurotransmitter dopamine may also be responsible for tonic inhibition of TSH release, as dopamine antagonists cause elevation of serum TSH levels in normal subjects. It is not known by what mechanism dopamine inhibits TSH; it may act via effects on somatostatin. Finally, glucocorticoids, when present at supraphysiological levels, lead to partial inhibition of TSH secretion.

Thyroid Autoregulation

Although TSH is the primary regulator of thyroid function, the thyroid is also capable of some degree of autoregulation (as discussed above in relation to iodide transport and organification). The autoregulatory responses appear to operate in a manner to maintain thyroid hormone stores in the thyroid gland. Thus, in a state of iodide deficiency the efficiency of iodide transport is enhanced, with the opposite occurring in the presence of iodide excess. This response occurs without a detectable change in TSH levels. Proof of the autoregulatory nature of the inverse effect of iodide availability on iodide transport is found in the persistence of the phenomenon in the hypophysectomized animal. As previously mentioned, the mediator of the autoregulatory effect appears to be organic iodine rather than inorganic iodine in the gland.

EFFECTS OF THYROID HORMONES

Mechanism of Thyroid Hormone Action

Although there is some evidence to support cell surface and mitochondrial sites of action of thyroid hormones, most of the characteristic biological effects of thyroid hormones are thought to be mediated by an interaction of T_3 with specific nuclear receptors. The mechanism of action of thyroid hormones is quite similar to that of steroid hormones in that the binding of the hormone is to a nuclear receptor, with resultant alteration of transcription of specific messenger RNAs (see Chapter 3). In contrast to steroid hormone receptors that may not be firmly anchored in the nucleus before hormone binding (and thus are found in cytosol fractions following cell disruption), thyroid hormone receptors are thought to be tightly associated with acidic nonhistone nuclear proteins.

This nuclear thyroid hormone receptor has a low capacity (about 1 pmol/mg DNA) and a high affinity for T_3 (about 10^{-10} M). The affinity of the receptor for T_4 is about 15-fold less. Initial studies of the nuclear receptor demonstrated a correspondence of receptor number and known responsiveness to thyroid hormones in a number of tissues. In the normal animal, about 85% of the total iodothyronine bound to liver and kidney nuclei is T_3 and the remaining 15% is T_4.

All of the major effects of thyroid hormones appear to be mediated by the nuclear receptor. The production of many major classes of messenger RNA rises in response to thyroid hormones. Thyroid hormones stimulate the cell membrane enzyme Na^+,K^+-ATPase and thus increase oxygen consumption. That this stimulation of ATPase activity is mediated through the nuclear receptor is indicated by the observation that the increased enzyme activity is due to an increased number of *pump units* rather than an alteration in preexisting enzyme molecules. Likewise, in studies of the effects of thyroid hormones on myocardial β-adrenergic receptors, the number but not the affinity of the receptors increased in response to thyroid hormones. The stimulation of uncoupling proteins in the inner mitochondrial membrane (see below) is also thought to be mediated by the nuclear receptor.

The thyroid hormone receptor (TR) belongs to the family of steroid-thyroid-retinoid of intracellular receptors (see Chapter 3) and is the product of the cellular homolog of the viral oncogene *erb-A*. There are multiple TRS divided into α- and β-forms on the basis of sequence similarities and chromosomal location (Fig. 13-7). The TRβ gene is on human chromosome 3. TRβ2 differs from TRβ1 in that it is not widely distributed and appears to be specific to pituitary, brain, and cochlea. TRα1 has been localized to human chromosome 17 and is widely distributed, like TRβ1. Alternative splicing of the TRα gene transcripts yields a species called *c-erb-Aα2*, which is identical to TRα1 for the first 370 amino acids, including the DNA-binding domain, and then diverges completely (Fig. 13-7). This latter *c-erb-Aα* does not bind T_3 and is thus not a TR. However, it is widely distributed and demonstrates regulation by T_3, as do the true TRs.

In addition to binding T_3, a true TR must also be able to bind to a thyroid hormone response element (TRE), a specific DNA sequence in the promoter region of thyroid-responsive genes. Generally, binding of T_3 and the TRE by TRs results in alteration (either activation or suppression) of gene transcription. TRβ1, TRβ2, and TRα1 all bind T_3 in a similar manner. The binding of TRs to TREs is independent of T_3. All three TRs are able to confer T_3 responsiveness when expressed in cells that normally do not respond to T_3. In contrast, *c-erb-Aa2* does not produce a T_3 dependency of transcription of genes bearing TREs. Instead, it appears to inhibit

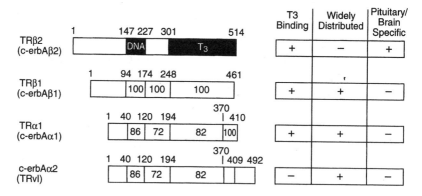

Fig. 13-7 Thyroid hormone receptors and the carboxy-terminal variant *c-erb-Aa2*. The sequences deduced from rat cDNAs are depicted with the amino acids numbered above. Putative DNA- and T_3-binding domains are indicated. Numbers in boxes indicate percent identity with TRβ2.

the action of TRs in a concentration-dependent manner. Although it may regulate thyroid hormone action, the exact *in vivo* functions of *c-erb-Aa2* have not been defined. In the absence of T_3, a TRE-bound TR may actually decrease basal T_3-responsive gene expression.

Based on evidence of heterodimer formation of TRs with the closely related retinoid-X receptor (RXR) and the enhanced stability of the TR:RXR heterodimer binding to most TREs compared to TR monomers or homodimers, the TR:RXR heterodimer is thought to be the most important complex *in vivo*. TRβ knockout mice have deafness, a decreased feedback effect of thyroid hormones on the hypothalamus and pituitary, and resultant high levels of TSH and thyroid hormones similar to those in humans with generalized resistance to thyroid hormone known to be associated with TRβ mutations. TRα-1 knockout mice have bradycardia and hypothermia.

Physiological Effects

Thyroid hormones have effects in almost all tissues of the body. In many respects, thyroid hormones may be viewed as tissue growth factors. Indeed, normal overall whole body growth does not occur in the absence of thyroid hormones despite adequate levels of growth hormone. In amphibians the effects of thyroid hormones on differentiation are dramatically evidenced by the failure of metamorphosis to occur in their absence.

Thyroid hormones have specific tissue effects that are perhaps best exemplified by the effects of thyroid hormone deficiency and excess (see below). These effects are mediated by the action of thyroid hormones on the concentration and activity of enzymes; the metabolism of substrates, vitamins, and minerals; and the function of other endocrine systems. The earliest recognized physiological effect of thyroid hormones is their ability to stimulate the basal metabolic rate or calorigenesis. Thyroid hormones stimulate oxygen consumption in the whole animal and in isolated tissues *in vitro*.

The stimulation of synthesis of membrane Na^+,K^+-ATPase is thought to contribute to the increased energy expenditure in going from the thyroid-deficient to the normal (euthyroid) state. This ability of thyroid hormones to enhance ATPase activity can be detected in many but not all tissues, and it is thought to account for only a small fraction of the effects of thyroid hormone on calorigenesis. Thyroid hormones exert effects on thermogenesis and temperature regulation that are related to their effects on energy metabolism. Rats deficient in thyroid hormones are unable to survive in a cold environment.

Because of the central role mitochondria play in cellular energy transduction, effects of thyroid hormones on mitochondrial oxidative phosphorylation are thought to be the primary mechanism for thyroid hormone to stimulate calorigenesis. Uncoupling protein 1 (UCP1) was initially described in the brown adipose tissue of the rodent as a molecule that allowed the return of protons to the mitochondrial matrix, bypassing ATP synthase and therefore uncoupling oxidative phosphorylation. Thus, fatty acids can be oxidized with generation of heat but not ATP. Because thyroid hormone stimulates UCP, this was considered a potential site of regulation of energy metabolism. However, very little brown adipose tissue is present in humans.

Additional UCPs—UCP2, UCP3, BMCP1 (brain mitochondrial carrier protein 1) or UCP5, and UCP4—have been identified. Uncoupling protein 3 is predominantly expressed in skeletal muscle, and it is also present in heart and brown adipose tissue. The proteins BMCP1/UCP5 and UCP4 are predominantly expressed in brain, whereas UCP2 is more widely expressed. Studies in hypothyroid rodents suggest that T_3 stimulates UCP3 in skeletal muscle and heart, and that the resulting mitochondrial uncoupling occurs in a time course consistent with UCP3 serving as a molecular determinant for regulation of the resting metabolic rate by thyroid hormone.

Protein synthesis and degradation are stimulated by thyroid hormones. Stimulation of protein synthesis may be responsible for a portion of the calorigenic effect of thyroid hormones. The positive influence of thyroid hormones on normal body growth is derived largely from stimulation of protein synthesis. In the presence of a large excess of thyroid hormones there is accelerated protein catabolism, leading to increased nitrogen excretion.

Thyroid hormones affect most aspects of carbohydrate metabolism. They appear to enhance the actions of epinephrine in stimulating glycogenolysis and gluconeogenesis and to potentiate the actions of insulin on glycogen synthesis and glucose utilization. As with thyroid hormone effects on protein metabolism, a biphasic action of thyroid hormones on carbohydrate metabolism can be detected. Thus, low doses of thyroid hormones given to animals enhance glycogen synthesis in the presence of insulin, whereas large doses stimulate glycogenolysis. Thyroid hormones also enhance the rate of intestinal absorption of glucose and its rate of uptake by adipose tissue and muscle.

Thyroid hormones have multiple effects on lipid metabolism. Cholesterol synthesis and its metabolic conversions are depressed in thyroid hormone deficiency. However, as degradation is affected to a greater extent than synthesis, serum cholesterol levels increase in the thyroid-deficient state, and serum levels of cholesterol, phospholipids, and triglycerides decrease with thyroid hormone excess. One mechanism that may partially account for enhanced cholesterol metabolism in response to thyroid hormones is the ability of thyroid hormones to increase the number of low-density lipoprotein receptors on the cell surface (see Chapter 16). Fatty acid metabolism is affected by thyroid hormones that enhance lipolysis in adipose tissue.

Effects of Thyroid Hormone Deficiency

Severe thyroid hormone deficiency in infancy is termed *cretinism* and is characterized by mental as well as growth retardation. The developmental milestones of the infant such as sitting and walking are delayed. Linear growth impairment may lead to dwarfism, characterized by limbs that are disproportionately short compared with the trunk. When thyroid hormone deficiency begins later in childhood, mental retardation is less prominent and impairment of linear growth is the major feature. The result is a child who appears younger than his or her chronological age. Epiphyseal development is delayed so that bone age is less than chronological age.

The onset of thyroid hormone deficiency in the adult is usually insidious; the symptoms and signs gradually appear over months or years. The early symptoms are nonspecific. Fatigue and lethargy are common, and constipation may develop or worsen. Eventually there is an overall slowing of mental function and motor activity. Although some weight gain usually occurs, appetite is usually decreased so that gross obesity is rare. Cold intolerance may be the first manifestation of thyroid hormone deficiency, with the individual complaining of feeling cold in a room in which others are comfortable. Women may experience abnormalities of menstrual function, with increased menstrual flow being more common than cessation of menses. Decreased clearance of adrenal androgens may facilitate extraglandular estrogen formation leading to anovulatory cycles with infertility. Hair loss may occur, as may brittle nails and dry, coarse skin. The voice may become hoarse.

When thyroid hormone deficiency is long-standing and severe, there is an accumulation of mucopolysaccharides in subcutaneous tissues and other organs, termed *myxedema*. Dermal infiltration results in thickened features, periorbital edema, and swelling of the hands and feet that does not indent with pressure. Stiffness and aching of muscles may be followed by muscle swelling as an early manifestation. Delayed muscle contraction and relaxation lead to slow movement and delayed tendon reflexes. Both stroke volume and heart rate are reduced so that cardiac output decreases. The heart may enlarge, and a pericardial effusion develops. Pleural and peritoneal fluids rich in protein and mucopolysaccharides may accumulate. The slowing of mental function is characterized by impaired memory, slow speech, decreased initiative, and eventually somnolence. Mild hypothermia may lead to more severe hypothermia if there is environmental exposure. Eventually, coma may develop in conjunction with hypoventilation.

Effects of Thyroid Hormone Excess

The earliest manifestations of thyroid hormone excess are usually nervousness, irritability or emotional instability, a feeling that the heart is pounding, fatigue, and heat intolerance. As with thyroid hormone deficiency, the last may be manifested as discomfort in a room in which others are comfortable and lead to resetting the thermostat or requiring lighter clothing. Increased sweating is commonly noticed. Although fatigue invariably occurs, the nervousness and irritability may give the impression of increased energy. Weight loss despite normal or increased food intake is one of the most common manifestations. The increased food intake occasionally can be so great as to overcome the hypermetabolic state and result in weight gain. Interestingly, most patients state that their increased caloric intake is predominantly in the form of carbohydrates. Women have decreased or absent menstrual flow. The number of bowel movements per day often increases, but true watery diarrhea is rare. Physical findings may include warm, moist skin with a velvety texture often compared to that of a newborn; a change in the fingernails, termed *onycholysis*, involving separation of the nail from the nail bed; and proximal muscle weakness, often making it difficult for the patient to rise from a sitting or squatting position. In contrast to thyroid hormone deficiency, the hair has a very fine texture, but hair loss may similarly occur. On extending the fingers of an outstretched hand a fine tremor may be seen. The eyelids may retract, leading to the impression that the patient is staring. Tachycardia that persists during sleep is characteristic, and atrial arrhythmias and congestive heart failure may develop.

CLINICAL ASSESSMENT OF THYROID STATUS

To assess thyroid status, one must search the medical history for symptoms of thyroid hormone deficiency or excess and examine the patient for thyroid enlargement as well as other physical findings typical of thyroid disease (see above). Because thyroid disease is relatively common and the clinical manifestations may be subtle, laboratory tests are widely used to screen for the presence of thyroid dysfunction and to confirm the suspected diagnosis.

Measurement of Serum Thyroid-Stimulating Hormone

With the development of immunometric assays (see Chapter 5), measurement of the serum TSH has become the best initial test in clinical assessment of thyroid status in most situations. The previous (or first-generation) TSH assays were radioimmunoassays that did not have sufficient sensitivity to differentiate low values from normal values. The current second- and third-generation TSH assays have increased sensitivity (0.1 and 0.01 mU/ml, respectively). The typical range of serum TSH in a normal population is 0.4–4.5 mU/ml. Because the overwhelming majority of patients with thyroid disease have primary disease of the thyroid rather than abnormalities of the hypothalamus or pituitary (see below), the usual clinical laboratory second-generation TSH assay can distinguish thyroid hormone deficiency or excess by the response of the hypothalamic–pituitary axis. Thyroid hormone deficiency results in increased serum TSH levels if the axis is intact, and thyroid hormone excess results in low TSH levels (Fig. 13-8). If hypothalamic–pituitary function is not normal—as in the patient with hypopituitarism or a TSH-producing pituitary tumor (see Chapter 6)—the TSH is not a reliable indicator of thyroid status. The serum TSH may also be unreliable in some patients with nonthyroidal illness (see below).

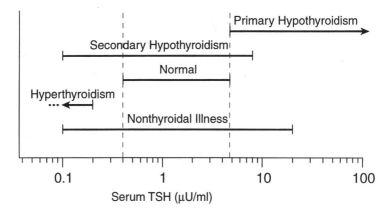

Fig. 13-8 The range of serum thyroid-stimulating hormone (TSH) values encountered in various thyroid states and nonthyroidal illness. The usual sensitivity of the second-generation immunometric TSH assay of 0.1 mU/ml is shown. Patients with hyperthyroidism are shown as having values that may be undetectable not only in this assay but also in more sensitive assays.

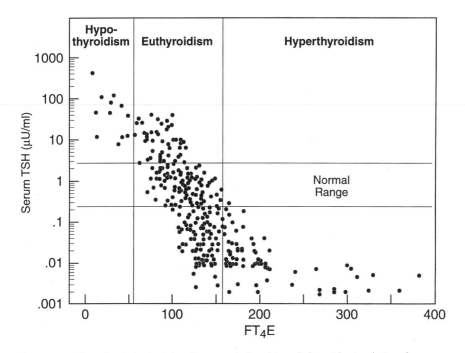

Fig. 13-9 The physiological log/linear relationship of thyroid-stimulating hormone (TSH) to the free T₄ estimate (FT₄E). The FT₄E is given in arbitrary units. A 2-fold change in the serum FT₄E results in a 160-fold change in serum TSH. (Redrawn from Spencer C: Kodak Thyroid Information Service 1992, p. 17.)

The reason that the serum TSH is particularly useful in assessment of thyroid status is the log-linear relationship that exists between serum TSH and the free thyroid hormone estimate (Fig. 13-9). A small change in the free thyroid levels results in a much greater proportional change in TSH levels. For example, a 2-fold change of the free T_4 concentration results in a greater than 50-fold change in the serum TSH level (Fig. 13-9).

Measurement of Circulating Thyroid Hormones

Measurement of total T_4 and T_3 concentrations in the plasma is accomplished by immunoassay. As discussed above, both hormones are largely bound to serum proteins, and the bioavailable component would appear to be the most desirable fraction to measure. However, the bioavailable fraction is different for T_4 and T_3 and varies in different tissues.

Although the actual bioavailable thyroid hormone fraction is greater than the free or unbound fraction in the plasma (see above), clinical states of thyroid hormone deficiency and excess correlate reasonably well with the free iodothyronine concentrations. Thus, attempts have been made to assess the free T_4 and T_3 concentrations. The reference test for free thyroid hormone levels is equilibrium dialysis. In this test radiolabeled iodothyronine is added to the patient's serum, and the percentage that is able to pass through a dialysis membrane is determined. This percentage is then multiplied by the total iodothyronine concentration measured by immunoassay to obtain a free iodothyronine concentration. The free T_4 concentration by dialysis in a normal population is about 0.8–1.5 ng/dl.

Because determination of the free T_4 by equilibrium dialysis is laborious and not routinely available in clinical laboratories, several approaches in obtaining an approximation of the free T_4 (or T_3) have been developed. These free T_4 and T_3 estimates are primarily important for correcting for variations in the concentration of TBG (see below).

Until recently, the most commonly used method for estimating free T_4 and T_3 levels was the correction of the measured total T_4 or T_3 by an *in vitro* test to assess total available binding sites for thyroid hormone in the serum and calculate a free T_4 or T_3 index. The ranges for the total T_4 and T_3 concentrations in a normal population are 5–12 mg/dl and 60–180 ng/dl, respectively. The *in vitro* test used to adjust the total iodothyronine concentrations is termed the *T_3-resin uptake* or *T_3-uptake ratio* and is performed by incubating a serum sample with radioactive T_3. After equilibration a resin or other substance is added to the mixture to bind the radioactive T_3 not bound to serum proteins. The percentage of the total radioactive T_3 bound to the resin is related in a reciprocal manner to the thyroid hormone-binding capacity in the sample. There are two possible interpretations of both an increased and a decreased T_3-resin uptake. An increased T_3-resin uptake (i.e., more T_3 bound to the resin and less to the serum-binding proteins) could be due to greater saturation of a normal amount of TBG secondary to increased thyroid hormone production (i.e., thyroid hormone excess). Alternatively, because of a decreased concentration of TBG with normal thyroid hormone production, there could be fewer available binding sites, resulting in more T_3 being bound to the resin.

Conversely, decreased T_3-resin uptake (i.e., less T_3 bound to the resin and more to the serum-binding proteins) could be due to decreased saturation of a normal amount of TBG because of decreased thyroid hormone production (i.e., thyroid hormone deficiency). Alternatively, because of an increased concentration of TBG with normal thyroid hormone production, there could be more available binding sites, resulting in less T_3 being bound to the resin. The value of the T_3-resin uptake is either reported as a percentage or compared to the T_3-resin uptake of a normal serum pool and reported as a T_3-uptake ratio, with the normal being unity. The free T_4 index is the product of the serum total T_4 and the T_3-resin uptake. This calculation is usually made only for the total T_4, but it can also be made for the total T_3.

The effect of pregnancy and other conditions that alter the level of TBG (Table 13-2) is to increase or decrease total T_4 and T_3 concentrations without changing the level of free, unbound hormone in the steady state. For example, if TBG increases in concentration, the amount of free hormone decreases temporarily until compensatory mechanisms result in a new steady state with an increased total hormone concentration but normal free hormone. The correction of the increased total T_4 by the decreased T_3-resin uptake results in a normal free T_4 index. Thus, changes in the T_3-resin uptake are reciprocal to the changes in the number of available binding sites on TBG and the total T_4 when the primary abnormality is a change in binding proteins. When there is a primary alteration in thyroid hormone

Table 13-2 Conditions and Hormones That Alter the Level of Thyroid Hormone–Binding Globulin (TBG)

Increased TBG	Decreased TBG
Pregnancy	Androgens and anabolic steroids
Newborn state	Large dose of glucocorticoids
Oral contraceptives and other sources of estrogens	Chronic liver disease
Infectious and chronic active hepatitis	Severe systemic illness
Genetically determined	Active acromegaly
	Kidney disease with proteinuria
	Genetically determined

production, the change in the T_3-resin uptake is in the same direction as the change in the total T_4 level.

An alternative to calculation of the free T_4 index as an estimate of the free T_4 concentration is one of the newer assays to measure the free T_4 either indirectly or directly. In the indirect approach, a two-step method of preincubation of the serum with an anti-T_4 antibody–coated tube is followed by addition of labeled T_4. In the direct approach, a one-step incubation of a labeled T_4 analog is incubated with an anti-T_4 antibody–coated tube. In each assay the amount of labeled iodothyronine bound is inversely proportional to the free T_4 level in the test specimen. In persons with marked alteration of TBG, these free T_4 estimates may correlate better than the free T_4 index with the clinical thyroid state. However, these free T_4 assays are still subject to spurious results in the setting of extreme alterations in serum proteins, confounding antibodies, and nonthyroidal illness (see below).

Effect of Nonthyroidal Illness on Thyroid Function Tests

Abnormal results on thyroid function tests are frequently encountered in the evaluation of patients without obvious thyroid disease. Some of these abnormal results are caused by altered levels of TBG (see above). In the remainder, it is necessary to decide whether a subtle thyroid hormone deficiency or excess exists or whether the abnormal values are somehow spurious. The T_4 and free T_4 estimates may be either decreased or increased in subjects who are actually euthyroid but suffer from acute or chronic nonthyroid illness. As discussed in the section on thyroid hormone metabolism, the most common effect of nonthyroidal illness on thyroid function tests is to lower T_3 levels.

In addition to the low T_3 levels, some patients with nonthyroidal illness have decreased total T_4 and free T_4 estimates. These are often the more critically ill patients. Studies have shown that the decreased level of T_4 is due to circulating inhibitors of thyroid hormone binding to serum-binding proteins. Because the inhibitors are not detected in the T_3-resin uptake test, the decreased total T_4 is not adjusted in calculations of the free T_4 index. These inhibitors of thyroid hormone binding can also result in spuriously low direct free T_4 estimates. The free T_4 concentrations by equilibrium dialysis are not usually decreased in such patients with nonthyroid illness, and the T_4 production rate is usually normal. All of the abnormalities of iodothyronine levels revert to normal on recovery from the illness.

The serum TSH may be helpful in confirming that the thyroid status of an ill individual with a low free T_4 estimate is normal. However, current sensitive TSH assays have also been found to be temporarily abnormal in patients with nonthyroidal illness, especially acutely ill hospitalized patients (Fig. 13-8). In some instances, administration of high-dose glucocorticoids or dopamine lowers TSH levels below the lower reference range with a brief rebound elevation above the upper reference range once the drug is discontinued. In other patients the nonthyroidal illness itself, perhaps by cytokines inhibiting TRH synthesis, lowers TSH levels. During recovery from the illness, the patient's TSH levels may transiently rise above normal.

DERANGED THYROID PHYSIOLOGY

Deranged thyroid physiology may involve altered thyroid growth, in either a diffuse or a nodular pattern, while thyroid hormone production remains normal. Although this simple increase in thyroid size, termed *euthyroid goiter*, is common in the population, the physiological derangement(s) leading to its development in areas of iodide sufficiency are poorly understood. Thus, to illustrate the effects of thyroid hormones and pathophysiological mechanisms of thyroid hormone secretion, only hypothyroidism and hyperthyroidism will be considered here.

Hypothyroidism

Hypothyroidism is a clinical state resulting from decreased production of thyroid hormones. It may begin *in utero* or later in life, resulting in a different set of clinical features, as we saw in the discussion of thyroid hormone deficiency.

Hypothyroidism is relatively common, occurring in about 2% of adult women in a clinically overt form. It is much less common in men. Spontaneous hypothyroidism may be due to disorders of the thyroid (primary hypothyroidism), of the anterior pituitary or hypothalamus (secondary hypothyroidism), or, rarely, of peripheral target tissues (severe generalized thyroid hormone resistance). Primary hypothyroidism accounts for over 95% of patients with hypothyroidism. In rare congenital forms of hypothyroidism, enzyme defects in thyroid hormone formation or mutations in the NIS may result in hypothyroidism with goiter, or inactivating mutations in the TSH receptor may cause congenital hypothyroidism without thyroid enlargement.

Primary hypothyroidism developing later in life also may be associated either with a decrease in thyroid tissue or with thyroid enlargement. Both the nongoitrous and goitrous forms are commonly the result of an autoimmune thyroiditis leading to destruction of thyroid parenchyma. In those who have goiters, lymphocytic infiltration of the thyroid is seen and the condition is termed *Hashimoto's disease*. This autoimmune destruction of the thyroid may be part of a polyglandular endocrine deficiency syndrome in which the adrenals, parathyroids, gonads, pancreatic islets, and stomach parietal cells are variably involved but the hypothyroidism is usually an isolated finding. The most common cause of primary hypothyroidism in adults is destruction of the thyroid tissue by prior surgery or radioactive iodine treatment for hyperthyroidism.

In areas in which iodine is not sufficient, goitrous hypothyroidism may be due to endemic iodine deficiency. This is rare in North America but quite common in many other parts of the world. The incidence of endemic goiter has been greatly reduced in many areas by the introduction of iodized salt.

Secondary hypothyroidism is due to decreased TSH secretion. Although an isolated abnormality of TSH release has been described, most secondary hypothyroidism is due to pituitary insufficiency involving multiple anterior pituitary hormones (see Chapter 6). The pituitary may be affected directly or indirectly as a result of hypothalamic disease inhibiting the delivery of releasing factors.

As with almost all hormones, resistance to the action of thyroid hormones has been described as a disease mechanism. In more severely affected individuals the resistance is present in all target tissues. This leads to increased thyroid hormone production in the absence of symptoms of thyroid hormone excess and occasionally in the face of symptoms of thyroid hormone deficiency (delayed bone age, epiphyseal stippling, and decreased hydroxyproline excretion). In such patients the serum TSH is normal. The defect in most instances is due to a $TR\beta$ mutation.

Most patients with clinical hypothyroidism have a free T_4 estimate below the lower range of normal. Because the normal range is relatively broad, some hypothyroid patients may have T_4 levels that are within the low normal range. As most patients with hypothyroidism have primary disease of the thyroid gland rather than secondary hypothyroidism resulting from hypothalamic or pituitary disease, the serum TSH is the most useful screening test (see above). The serum TSH in patients with primary hypothyroidism can range from values just slightly above the normal range in patients with mild disease to values ranging from 20 to more than 100 μU/ml in patients with more severe and long-standing thyroid deficiency (Fig. 13-8).

The TSH level is usually inappropriately normal in the presence of a low free T_4 estimate in patients with hypothalamic or pituitary disorders resulting in secondary hypothyroidism. However, the TSH is occasionally low or even elevated in such patients (Fig. 13-8). Altered glycosylation of TSH resulting in a prolonged half-life and reduced biological activity is thought to account for the mildly increased TSH levels observed in some patients with hypopituitarism.

The thyroid radioactive iodine uptake (RAIU) is a direct test of thyroid function; a tracer dose of ^{123}I is given orally, and the percentage accumulation in the thyroid is measured, usually at 24 hours. The RAIU varies directly with the functional activity of the thyroid. However, this test is not useful in suspected hypothyroidism because many normal subjects have RAIUs in the range observed in patients with hypothyroidism.

Hyperthyroidism

Hyperthyroidism is the clinical state resulting from increased circulating levels of available thyroid hormones. The manifestations are, in general, an exaggeration of the normal physiological actions of thyroid hormones. In fact, except for the specific form of eye changes, termed *ophthalmopathy*, certain skin changes (which may or may not be present, depending on the cause of the hyperthyroidism), and goiter, all of the clinical manifestations can be related to excess thyroid hormone. In contrast to hypothyroidism, which tends to be insidious in onset and slowly progressive in course, hyperthyroidism usually results in recognized symptoms and may (in the case of the most common cause, Graves' disease) undergo periods of exacerbation and remission. The clinical manifestations common to all forms of hyperthyroidism were described in the section on thyroid hormone excess.

Like hypothyroidism, hyperthyroidism is relatively common, occurring in 2% of women but only one-tenth as many men. The predominant cause is diffuse toxic goiter, usually termed *Graves' disease*. The mechanism of the autonomous thyroid hormone secretion in Graves' disease is stimulation of the gland by an IgG immunoglobulin that interacts with the TSH receptor. In contrast to most antireceptor antibodies, this antibody does not inhibit but profoundly activates the receptor. Most patients with Graves' disease have a palpably enlarged thyroid gland. A specific infiltrative ophthalmopathy is seen only in Graves' disease. The eyes become protuberant due to infiltration of the extraocular tissues with mucopolysaccharides. Trapping of extraocular muscles in the confined space of the orbit may result in paralysis of eye movement and double vision. In some patients the ophthalmopathy may be the most severe manifestation of Graves' disease. The specific cause of the infiltrative ophthalmopathy of Graves' disease is unknown.

Other causes of hyperthyroidism, such as toxic uninodular or multinodular goiters or inflammation of the thyroid gland (thyroiditis), account for only 10%–15% of patients. Recently, patients with toxic uninodular and multinodular goiters have been found to have somatic mutations in the TSH receptors in the hyperfunctioning nodules, which result in constitutive activation of the receptor. Similar germline mutations cause familial nonautoimmune diffuse toxic goiter. Excess dietary or medication iodide may lead to a low-RAIU form of hyperthyroidism, and ingested thyroid hormones may mimic endogenous hyperthyroidism.

The appropriate initial test in patients with suspected hyperthyroidism is the serum TSH. In patients with mild thyroid hormone excess, as in older individuals with autonomous function of a multinodular goiter or a patient slightly overmedicated with thyroid hormone, the TSH level may be below the lower limit of a reference population but still detectable. However, in almost all subjects with symptomatic thyroid hormone excess, the serum TSH is below the limit of detection (less than 0.1 μU/ml in the usual second-generation assay) (Fig. 13-8). Before the availability of sensitive TSH assays, which can distinguish low from normal values, the TRH test was used to identify some patients with subtle thyroid excess and equivocal clinical findings (see Fig. 13-10). Inhibition of the response of serum TSH to an intravenous injection of TRH was consistent with thyroid excess.

After finding a low serum TSH, it is necessary to assess whether there are elevations in thyroid hormone levels to confirm overt hyperthyroidism. Because the average increase in circulating T_4 in patients with the common form of hyperthyroidism is approximately twofold, whereas T_3 levels increase threefold or fourfold, the measurement of the total serum T_3 concentration is useful in patients in whom the free T_4 estimate is not clearly elevated.

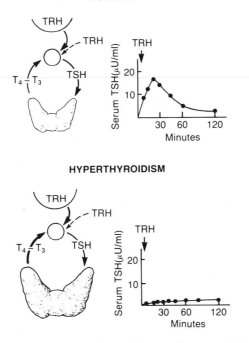

NORMAL

HYPERTHYROIDISM

Fig. 13-10 Hypothalamic–pituitary–thyroid interactions and the serum thyroid-stimulating hormone (TSH) response to thyrotropin-releasing hormone (TRH) injection in normal subjects and patients with hyperthyroidism. The increased thyroid hormone levels in the hyperthyroid patients inhibit the TSH response to TRH. T_4, thyroxine; T_3, 3,5,3'-triiodothyronine. (Adapted from Kaplan MM and Utiger RD: Clin Endocrinol Metab 7:97, 1978, with permission.)

Finally, although the thyroid RAIU is of limited value in the evaluation of suspected hypothyroidism, it has a role in the assessment of hyperthyroidism. Elevation of the RAIU above the normal range indicates thyroid hyperfunction. However, some patients with endogenous thyroid hormone excess have RAIUs in the normal or low range.

SUGGESTED READING

Abramowicz MJ, Duprez L, Parma J, Vassart G, and Heinrichs C: Familial congenital hypothyroidism due to inactivating mutation of the thyrotropin receptor causing profound hypoplasia of the thyroid gland. J Clin Invest 99:3108–3124, 1997.

Amma LL, Campos-Barros A, Wang Z, Vennstrom B, and Forrest D: Distinct tissue-specific roles for thyroid hormone receptors β and $\alpha 1$ in regulation of type 1 deiodinase expression. Mol Endocrinol 15:467–475, 2001.

Bianco AC, Salvatore D, Gereben B, Berry MJ, and Larsen PR: Biochemistry, molecular biology, and physiological roles of the iodothyronine selenodeiodinases. Endocr Rev 23:38–89, 2002.

Bodenner DL and Lash RW: Thyroid disease mediated by molecular defects in cell surface and nuclear receptors. Am J Med 105:524–538, 1998.

de Lange P, Lanni A, Beneduce L, Moreno M, Lombardi A, Silvestri E, and Goglia F: Uncoupling protein-3 is a molecular determinant for the regulation of the resting metabolic rate by thyroid hormone. Endocrinology 142:3414–3420, 2001.

Dohan O, De la Vieja A, Paroder V, Riedel C, Artani M, Reed M, Ginter CS, and Carrasco N: The sodium/iodide symporter (NIS): characterization, regulation, and medical significance. Endocr Rev 24:48–77, 2003.

Gershengorn MC: Mechanism of thyrotropin releasing hormone stimulation of pituitary hormone secretion. Annu Rev Physiol 48:515–526, 1986.

Gruters A, Schoneberg T, Biebermann H, Krude H, Krohn HP, Dralle H, and Gudermann T: Severe congenital hyperthyroidism caused by a germ-line neo-mutation in the extracellular portion of the thyrotropin receptor. J Clin Endocrinol Metab 83:1431–1436, 1998.

Hamburger JI: The various presentation of thyroiditis: diagnostic considerations. Ann Intern Med 104:219–224, 1986.

Hennemann G, Docter R, Friesema CH, de Jong M, Krenning EP, and Visser TJ: Plasma membrane transport of thyroid hormones and its role in thyroid hormone metabolism and bioavailability. Endocr Rev 22:451–476, 2001.

Hollowell JG, Staehling NW, Hannon WH, Flanders DW, Gunter EW, Maberly GF, Braverman LE, Pino S, Miller DT, Garbe PL, DeLozier DM, and Jackson RJ: Iodine nutrition in the United States. Trends and public health implications: iodine excretion data from National Health and Nutritional Surveys I and III (1971–1974 and 1988–1994). J Clin Endocrinol Metab 83:3401–3408, 1998.

Klee GG and Hay ID: Biochemical testing of thyroid function. Encodrinol Metab Clin North Am 26:763–775, 1997.

Lanni A, Moreno M, Lombardi A, de Lange P, and Goglia F: Control of energy metabolism by iodothyronines. J Enocrinol Invest 24:897–913, 2001.

Larsen PR: Thyroid–pituitary interaction. Feedback regulation of thyrotropin secretion by thyroid hormones. N Engl J Med 306:23–32, 1982.

Larsen PR, Davies TF, Schlumberger MJ, and Hay ID: Thyroid physiology and diagnostic evaluation of patients with thyroid disorders. In: *Williams Textbook of Endocrinology*, 10th ed., PR Larsen, HM Kronenberg, S Melmed, and K Polonsky, eds., Saunders, Philadelphia, pp. 331–368, 2003.

Lazar MA: Thyroid hormone receptors: multiple forms, multiple possibilities. Endocr Rev 14:184–193, 1993.

Nicoloff JT and Spencer CA: The use and misuse of the sensitive thyrotropin assays. J Clin Endocrinol Metab 71:553–558, 1990.

Ribeiro RCJ, Aprilette JW, Wagner RL, West BL, Fend W, Huber R, Kushner PJ, Nilsson S, Scanlan T, Fetterick RJ, Schaufele F, and Baxter JD: Mechanisms of thyroid hormone action: insights from x-ray crystallographic and functional studies. Recent Prog Horm Res 53:351–394, 1998.

Spitzweg C, Heufelder AE, and Morris JC: Thyroid iodine transport. Thyroid 10:321–330, 2000.

14

The Adrenal Glands

KEITH L. PARKER
WILLIAM E. RAINEY

The basic function of the adrenal glands is to protect the organism against acute and chronic stress, a concept popularized as the *fight-or-flight* response for the medulla and as the *alarm* reaction for the cortex. The steroid hormones of the cortex and the catecholamines of the medulla probably developed as protection against immediate stress or injury and more prolonged deprivation of food and water. In acute stress, catecholamines mobilize glucose and fatty acids for energy and prepare the heart, lungs, and muscles for action, while glucocorticoids protect against overreactions from the body's responses to stress. In the more chronic stress of food and fluid deprivation, adrenocortical steroid hormones stimulate gluconeogenesis to maintain the supply of glucose and increase sodium reabsorption to maintain body fluid volume.

Based on the widespread effects of its secreted products in multiple tissues, adrenal dysfunction is associated with protean manifestations. Diseases associated with adrenocortical hypofunction are relatively rare, while those associated with adrenocortical hyperfunction are slightly more common. However, both of these conditions are life-threatening if untreated, and a high index of suspicion must therefore be maintained. Subtle increases in cortisol secretion or tissue sensitivity to glucocorticoids may be involved in many of the devastating effects of chronic stress, including visceral obesity, hypertension, diabetes mellitus, dyslipidemia, and depression. Moreover, exogenous glucocorticoids are widely used to treat numerous diseases and, when used in supraphysiological doses, can induce all of the manifestations of glucocorticoid excess.

Perhaps because the adrenal medulla accounts for only 10% of total sympathetic nervous activation, we can live quite well without it and syndromes due to hypofunction are not clinically significant. Conditions of excess catecholamine output due to tumors called *pheochromocytomas* are a rare but potentially life-threatening cause of secondary hypertension.

ANATOMY

The adrenal glands are located above the kidneys (Fig. 14-1), hence their other name: *suprarenal glands*. In keeping with their essential function, they are liberally sup-

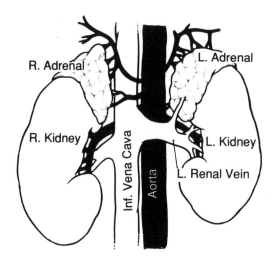

Fig. 14-1   Gross anatomy of the adrenal glands.

plied with arterial blood from branches of the aorta, the renal arteries, and the phrenic arteries, receiving on a per gram basis perhaps the highest rate of blood flow in the body. Arterial blood enters the outer cortex, flows through fenestrated capillaries between the cords of adrenocortical cells, and drains inwardly into venules in the medulla. On the right, the adrenal vein directly enters the inferior vena cava; on the left, it usually drains into the left renal vein. An understanding of this anatomy is important when attempts are made to obtain blood from or inject radiographic dye into the adrenals for the diagnosis of adrenal disorders.

Anatomical Zonation

The adrenal cortex is derived from mesoderm and comprises 90% of the gland. Beneath its fibrous capsule, it contains three zones that make different steroid hormones and are subject to different regulation (Fig. 14-2, Table 14-1). The outer zona glomerulosa makes mineralocorticoids under regulation by the renin–angiotensin system, the middle zona fasciculata secretes cortisol under regulation by corticotropin (ACTH), and the inner zona reticularis makes the androgen precursors dehydroepiandrosterone (DHEA) and its sulfated derivative (DHEA-S).

The medulla, which arises from neuroectodermal cells derived from the neural crest, synthesizes and secretes catecholamines. Whereas norepinephrine is the primary neurotransmitter secreted by sympathetic ganglia and neurons, the adrenal medulla secretes mostly ($\sim$80%) epinephrine, reflecting its predominant expression of the enzyme phenylethanolamine-N-methyltransferase (PNMT), which converts norepinephrine into epinephrine.

Relative to body size, the human fetal adrenal is considerably larger than the adult gland, approaching at term the size of the fetal kidney. The fetal adrenal gland has an outer subcapsular zone—the *neocortex*—which represents the presumptive precursor of the three zones of the postnatal cortex, and a much larger inner region

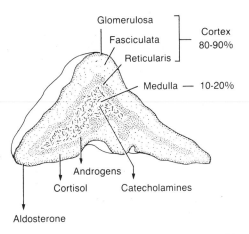

Fig. 14-2 Organization of the adrenal gland and adrenocortical hormones produced by the different zones of the adrenal cortex and by the medulla. (From Guyton AC: *Textbook of Medical Physiology,* Saunders, Philadelphia, p. 909, 1986.)

comprising ~80% of the gland termed the *fetal zone.* The cells of the fetal zone are highly active steroidogenically, but do not express 3β-hydroxysteroid dehydrogenase and therefore make neither glucocorticoids nor mineralocorticoids. Rather, they produce large quantities of DHEA and DHEA-S, which serve as precursors for the synthesis of estrogens by the placenta (see Chapter 11), and also can serve as precursors for androgens in certain disease states. Postnatally, the fetal zone involutes rapidly, while the outer neocortex zone differentiates into the three zones of the postnatal adrenal cortex.

Functional Zonation

Although adrenocortical zonation is critical for the differential regulation of mineralocorticoids and glucocorticoids, its molecular basis remains poorly understood. Subcapsular cells are capable of regenerating all three cortical zones, and one theory of zonation proposes that the subcapsular region contains adrenocortical progenitor cells that modulate their phenotype as they migrate centripetally from the zona glomerulosa to the zona fasciculata to the zona reticularis. Consistent with this model, cells of the inner zona reticularis have lower rates of cell division and exhibit increased pigmentation and other signs of a progressive loss of functional activity.

Table 14-1 Functional Zonation of the Adrenal Cortex

Zone	Major secretion	Major control mechanism
Zona glomerulosa	Aldosterone (mineralocorticoid)	Renin–angiotensin
Zona fasciculata	Cortisol (glucocorticoid)	ACTH
Zona reticularis	Dehydroepiandrosterone (androgen precursor)	? (ACTH)

ACTH, corticotropin.

As outlined in the steroidogenic pathway, a key component of functional zonation clearly is the zone-specific expression of cytochrome P450 (CYP) enzymes that catalyze different modifications of steroid precursors (Fig. 14-3). The outer zona glomerulosa expresses aldosterone synthase (CYP11B2), which catalyzes three separate reactions to convert 11-deoxycorticosterone to aldosterone: 11β-hydroxylation, 18-hydroxylation, and oxidation of the 18-hydroxyl to an aldehyde moiety. (The last two activities are sometimes referred to as *corticosterone methyloxidase I* and *II*). In contrast, steroid 11β-hydroxylase (CYP11B1) in the zona fasciculata carries out a single 11β-hydroxylation to convert 11-deoxycortisol to cortisol. Similarly, the zona glomerulosa does not express steroid 17α-hydroxylase (CYP17), which is expressed by the zona fasciculata and zona reticularis Of note, the same CYP17 enzyme predominantly catalyzes only 17α-hydroxylation in the zona fasciculata while catalyzing both 17α-hydroxylation and cleavage of the C17-20 bond (17,20-lyase activity) in the zona reticularis. As discussed below, defects in the zone-specific expression of the steroidogenic enzymes can cause clinical disorders of steroidogenesis.

The distribution of blood flow from the outer cortex to the inner medulla also supports high levels of synthesis and secretion of epinephrine, the major cate-

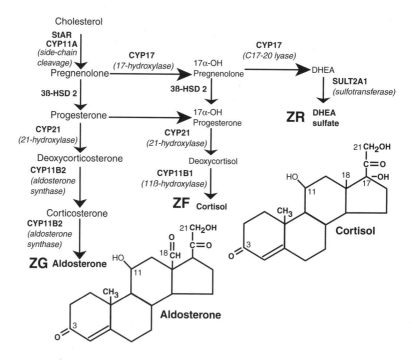

Fig. 14-3 Pathways of adrenal steroidogenesis. Gene products mediating each biosynthetic step are boxed, with the corresponding enzymatic activity listed in parentheses. The planar structures of the mineralocorticoid aldosterone and the glucocorticoid cortisol are shown. 3β-HSD, 3β-hydroxysteroid dehydrogenase; DHEA, dehydroepiandrosterone; StAR, steroidogenic acute regulatory protein; ZF, zona fasciculata; ZG, zona glomerulosa; ZR, zona reticularis.

cholamine required for the acute response to stress. PNMT, the enzyme that converts norepinephrine to epinephrine, is specifically induced by cortisol. Therefore, after the immediate release of stored epinephrine in response to stress, cortisol secretion ensures continued production of epinephrine.

The traditional view of a complete separation of adrenal zones and secretions described above has recently been challenged. In particular, it is proposed that the integrated control of adrenal function involves direct innervation, control of the blood supply, and direct cell-to-cell interactions via regulatory peptides, neurotransmitters, cytokines, and growth factors that provide complex intra-adrenal regulatory networks. These regulators include a number of secretory products of chromaffin cells, which thereby can affect function in the adrenal cortex rather than being sequestered within the medulla. With the rich blood supply to the adrenals, virtually every cell also is adjacent to an endothelial cell, thereby exposing adrenal cells to the multiple endothelium-derived secretions, including nitric oxide, adrenomedullin, and endothelin (see Chapter 7). Finally, an intra-adrenal renin–angiotensin system likely is involved in certain aspects of aldosterone synthesis by the zona glomerulosa.

Although this revised scheme of intra-adrenal communication and regulation may delineate additional levels of regulation, the basic concepts of the regulation of adrenal steroidogenesis described here remain valid.

ADRENAL CORTEX

There are three major classes of secretory products of the adrenal cortex (Table 14-2), but the biosynthetic pathways for all three zones share many common features that first are examined together. Of note, relatively small amounts of steroid hormones are stored in the adrenal gland. Thus, the biosynthetic pathway for *de novo* steroidogenesis described below must be activated when more is needed.

Steroidogenesis

All adrenal steroids are derived from cholesterol by sequential, enzymatically mediated modifications of its structure (Fig. 14-3). Cholesterol can be synthesized

Table 14-2 Secretion Rates and Plasma Concentrations of Major Adrenocortical Hormones

Class	Steroid	Secretion rate	Plasma concentration[a]
Glucocorticoid	Cortisol	10–15 mg/day	8–25 μg/dl
	Corticosterone	1–4 mg/day	0.2–0.6 μg/dl
Mineralocorticoid	Aldosterone	5–20 ng/day	5–15 ng/dl
	Deoxycorticosterone	0.1–0.6 mg/day	5–20 ng/dl
Androgen[b]	DHEA	3–7 mg/day	0.1–1.5 μg/dl
	DHEA-S	7–15 mg/day	40–300 μg/dl
	Androstenedione	2–3 mg/day	100–200 ng/dl

[a]Plasma concentrations vary with time of day.

[b]Secretion rates vary with sex.

DHEA, dehydroepiandrosterone; DHEA-S, sulfated DHEA.

within the adrenal cortex from acetyl-coenzyme A, but is obtained predominantly from the blood by specific plasma membrane receptors that bind cholesterol-rich low-density lipoproteins (LDL) and high-density lipoproteins (HDL). Lipoprotein-bound cholesterol enters the cell, and the cholesterol is then esterified and stored in cytoplasmic vacuoles. Stimulation by corticotropin (ACTH) activates cholesterol esterase, which releases free cholesterol from these storage depots to provide substrate for steroid synthesis. The rate-limiting step in steroid biosynthesis is the transfer of cholesterol from the outer mitochondrial membrane to the inner mitochondrial membrane, where the cholesterol side-chain cleavage enzyme (CYP11A) resides. This transfer is mediated by the steroidogenic acute regulatory protein (StAR), and ACTH stimulates the levels of StAR as part of its acute induction of steroidogenesis.

The synthesis of the various corticosteroid hormones involves several enzymes, most of which catalyze steroid hydroxylations. CYP11A converts cholesterol into pregnenolone, and all stimulators of steroidogenesis, including ACTH, increase cholesterol delivery to CYP11A. After pregnenolone is formed, it exits the mitochondria and is sequentially modified by dehydrogenases and hydroxylases within the endoplasmic reticulum and mitochondria to form the three major classes of adrenocortical steroids.

Glucocorticoids

Cortisol is the primary glucocorticoid in humans and most mammals, while corticosterone serves this function in some rodents.

Regulation of Glucocorticoid Secretion

As described in Chapter 6, the hypothalamic–pituitary axis controls adrenocortical function through the release of ACTH. After binding to its plasma membrane receptor, the melanocortin 2 receptor (MC2-R), ACTH activates cyclic adenosine monophosphate (AMP)-dependent protein kinase and increases cyclic AMP, thereby activating protein kinase A. This, in turn, increases the conversion of cholesterol esters to free cholesterol that can enter the steroidogenic pathway. In concert, ACTH stimulates the expression of StAR to increase the rate-limiting transport of cholesterol into mitochondria, increasing the conversion of cholesterol to pregnenolone and starting the biosynthetic cascade to cortisol (Fig. 14-3).

Plasma levels of cortisol rise within minutes of the intravenous infusion of ACTH, increasing two to five times by 30 minutes. With chronic ACTH stimulation, as in severe stress, the mass of adrenal tissue actually increases, so that cortisol secretion may reach 200–250 mg/day, some 10 to 20 times the basal level.

Secretion. Normally, daily secretion of cortisol is both episodic and variable (Fig. 14-4). Peaks of secretion follow by 15–30 minutes those of plasma ACTH, with the major burst of activity at around 8:00 A.M. Thereafter, the release of ACTH from the pituitary and cortisol from the adrenal generally occur only in brief bursts, 7–15 episodes per day. After each episode, plasma cortisol rises enough to suppress further ACTH release. Circulating levels of cortisol then fall progressively, ultimately reaching the set point of hypothalamic–pituitary negative feedback control so that more corticotropin-releasing hormone (CRH) and ACTH are released.

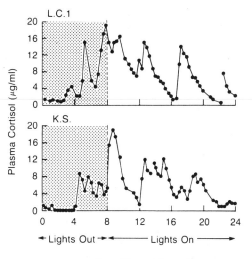

Fig. 14-4 Typical pattern of cortisol secretion during the 24-hour day. Note the oscillations in secretion as well as the major secretory surge at around the time of awakening in the morning. (From Weitzman ED, Fukushima D, Noseire C, Roffwarg H, Gallagher TF, and Hellman L: J Clin Endocrinol Metab 33:14, 1971.)

The normal fine-tuning of hypothalamic–pituitary control of cortisol secretion may be interrupted by administration of supraphysiological doses of glucocorticoids. In keeping with their actions as described in the next section, glucocorticoids typically are used to control serious inflammatory or immune reactions. Various synthetic steroids are available with substitutions that enhance their glucocorticoid activity and reduce their mineralocorticoid activity (Table 14-3).

In the setting of acute adrenal insufficiency (see below), exogenous glucocorticoids are initially administered in doses equal to the normal maximal daily secretion of 200–300 mg of cortisol or equivalent per day. With high-dose therapy, or

Table 14-3 Relative Glucocorticoid and Mineralocorticoid Potency of Natural Adrenal Steroids and Some Derivatives in Bioassays

Steroid	Glucocorticoid activity	Mineralocorticoid activity
Cortisol	1.0	1.0
Prednisone (1,2 double bond)	4	0.5
6α-Methylprednisone	5	0.5
9α-Fluoro-16α-hydroxyprednisolone (triamcinolone)	5	<0.1
9α-Fluoro-16α-methylprednisolone (dexamethasone)	30	<0.1
Aldosterone	0.25	500
Deoxycorticosterone	0.01	30
9α-Fluorocortisol	10	500

indeed with chronic therapy at any daily dose that significantly exceeds the 10–15 mg of cortisol that normally is secreted, the hypothalamic–pituitary axis remains suppressed. In the prolonged absence of ACTH stimulation, the adrenals atrophy both in function and in structure.

As long as the patient receives exogenous steroid, suppression of the hypothalamic–pituitary–adrenal system is irrelevant. When the exogenous steroid is discontinued, however, the hypothalamic–pituitary–adrenal axis may remain suppressed such that the patient is unable to produce cortisol normally. Therefore, prolonged adrenal suppression renders the patient susceptible to developing adrenal insufficiency if stressed. After exogenous steroids are stopped, the capacity for ACTH synthesis returns first, and because the adrenal remains unresponsive, the ACTH level transiently rises above normal. Cortisol production takes considerably longer to return to normal, and there are documented examples of impaired adrenal reserve for up to 1 year after cessation of glucocorticoid therapy.

Metabolism. Once in the circulation, cortisol is largely bound to a specific glucocorticoid binding α2-globulin called *corticosteroid-binding globulin* (CBG). The normal level of CBG, 3–4 mg/dl, is saturated when the cortisol level reaches approximately 28 μg/dl. Thus, in the setting of excess cortisol production, the free cortisol rises disproportionately after this level is exceeded. Of the circulating cortisol that is not bound to CBG, 15%–20% is bound less tightly to albumin, leaving only about 5% unbound. This small fraction, however, is critical because only the free form of cortisol is able to enter cells and mediate glucocorticoid action.

In a manner similar to that of thyroid-binding globulin (TBG) and other hormone carrier proteins, hepatic synthesis of CBG is increased by estrogen. As a result, women taking exogenous estrogen or with high endogenous levels during pregnancy have elevated plasma cortisol levels but lack manifestations of cortisol excess since their free cortisol levels are normal. In contrast, CBG levels are lower in diseases with reduced blood protein concentrations, such as cirrhosis of the liver. Here again, the free cortisol is normal.

The half-life of cortisol in circulation is ~70–90 minutes. As shown in Figure 14-5, cortisol (sometimes called *compound F*) can be interconverted to its inactive 11-keto analog, cortisone (*compound E*), by the type 2 isozyme of 11β-hydroxy-

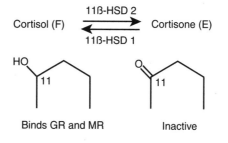

Fig. 14-5 Interconversion of active cortisol and inactive cortisone by the type 1 and type 2 isozymes of 11β-hydroxysteroid dehydrogenase (11β-HSD). GR, glucocorticoid receptor; MR, mineralocorticoid receptor.

steroid dehydrogenase (11β-HSD2; see further discussion below). Both cortisol and cortisone are reduced in the liver to tetrahydro derivatives and then conjugated to glucuronides, yielding more hydrophilic derivatives that are excreted into the urine.

The 24-hour urinary excretion of unmetabolized cortisol (i.e., the urinary free cortisol) is a useful test for diagnosing cortisol excess. Because only free cortisol is excreted into the urine, the total urinary free cortisol in normal individuals is below 50 μg/day (the absolute value varies depending on the assay that is used). However, if the cortisol level rises above 25–30 μg/dl, thereby exceeding the binding capacity of CBG, a progressively larger share will remain free to be available for filtration and excretion into the urine.

Molecular Mechanisms of Corticosteroid Action

As described in Chapter 3, adrenal corticosteroids enter target cells by passive diffusion and are bound to specific steroid hormone receptors. The glucocorticoid receptor (GR) is a single-chain polypeptide of approximately 94 kDa that binds glucocorticoids with high affinity in a specific, saturable manner. Unliganded GR resides in the cytosol, complexed with other proteins including heat-shock protein 90. After glucocorticoid binding, the hormone–receptor complex translocates to the nucleus and binds to DNA (see Fig. 3-8). By interacting with specific regulatory DNA sequences called *glucocorticoid-responsive elements*, GR affects the transcription of specific genes and thereby changes the cellular synthesis of specific proteins. The GR does not mediate these effects by itself, but recruits transcriptional coactivators and corepressors to affect the transcription of target genes. Moreover, although many of the best-characterized effects of GR involve transcriptional activation, inhibiting gene expression also is a key component of glucocorticoid action. In immune cells, for example, GR inhibits the action of NF-κB, a transcription factor that regulates the expression of several cytokine pathways, thereby exerting multifaceted effects to inhibit the immune response.

Mineralocorticoids are bound by the mineralocorticoid receptor (MR), a related steroid receptor, which is expressed in classical mineralocorticoid target tissues such as kidney, colon, and salivary glands. When the MR was isolated, it became apparent that its affinity for cortisol equals that for aldosterone. As the circulating cortisol concentration exceeds that of aldosterone by ~100-fold, this raised the question of how the MR is protected from activation by cortisol. We know now that the type 2 isozyme of 11β-HSD2) in aldosterone target tissues protects the MR from being overwhelmed by cortisol. The 11β-HSD2 converts cortisol—which binds both MR and GR with high affinity—into the inactive cortisone (see Fig. 14-5). Despite the much higher concentration of cortisol in the glomerular filtrate, its conversion to cortisone by 11β-HSD2 prevents MR activation.

Patients with the syndrome of apparent mineralocorticoid excess lack 11β-HSD2; because they cannot inactivate cortisol, they exhibit severe manifestations of mineralocorticoid excess despite having very low aldosterone levels. In addition, 11β-HSD2 can be inhibited by glycyrrhizic acid present in licorice, and individuals who consume large amounts of licorice may manifest a syndrome with all of the features of mineralocorticoid excess. In contrast, 11β-HSD1 converts inactive cortisone into active cortisol. In one mouse model, overexpression of this enzyme in adipocytes is associated with obesity, suggesting that increased activation of cortisol can cause manifestations of hypercorticism on a local basis.

Functions

Cortisol, the primary glucocorticoid, is essential for life, but we still do not fully understand why. In a simplistic way, cortisol is necessary to maintain critical processes at times of prolonged stress and to contain the reactions to inflammation. Most of its effects are permissive; that is, cortisol does not directly initiate metabolic or circulatory processes but rather is necessary to permit their full expression.

Intermediary Metabolism. The name *glucocorticoid* derives from the effect of these steroids on intermediary metabolism. Glucocorticoids exert both anabolic and catabolic effects (Fig. 14-6), with the catabolic effects predominating. The major catabolic effect is to facilitate the conversion of protein in skeletal muscle and connective tissue into glucose and glycogen. This diversion of peripheral intermediates to hepatic gluconeogenesis involves both the increased degradation of protein already formed and the decreased synthesis of new protein. Gluconeogenesis is critical during prolonged fasting, as stores of liver glycogen will otherwise be depleted in less than 24 hours, resulting in hypoglycemia.

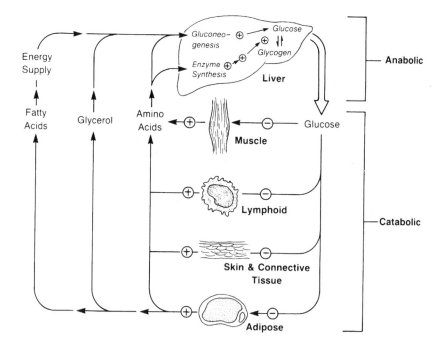

Fig. 14-6 Glucocorticoid influences on peripheral tissues. +, stimulation; −, inhibition. (From Baxter JD and Tyrrell JB: In: *Endocrinology and Metabolism*, 2nd ed., P Felig, JD Baxter, AE Broadus, and LA Frohman, eds., McGraw-Hill, New York, p. 545, 1987.)

Carbohydrate Metabolism. Cortisol not only increases the supply of glucose through hepatic gluconeogenesis but also decreases the utilization of glucose by cells elsewhere in the body. The former effect likely reflects increased hepatocyte expression of various enzymes involved in the conversion of amino acids into glucose and glycogen. The decreased utilization of glucose by other cells involves direct inhibition of glucose transport into these cells. Consistent with these effects, cortisol deficiency increases the susceptibility to and decreases the recovery from hypoglycemia, while an excess of cortisol decreases insulin sensitivity and raises the blood sugar level.

Protein Metabolism. As noted above, cortisol reduces the utilization of amino acids for protein synthesis everywhere except in the liver. Extrahepatic protein stores are reduced and amino acid levels in the blood increase. Extrahepatic utilization is decreased because amino acids are not transported into muscle cells, thereby reducing protein synthesis. Breakdown of cellular proteins continues, further increasing plasma amino acids. In the liver, circulating amino acids are transported more avidly into hepatic cells, where they are utilized for gluconeogenesis, glycogen formation, and protein synthesis. While a deficiency of cortisol is not followed by any measurable increase in protein synthesis, cortisol excess is associated with progressive loss of protein, atrophy and weakness of muscles, thinning of skin, and loss of bone matrix and mass. Bone formation is reduced, and less calcium is absorbed in the gut and more is excreted into the urine.

Fat Metabolism. Cortisol also increases the mobilization of fatty acids and glycerol from adipose tissue, increasing their concentration in the blood and providing energy stores for gluconeogenesis. Not only is fat broken down but less fat is formed, perhaps because less glucose is transported into fat cells. The actions of cortisol on fat metabolism are not entirely lipolytic: it also stimulates appetite and the deposition of additional fat in the central or truncal areas. With cortisol excess, the extremities lose fat and muscle, whereas the trunk and face become fatter; the mechanism for this fat redistribution is unknown. These effects of cortisol on intermediary metabolism help to maintain blood glucose during food deprivation and to mobilize extra glucose during stress, at the cost of decreased protein and redistributed fat.

Cardiovascular System. Cortisol is needed to maintain normal vascular integrity and responsiveness, as well as to preserve the volume of body fluids. In its absence, abnormal vasodilation occurs, such that vascular volume is reduced and blood pressure falls even without an external loss of fluid. In addition, normal renal function requires cortisol, and glomerular filtration and free water excretion are impaired in its absence. As discussed above, cortisol also has a mineralocorticoid effect that, to the extent that it escapes inactivation by 11β-HSD2, stimulates sodium retention and potassium excretion via the MR. Of course, when blood pressure or intravascular volume is reduced, the renin–angiotensin system (described in the next section) is activated to stimulate aldosterone rather than cortisol. Thus, when extra mineralocorticoids are needed, aldosterone and not cortisol serves that function.

Inflammatory and Immune Responses. Glucocorticoids suppress inflammation and immune reactions. As described in Chapter 4, inflammation and immune reactions induce the synthesis of multiple cytokines, and the suppressive effects of glucocorticoids have logically been assumed to reflect their ability to inhibit the expression of multiple genes involved in the synthesis of proinflammatory cytokines. Glucocorticoids have also been shown to increase the transcription of genes coding for antiinflammatory proteins, including lipocortin-1, interleukin-10, and neutral endopeptidase. Finally, glucocorticoids induce the expression of various cytokine receptors, such that glucocorticoids and cytokines in combination may act synergistically.

These divergent effects may explain one clinical scenario wherein glucocorticoid administration has experimental support but clinical failure: the treatment of shock due to overwhelming sepsis. In animal models, glucocorticoids—given before the sepsis-inducing agent so that they inhibit the production of cytokines—are protective. Clinically, glucocorticoids have been administered to patients only after the onset of septic shock, when levels of proinflammatory cytokines already are high. In this setting, glucocorticoids generally have shown no protection and, perhaps because they induce cytokine receptors, have even worsened the outcome in some studies.

Most anti-inflammatory effects require supraphysiological doses of glucocorticoids. Synthetic glucocorticoids with greater glucocorticoid selectivity are widely used clinically in the treatment of diseases in which the inflammatory reactions are harmful or in which there is a need to block the immune response. The treatment of rheumatoid arthritis is an example of the former, while the prevention of transplant rejection is an example of the latter use of glucocorticoids.

Central Nervous System. In addition to the physiological negative feedback control of hypothalamic–pituitary release of ACTH, cortisol modulates perception and emotion. Cortisol deficiency accentuates the senses of taste, hearing, and smell, while cortisol excess may initially cause euphoria but subsequently is associated with depression and a lowered threshold for seizure activity.

Developmental Effects. Cortisol is important for the maturation of various fetal organs, again acting in a permissive manner. It is involved in the maturation of intestinal enzymes, as well as in the synthesis of surfactant, a phospholipid that maintains alveolar surface tension in the lungs. Because of their action to induce surfactant production, glucocorticoids frequently are employed in the setting of preterm labor in an effort to increase lung maturation and avoid respiratory distress syndrome. Studies in animal models and epidemiological studies in humans have raised concerns that fetal exposure to glucocorticoids—whether exogenous or endogenous due to fetal stress—is associated with deleterious postnatal consequences, including hypertension, coronary artery disease, and obesity. These studies mandate a careful consideration of risks and benefits when using antenatal glucocorticoids. After birth, glucocorticoids in pharmacological doses inhibit linear skeletal growth by producing direct effects on bone and connective tissue, again mandating caution before initiating long-term glucocorticoid therapy in children.

Disorders of Adrenocortical Function

Syndromes of Congenital Enzymatic Deficiency

The adrenal cortex also secretes lesser amounts of precursors of the major steroid products, but these have limited biological activity. However, congenital deficiencies of various adrenal enzymes impede the normal biosynthetic pathway, causing the accumulation of precursors upstream of the enzymatic block. This buildup tends to be progressive, since the impaired cortisol synthesis resulting from the enzyme deficiency prevents the normal negative feedback at the hypothalamic and pituitary levels. Thus, high levels of ACTH continue to drive the production of steroid intermediates and to stimulate the proliferation of the adrenocortical cells. The resulting hyperplasia of the gland provides the generic name for these relatively rare congenital syndromes: *congenital adrenal hyperplasia* (CAH).

The most common form of CAH, accounting for ~95% of all cases, results from mutations in steroid 21-hydroxylase (CYP21). CYP21 is needed to convert 17-hydroxyprogesterone to 11-deoxycortisol, the precursor of cortisol, and progesterone to 11-deoxycorticosterone (DOC), the precursor of aldosterone (Fig. 14-7). The deficiency of aldosterone in severely affected cases can result in salt-wasting crises that present with severe volume depletion, hyponatremia, and hyperkalemia. Because cortisol is deficient, increasing amounts of ACTH stimulate the gland to overproduce precursors upstream of the 21-hydroxylation step, most strikingly 17α-hydroxyprogesterone. Some of these precursors can be converted into androgens,

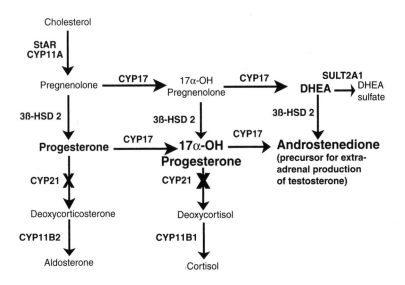

Fig. 14-7 Schematic representation of the effects of 21-hydroxylase deficiency on the pathway of adrenal steroidogenesis. Wide arrows denote pathways with increased synthesis proximal to the block. Thinner arrows denote pathways with decreased or absent steroid synthesis. Specific conversions that are blocked by the deficiency of 21-hydroxylase are shown. 3β-HSD 2, 3β-hydroxysteroid dehydrogenase 2; DHEA, dehydroepiandrosterone; StAR, steroidogenic acute regulatory protein.

leading to androgen excess and, in many cases, virilization. In girls, this usually is obvious at birth because of enlargement of the clitoris and fusion of the labia. However, the enzymatic deficiency is variable; some girls with milder defects manifest only excessive hair growth with menstrual irregularities in adult life, whereas others may have a defect so severe as to cause completely virilized external genitalia including a penile urethra and a "scrotum," resulting in incorrect sex assignment at birth (see also Chapter 8).

In affected males, virilization usually is not clinically apparent until after age 2 and sometimes not until age 10. The manifestations include accelerated growth and early maturation of secondary sex characteristics such as penile growth and pubic hair. Because the diagnosis in males may be missed, neonatal screening for serum 17-hydroxyprogesterone is routinely done in many regions.

Virilization of equal or even greater severity is seen in individuals who have mutations of CYP11B1, which is also required for cortisol production in the zona fasciculata. In this case, however, the enzymatic block permits the overproduction of 11-deoxycorticosterone, which has intrinsic mineralocorticoid activity and thus can cause mineralocorticoid excess and hypertension.

Considerably less common are those congenital enzyme deficiencies involving other components of the adrenal biosynthetic pathway. If the defect is early, as with lack of functional StAR or CYP11A in lipoid CAH, all steroids will be deficient and patients will manifest both adrenal insufficiency and impaired formation of sex steroids. If the defect involves steroid 17α-hydroxylase (CYP17), mineralocorticoid activity again may be high, since 11-deoxycorticosterone is over-produced. If the defect involves aldosterone synthase (CYP11B2), aldosterone will be deficient with normal cortisol. Thus, with knowledge of the normal steroidogenic pathway and the physiological actions of the various steroids and intermediates, the clinical expression of each enzyme deficiency can be rationalized.

Glucocorticoid-Remediable Aldosteronism—An Example of Aberrant Zonation

As noted above, we do not fully understand at a molecular level how the adrenal cortex differentially modulates steroid production in the different zones. An inherited disorder called *glucocorticoid-remediable aldosteronism* vividly illustrates the importance of this zonation in adrenocortical function. CYP11B1 and CYP11B2 are encoded by tandemly duplicated genes on the long arm of chromosome 8 (8 q21-q22). An autosomal dominant form of hypertension results from an unequal crossover that fuses the 5′ end of CYP11B1, including regulatory sequences, with the 3′ end of CYP11B2. This chimeric gene results in the ectopic expression in the zona fasciculata of a protein that produces mineralocorticoids under ACTH stimulation, ultimately leading to mineralocorticoid excess, hypokalemia, and hypertension. Because ACTH regulates the production of these mineralocorticoids by the zona fasciculata, administration of glucocorticoids will lower ACTH and ameliorate the process, leading to the name *glucocorticoid-remediable aldosteronism.*

Glucocorticoid Insufficiency

The classic features of cortisol deficiency (Table 14-4) are seen with primary hypofunction of the adrenal glands (Addison's disease). Historically, this usually re-

Table 14-4 Major Functions of Cortisol and Their Clinical Expression

	Clinical expression	
Effect	Cortisol deficiency	Cortisol excess
Carbohydrate metabolism		
Increased gluconeogenesis, decreased glucose utilization	Hypoglycemia	Hyperglycemia
Decreased sensitivity to insulin	Insulin sensitivity	Insulin resistance
Protein metabolism		
Decreased extrahepatic amino acid utilization	Hypoglycemia	Decreased protein structure of bone, skin, muscle
Increased gluconeogenesis		Poor wound healing
Fat metabolism		
Increased lipolysis, decreased lipogenesis	Weight loss	Hyperlipemia
Distribution of fat		Redistribution of body fat, truncal obesity
Circulatory		
Maintain ECF volume	Vasodilation, hypotension	Hypertension
Maintain capillary integrity		
Mineralocorticoid		
Sodium retention	Hypovolemia Hyponatremia	Hypervolemia Hypernatremia
Potassium excretion	Hyperkalemia	Hypokalemia
Inflammatory and immune responses		
Stabilize lysosomes	Propensity	Decreased inflammatory response
Suppress synthesis of antibodies	toward	Increased susceptibility to infection
Decrease capillary permeability	autoimmune	Decreased fibrous tissue formation
Decrease phagocytosis	disease	
Hematopoietic		
Stimulate red cell production	Anemia	Erythrocytosis
Lympholysis	Lymphocytosis	Lymphopenia
Inhibit neutrophil accumulation at inflammatory sites		Leukocytosis
Central nervous system	Anorexia Fatigue	Euphoria Depression
Hypothalamic–pituitary feedback control of ACTH	Increased ACTH secretion Pigmentation	Decreased ACTH secretion If excess is 2° to hypothalamic–pituitary drive, ACTH increased

ACTH, corticotropin; ECF, extracellular fluid.

sulted from destruction of the glands by tuberculosis; in developed nations, this condition today usually is associated with anti-adrenal antibodies due to an autoimmune process, and detection of antibodies against CYP21 is useful in diagnosing this autoimmune form of primary adrenal insufficiency.

Hypofunction of the adrenals also can be secondary to a deficiency of ACTH due to impaired hypothalamic–pituitary function. Clinically, secondary adrenal insufficiency is seen most frequently in patients who have been treated chronically with pharmacological doses of glucocorticoids, thereby suppressing the hypothalamic–pituitary–adrenal axis and preventing normal production when steroids are discontinued. Secondary adrenal insufficiency also results from intrinsic diseases of the hypothalamus or anterior pituitary, in which case the signs and symptoms of adrenal insufficiency usually are intermingled with manifestations of deficiencies of other glands that also are regulated by the hypothalamic–pituitary system (Table 14-5). Although most instances of pituitary insufficiency involve all of its hormones, isolated ACTH deficiency has been reported. Deficiency of ACTH, whether isolated or as part of panhypopituitarism, is rarely complete, so that cortisol deficiency typically is not usually as marked as in primary adrenal insufficiency. Moreover, because adrenal synthesis of aldosterone is not affected by the loss of ACTH, manifestations of mineralocorticoid deficiency usually do not arise.

Albeit rare, the two forms of adrenal insufficiency can pose some diagnostic dilemmas. In the setting of primary adrenal insufficiency, the plasma cortisol level—which should be measured in the early morning due to circadian variation—is very low, ACTH is elevated due to the loss of negative feedback regulation at hypothalamic–pituitary levels, and exogenous ACTH does not increase plasma cortisol secretion from the damaged glands. Conversely, in hypothalamic or pituitary disease, plasma ACTH is low and the adrenal becomes secondarily suppressed. The adrenals again will not respond to ACTH in the short-course ACTH stimulation test but will respond to prolonged treatment with ACTH. It is important to remember that it takes time before the effects of hypopituitarism lead to adrenal atrophy. Thus, patients with recent onset of pituitary dysfunction—such as after resection of a pituitary adenoma—may respond normally to exogenous ACTH even though their pituitary reserve is compromised.

Cortisol Excess (Cushing's Syndrome)

The syndrome of chronic cortisol excess, generically termed *Cushing's syndrome*, is caused most commonly by pharmacological uses of glucocorticoids for the management of various diseases. The multiple adverse effects of supraphysiological

Table 14-5 Distinction between Primary and Secondary Adrenal Insufficiency

	Primary	Secondary[a]
Site	Adrenal	Hypothalamic–pituitary
ACTH secretion	Increased	Decreased
Pigmentation	Increased	Decreased
Headaches, visual loss	Rare	Frequent
Body weight	Decreased	Variable
Other pituitary hormones		
Growth hormone	No change	Decreased
Gonadotropin	No change	Decreased
Adrenal hormones		
Aldosterone	Deficient	Normal
Androgens	Deficient	Variable
Cortisol	Markedly decreased	Moderately reduced
Response to exogenous ACTH	None	Sluggish

[a]Rare examples of isolated corticotropin (ACTH) deficiency have been reported with normal levels of other pituitary hormones.

doses of glucocorticoids may be diminished by intermittent therapy with prednisone, a synthetic steroid listed in Table 14-3 that remains in the circulation for about 36 hours. If glucocorticoids are given in somewhat larger doses once every 48 hours, much of the beneficial anti-inflammatory effect will be maintained, but the hypothalamic–pituitary axis will be suppressed to a lesser degree and the noninflamed body tissues will not be exposed to high levels of steroid for the last 12 hours.

Less commonly, endogenous disorders causing cortisol excess arise within the adrenal glands (i.e., ACTH-independent Cushing's syndrome) or from overproduction of ACTH, either by the pituitary or by ectopic ACTH-producing sources such as small cell lung carcinoma or carcinoid tumors (i.e., ACTH-dependent Cushing's syndrome) (Table 14-6). With some exceptions, the manifestations of cortisol excess (Table 14-4) are similar in both the ACTH-dependent and ACTH-independent forms of Cushing's syndrome. Moreover, the initial diagnostic workup also is similar (e.g., measurement of urinary free cortisol in a 24-hour urine sample or an overnight dexamethasone suppression test; see below).

Historically, endocrinologists have used suppression tests in an attempt to increase the specificity of initial screening for Cushing's syndrome and to differentiate between the various forms of this syndrome. Many experts still use an overnight suppression test employing the potent synthetic glucocorticoid dexamethasone as the initial screening test for Cushing's syndrome. In this regimen, 1 mg of dexamethasone (equivalent to approximately 20–25 mg of cortisol) is administered orally at bedtime, and serum cortisol is measured at 8 o'clock the next morning. Normal subjects will have a cortisol level of less than 5 μg/dl. As noted above, other experts prefer to use the 24-hour urine free cortisol for screening. Finally, some authorities advocate measuring cortisol—either via an indwelling catheter or in saliva—at 11 P.M., taking advantage of the fact that the cortisol level is normally very low at this time and that the circadian rhythm is lost in Cushing's syndrome of whatever cause.

After the diagnosis of Cushing's syndrome is confirmed biochemically, the maneuvers shown in Table 14-6 will usually differentiate between the two categories. The first goal is to determine if the condition is ACTH-dependent or ACTH-independent by measuring plasma ACTH. Thereafter, one proceeds with direct visualization of the appropriate site by computed tomography (CT) or magnetic resonance imaging (MRI) scans. If the Cushing's syndrome is ACTH-independent, then the problem lies in the adrenal gland, usually a tumor that can be visualized by CT

Table 14-6 Differential Diagnosis of Adrenal Hyperfunction

	Primary (30%)	Secondary (70%)	
Site	Adrenal	Hypothalamic–pituitary	Ectopic tumors
Adrenal pathology	Tumor	Bilateral hyperplasia	Bilateral hyperplasia
ACTH secretion	Decreased	Increased	Markedly increased
Suppression with exogenous glucocorticoid			
Low dose	None	Minimal	None
High dose	None	Marked	None

ACTH, corticotropin.

scan. In ACTH-dependent Cushing's syndrome, the ACTH hypersecretion can be from a pituitary adenoma (more specifically termed *Cushing's disease*) or an ectopic tumor. Because ACTH-dependent Cushing's syndrome usually arises from a pituitary adenoma, a pituitary MRI is the initial diagnostic test in most cases.

To elucidate further the nature of adrenal hyperfunction in patients with confirmed Cushing's syndrome, more prolonged suppression tests can be done. These tests are based on the fact that ACTH-secreting pituitary adenomas in Cushing's disease retain some capacity for negative feedback regulation, such that administration of high doses of a potent synthetic glucocorticoid (e.g., 2 mg dexamethasone given every 6 hours for 2 days) can still suppress cortisol production. Even at these high doses, however, an adrenal tumor will not be suppressed. In clinical practice, the ability of the formal dexamethasone suppression tests to define unambiguously the etiology of Cushing's syndrome is imperfect, and other tests such as direct sampling of ACTH levels in the perusal sinuses in response to corticotropin-releasing hormone (CRH) are sometimes employed when the source of excess ACTH is unclear.

Mineralocorticoids

Under normal conditions, aldosterone is the primary mineralocorticoid. It arises from the outer zona glomerulosa of the adrenal cortex and is regulated principally by angiotensin II and serum potassium, with lesser effects of ACTH. In its absence, fluid and electrolyte status are altered, although cortisol itself, if present in sufficient amounts, may exert a sufficient mineralocorticoid effect to prevent progressive depletion of body fluids.

Regulation of Mineralocorticoid Secretion

Because the major function of aldosterone is to control body fluid volume by increasing sodium reabsorption by the kidneys, it is appropriate that the major stimulus for aldosterone synthesis and secretion arises in the kidneys (Fig. 14-8). The juxtaglomerular apparatus consists of modified myoepithelial cells that surround the renal afferent arterioles, contiguous to the macula densa of the distal tubule. These cells, called *juxtaglomerular cells*, synthesize and secrete the proteolytic enzyme renin. Acting in the blood, renin mediates the rate-limiting step in the production of active angiogensin II, cleaving the circulating precursor angiotensinogen to release the 10-amino acid peptide, angiotensin I. Thereafter, inactive angiotensin I is converted rapidly to the potent octapeptide hormone angiotensin II by the action of angiotensin-converting enzyme, which is found in the plasma membrane of vascular endothelial cells throughout the body.

Angiotensin II exerts two major actions, one as a direct arteriolar vasoconstrictor and the other as a stimulus to aldosterone secretion. These two actions in concert maintain the volume and pressure of the arterial circulation, providing the major support to the circulation in times of fluid loss or falling blood pressure. Angiotensin II both acutely and chronically stimulates aldosterone production by the zona glomerulosa. It binds to the type 1 angiotensin receptor in the plasma membrane, which couples to several G proteins to activate phospholipase C and lipoxygenase. This activation results in increased levels of intracellular calcium and lipid

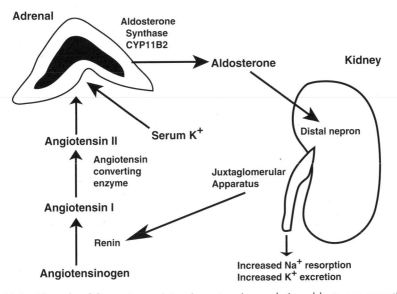

Fig. 14-8   The role of the renin–angiotensin system in regulating aldosterone secretion.

second messengers, ultimately stimulating StAR to facilitate cholesterol entry into the mitochondria. Chronically, angiotensin II increases the expression of the various steroidogenic enzymes, thus increasing the biosynthetic capacity of the zona glomerulosa.

All actions of renin apparently are mediated through its generation of angiotensin II, the primary stimulus to aldosterone synthesis. Aldosterone production is stimulated at multiple sites in the biosynthetic pathway.

Stimuli to Renin Release. The major stimulus to the release of renin is a decrease in the perfusion pressure of blood traversing the renal afferent arterioles, which is sensed by the juxtaglomerular apparatus functioning as a baroreceptor. When a decrease in either systemic blood volume or blood pressure leads to a fall in renal perfusion pressure, renin is secreted.

Renin secretion is also stimulated by other factors, including the concentration of sodium and chloride at the macula densa and the concentration of plasma electrolytes. Some of these factors act by stimulating renal sympathetic nerves that innervate the juxtaglomerular apparatus.

Other Stimuli for Aldosterone Secretion. Plasma potassium concentration and ACTH also stimulate aldosterone. Elevated plasma potassium depolarizes the zona glomerulosa cells, increasing intracellular calcium and activating calmodulin-dependent kinases to facilitate aldosterone production. This potassium effect appears appropriate, as aldosterone induces increased renal excretion of potassium. If levels of plasma potassium are suddenly raised, as after a large meal of potassium-rich foods, aldosterone is secreted and acts on the kidney to excrete the excess potassium load. As described below, however, the effects of aldosterone to increase renal sodium retention and potassium excretion require an hour or more; thus, there must be more rapid ways to remove high levels of potassium entering the circulation, because such levels could lead to instant and serious trouble. The rapid transfer of potassium from extracellular fluid into cells is accomplished by a combination of insulin and epinephrine effects on potassium transport across cell membranes.

The effect of ACTH on aldosterone biosynthesis is powerful but short-lived. Although the physiological role of ACTH in regulating aldosterone secretion is limited, prolonged ACTH deficiency may result in some atrophy of the zona glomerulosa, with a decreased response to other stimuli.

Secretion. Aldosterone is so potent a mineralocorticoid that very little is needed for its primary effect. Only 0.05–0.20 mg (50–200 μg) is produced each day. Because there is no specific aldosterone carrier protein in the blood, much of the circulating aldosterone is free and plasma concentrations are ~5–15 ng/dl. Acutely, renin levels are rapidly affected by postural changes, with upright levels approximating twice those observed under supine conditions. Chronically, secretion can be increased two- to sixfold by sodium depletion and even more by persistent shrinkage of effective arterial blood volume, as in cirrhosis of the liver with ascites and marked edema.

Metabolism. Due to the relatively large fraction of circulating aldosterone that is unbound, its half-life in circulation is only 15–20 minutes. Aldosterone is metabolized, predominantly in the liver, into a tetrahydroaldosterone derivative that is excreted in the urine as a glucuronide. Some is excreted as a glucuronide without being metabolized, and this acid-labile fraction, about 10% of total secretion, is what is usually measured. Therefore, a normal urine aldosterone level is 5–20 μg/day.

Functions

The primary action of aldosterone is to increase sodium reabsorption in the distal tubules. To do so, it first is bound to cytosolic MR; then the hormone–receptor complex is transferred to the nucleus. Once there, it initiates a sequence of events that includes the rapid induction of serum- and glucocorticoid-regulated kinase, which in turn phosphorylates and activates amiloride-sensitive epithelial Na^+ channels in the apical membrane. Thereafter, increased sodium influx stimulates the Na^+,K^+-ATPase in the basolateral membrane. In addition to these relatively rapid actions, aldosterone increases the synthesis of the individual components of these membrane proteins.

As aldosterone increases active sodium reabsorption, an electrochemical gradient is established that facilitates the passive transfer of potassium from tubular cells into the urine. Therefore, potassium is excreted not in a direct exchange for sodium, but rather in a manner that depends directly on the active reabsorption of sodium. If almost all sodium is reabsorbed more proximally, as in the presence of severe volume depletion, little will reach the distal reabsorptive site. Therefore, despite high levels of aldosterone, potassium excretion will be minimal in the absence of sodium delivery to the distal tubule. Conversely, a high sodium intake will increase potassium excretion. This is particularly true if the individual is receiving a diuretic that blocks part of the proximal reabsorption of sodium, causing even more sodium to reach the distal reabsorptive site.

Sodium Concentration. As sodium is reabsorbed in the kidney, an equivalent amount of water also is reabsorbed, thus preserving the normal concentration of sodium in the extracellular fluid. If water reabsorption is impaired and the concentration of sodium rises, the increase in osmotic pressure will activate the release of antidiuretic hormone, effectively increasing renal water reabsorption, and will increase water intake by stimulating thirst.

Aldosterone Escape. Normally, when mild sodium depletion leads to increased aldosterone secretion, the extracellular fluid volume reexpands as more sodium is reabsorbed. The degree of expansion should be adequate to replenish the shrinkage that initiated the process, so that further production of aldosterone is turned off. Under some circumstances, such as persistent leakage of effective blood volume into the abdomen in patients with cirrhosis of the liver and ascites, the stimulus to aldosterone never turns off. The extra sodium that is reabsorbed does not replenish the shrunken effective fluid volume because of the continuous leak. Therefore, very high levels of aldosterone—a condition called *secondary hyperaldosteronism*—are seen in chronic edematous states.

When aldosterone levels remain high in the absence of an ongoing fluid leak, as with exogenous administration of aldosterone or an aldosterone-secreting tumor, extracellular volume expands by a few liters but then stabilizes. This escape phenomenon likely results from a confluence of effects that include decreased proximal reabsorption of sodium, perhaps because of a natriuretic factor that arises in the hypothalamus; increased glomerular filtration, probably because of the actions of atrial natriuretic factor (see Chapter 7); and suppression of the renin–angiotensin system by increases in systemic blood pressure, renal perfusion pressure, and sodium content at the macula densa. As described below, however, these changes are sufficient to elevate blood pressure significantly. Moreover, although sodium reabsorption escapes, potassium excretion continues because more sodium is delivered to the distal tubule.

Extrarenal Effects. Aldosterone also increases the reabsorption of sodium in other places where it may be excreted—saliva, sweat, and stool. When physical activity is first begun in a hot climate, a great amount of sodium may be lost in the large volumes of sweat that are formed. The resulting shrinkage of fluid volume activates the renin–angiotensin system, increasing aldosterone secretion and causing more and more sodium to be retained, which is the process of acclimatization to a hot environment. After a few days, sweat will be sodium-free. Thus, there is no need to increase sodium intake beyond the usual amounts obtained in the diet when performing continued exercise in hot climates. Water intake should be adequate to replenish the volume of sweat.

Disorders of Mineralocorticoids

Primary Aldosterone Excess
Aldosterone excess due to benign tumors of the adrenal gland that autonomously secrete aldosterone (designated *Conn's syndrome*) has long been recognized as an unusual but interesting cause of secondary hypertension. The clinical hallmarks are

hypokalemia and hypertension. Blood pressure rises because plasma volume expands due to the aldosterone-mediated reabsorption of sodium. Even though *escape* occurs, the increased body fluid volume is sufficient to elevate the blood pressure. Similarly, as noted above, the increase in potassium excretion continues so that hypokalemia, with its various manifestations, is typical. The diagnosis is most easily made by finding high levels of aldosterone and low levels of renin in the blood. Some studies suggest that inappropriately high aldosterone levels may occur in up to 5%–10% of patients with *essential hypertension*, although the majority of these subjects do not have discrete adenomas but rather bilateral adrenal hyperplasia.

Secondary Aldosterone Excess

More common than aldosterone-secreting tumors are conditions in which effective arterial blood volume is diminished, provoking high levels of renin–angiotensin that persistently stimulate aldosterone synthesis to the point where bilateral adrenal hyperplasia may develop (Table 14-7). These include chronic edematous diseases such as severe heart failure, cirrhosis of the liver with ascites, and the nephrotic syndrome. Despite the high levels of renin–angiotensin and the secondarily increased aldosterone excess, fluid volume remains shrunken and the blood pressure is low-normal.

It is possible to block aldosterone's effects in the kidney with spironolactone, a nonmineralocorticoid steroidal compound that competes directly with aldosterone for binding to mineralocorticoid receptor (MR) in the renal tubule. Because it is more weakly bound than aldosterone, 50–500 mg/day is needed to competitively block the 0.5–10 mg aldosterone that may be secreted in secondary aldosteronism. This inhibition of aldosterone action is efficacious in conditions of secondary aldosteronism such as congestive heart failure and cirrhosis.

Genetic Disorders of Mineralocorticoid Action

Further insights into the roles of the mineralocorticoid receptor and its target genes in fluid and electrolyte balance have emerged from analyses of patients with rare genetic disorders of mineralocorticoid action, such as pseudohypoaldosteronism and pseudoaldosteronism. Despite elevated levels of mineralocorticoids, patients with pseudohypoaldosteronism present with clinical manifestations suggestive of deficient mineralocorticoid action (i.e., volume depletion, hypotension, hyperkalemia,

Table 14-7 The Two Major Forms of Aldosterone Excess

	Primary	Secondary
Pathology	Adrenal tumor	Adrenal hyperplasia
Mechanism	Autonomous hypersecretion	Driven hypersecretion (renin–angiotensin)
Effective arterial blood volume	Expanded	Shrunken
Total body fluid volume	Slightly expanded	Markedly expanded (edema)
Renin–angiotensin	Suppressed	Activated
Clinical expression	Hypertension Potassium wastage	Low-normal blood pressure Potassium wastage Edema

and metabolic acidosis). Molecular analyses have defined discrete subpopulations of patients with pseudohypoaldosteronism: one subset of patients has loss-of-function mutations in genes encoding subunits of the amiloride-sensitive epithelial Na^+ channel that have an autosomal recessive inheritance, whereas the other subset carries inactivating mutations in the mineralocorticoid receptor that cause an autosomal dominant disorder. Pseudoaldosteronism, also termed *Liddle's syndrome*, is an autosomal dominant disease that results from activating mutations in the amiloride-sensitive Na^+ channel. The constitutive activity of this channel leads to the manifestations of aldosterone excess described below despite low levels of plasma renin and aldosterone

Adrenal Androgens

The adrenal androgens represent the third class of adrenal steroids. Despite their designation, neither DHEA nor its sulfated derivative DHEA-S activates the androgen receptor. However, in peripheral tissues, they are precursors that can be converted to the potent androgen testosterone. Interestingly, the secretion of abundant amounts of androgen precursors by the zona reticularis is restricted to primates, in which circulating levels of DHEA and DHEA-S exhibit age- and sex-dependent profiles that are distinct from those of any other steroid hormone. As noted earlier, the fetal adrenal gland produces vast amounts of DHEA-S *in utero*, which are converted into estrogens by the placenta. After birth, DHEA-S production falls dramatically and remains low during infancy and early childhood. The resumption of DHEA-S production by the adrenal zona reticularis at ~7–8 years is termed *adrenarche*, and it is the resulting conversion of adrenal androgens to active androgens in target tissues that initiates the growth of pubic and axillary hair before the onset of gonadal steroidogenesis. Production continues to increase through the second decade of life but then decline progressively with aging. Although DHEA and DHEA-S have been implicated in a vast array of physiological and pathophysiological processes, adrenal androgens are not essential for life and are not routinely administered in replacement therapy for primary adrenal insufficiency. It should be noted, however, that DHEA is available in the United States as a nutritional supplement that may be taken without a physician's advice or supervision.

The precise physiological roles of adrenal androgens and the mechanisms that regulate their production remain poorly defined. It is known that ACTH can induce adrenal androgen production, but the characteristic changes in DHEA-S levels throughout life do not parallel changes in ACTH; thus, other extrinsic or intrinsic factors must also modulate the synthesis of adrenal androgens. Adrenal androgens are most prominent clinically in congenital adrenal hyperplasia, inherited defects in adrenal steroidogeneis that shuttle large amounts of precursors into the androgen pathway. As noted earlier in this chapter and in Chapter 8, the presence and degree of androgen excess or deficiency depend on the specific enzymatic defect.

ADRENAL MEDULLA

Catecholamines are the hormones secreted by the sympathetic nervous system. The two major catecholamine hormones are norepinephrine and epinephrine. Conceptually, it is useful to regard norepinephrine as a local neurotransmitter in the peripheral nerves that acts locally and reaches the general circulation only after intense activation of the sympathetic nervous system. In contrast, epinephrine is released from the adrenal medulla in response to stress and circulates throughout the body to prepare the organism for flight or fight. The effects of catecholamines are mediated via α- and β-receptors on effector tissues; these receptor classes often have antagonistic actions, such as α-vasoconstriction versus β-vasodilation.

Synthesis and Release of Epinephrine

The adrenal medulla, a modified sympathetic ganglion with postganglionic cells but no axons, is specialized to secrete catecholamines from chromaffin cells (so called because they take up chromium). One preganglionic fiber from the splanchnic nerve innervates a number of medullary cells, so that a few impulses can cause a massive catecholamine discharge.

Epinephrine is synthesized from norepinephrine in the adrenal medulla (and probably in certain brain neurons) by the action of PNMT (Fig. 14-9), an enzyme whose synthesis is induced by cortisol. As the adrenal medulla is cradled by the adrenal cortex, it is bathed with very high concentrations of cortisol, so that PNMT is highly expressed. Although 80% of adrenal medullary catecholamine secretion is

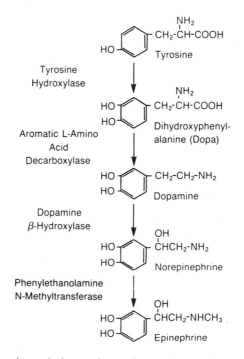

Fig. 14-9 Pathway of catecholamine biosynthesis. The rate-limiting step is catalyzed by tyrosine hydroxylase, while the reaction specific to the adrenal cortex is catalyzed by phenylethanolamine N-methyltransferase.

epinephrine and only 20% is norepinephrine, epinephrine makes up only 10% of circulating catecholamines, suggesting that extra-adrenal sources provide most of the circulating catecholamines.

Catecholamine synthesis is regulated by changes in the levels of the rate-limiting enzyme tyrosine hydroxylase. Acutely, tyrosine hydroxylase is activated by phosphorylation, as well as by the escape from end-product inhibition as neural activity causes a release of cytoplasmic catecholamines. With chronic stimulation, tyrosine hydroxylase expression is induced due to transcriptional and posttranscriptional effects.

Catecholamine release occurs by *stimulus–secretion coupling*: preganglionic nerve impulses release acetylcholine, which increases membrane permeability, thus depolarizing the cell membrane, and increases calcium influx. This induces exocytosis of the secretory granules.

Accurate assays are now available for the very small quantities of circulating catecholamines. Increased levels under various clinical circumstances reflect the involvement of epinephrine in cardiovascular, metabolic, and other responses to stress. Repetitive sympathetic activation may eventuate in persistently high blood pressure and also may potentiate atherosclerosis.

Fate of Secreted Catecholamines

Catecholamines are rapidly ($t_{1/2} < 1$ minute) removed from the synapses and circulation by a number of processes:

1. Reuptake by catechol-secreting cells for reuse or metabolism (i.e., presynaptic uptake).
2. Uptake by receptors on effector cells.
3. Metabolism by inactivating mechanisms, mainly in the liver, involving the catecholamine-*O*-transferase and monamine oxidase enzymes. The products are mainly excreted through the kidney as metanephrines or vanillymandelic acid (VMA) (Fig. 14-10).

Action of Epinephrine

α- and β-Adrenergic receptors are present in many tissues, ensuring widespread actions of catecholamine hormones. Initially, distinct classes of adrenergic receptors were characterized based on the apparent differential actions of epinephrine and norepinephrine and the behavior of agonists and antagonists. Traditionally, postsynaptic α-receptors on effector cells were designated $\alpha 1$, while $\alpha 2$ receptors were expressed on presynaptic sympathetic neurons. Thus, $\alpha 1$ receptors mediate the classic effects of α-agonists such as vasoconstriction, while the $\alpha 2$-receptors inhibit the release of norepinephrine from sympathetic nerves. The β-receptors mediate events such as vasodilation, increased heart rate and contractile function, bronchodilation, and lipolysis.

The cloning of the genes encoding adrenergic receptors has revealed surprising complexity, with three distinct genes encoding β-receptors ($\beta 1$, $\beta 2$, and $\beta 3$),

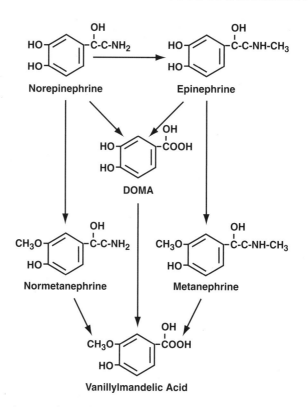

Fig. 14-10 Pathways of catecholamine metabolism.

three genes encoding α1-adrenergic receptors, and three genes encoding α2-adrenergic receptors. Both epinephrine and norepinephrine stimulate both α- and β-adrenergic receptors, with the response of a given system largely determined by the relative expression of the various adrenergic receptors (Table 14-8). All β-adrenergic receptor subtypes couple via Gαs to activate adenylyl cyclase, thereby activating cyclic AMP–dependent protein kinase. The α2-adrenergic receptors generally couple via Gαi to inhibit adenylyl cyclase, although they also activate potassium channels to depolarize cells and activate mitogen-activated protein kinases. Finally, the α1-adrenergic receptors couple to Gαq, thereby increasing the generation of phosphoinositides via activation of phospholipase C and mobilizing intracellular calcium stores.

The major actions of epinephrine will now be considered.

Arousal

These actions include alerting, pupillary dilation, piloerection, sweating, bronchial dilation, tachycardia, inhibition of smooth muscle in the gastrointestinal tract, constriction of sphincters, and relaxation of uterine muscles.

Table 14-8   Adrenergic Receptors and Function

α-Receptor	β-Receptor
Vasoconstriction	Vasodilatation (β_2)
Iris dilatation	Cardioacceleration (β_1)
Intestinal relaxation	Increased myocardial strength (β_1)
Intestinal sphincter contraction	Intestinal relaxation (β_2)
	Uterus relaxation (β_2)
Pilomotor contraction	Bronchodilatation (β_2)
Bladder sphincter contraction	Calorigenesis (β_2)
	Glycogenolysis (β_2)
	Lipolysis (β_3)
	Bladder wall relaxation (β_2)

Source: Guyton AC: *Textbook of Medical Physiology*, Saunders, Philadelphia, p. 671, 1991.

Metabolic Actions

In keeping with the need for ready fuel, epinephrine's actions provide more glucose and free fatty acids. This occurs through the release of glucose from glycogen (glycogenolysis) by activation of phosphorylase in the liver and muscle via the Cori cycle (see Chapter 16). In muscle, without glucose-6-phosphatase, the glucose is metabolized to lactate. Epinephrine also stimulates lipolysis in adipose cells by activating the lipase that converts triglycerides into free fatty acids and glycerol. As a result of these calorigenic effects, the metabolic rate increases by 20%–30%.

Cardiovascular Actions

In addition to directly stimulating heart rate and vasoconstriction, repeated bursts of epinephrine have been hypothesized to result in permanent hypertension via a number of possible effects.

Both agonists and antagonists of α- and β-adrenergic receptors are widely used in clinical medicine. Examples include the use of β-agonists such as isoproterenol to dilate bronchi for the treatment of asthma and of β-antagonists such as propranolol to decrease cardiac output for the treatment of hypertension. In addition, the endogenous compounds are used clinically, (e.g., epinephrine for allergic reactions and norepinephrine to increase blood pressure).

Features of Catecholamine Excess

Pheochromocytomas are usually benign tumors arising from the adrenal medulla, with clinical features that reflect the effects of epinephrine and norepinephrine (shown in Table 14-9) in excess. Thus, most patients have paroxysms of hypertension, tachycardia, sweating, tremor, palpitations, and nervousness. Most lose weight and are hyperglycemic. The diagnosis, if entertained, is made by measuring either plasma free catecholamines or urinary levels of metanephrines or fractionated catecholamines, followed by direct visualization of the typically large adrenal tumors, usually by CT scan.

Table 14-9   Assessments of Adrenal Function

	Hypofunction		Hyperfunction	
	Screening	Definitive	Screening	Definitive
Cortical				
Glucocorticoid	Low cortisol, high ACTH Response to single ACTH injection	Response to repeated ACTH injections	High cortisol Response to single dose of glucocorticoid	Response to repeated doses of glucocorticoid
Mineralocorticoid	Low aldosterone, high renin Response to acute volume depletion	Response to chronic volume depletion	High aldosterone, low renin Response to acute volume expansion	Response to chronic volume expansion
Androgen	Low plasma levels	—	High plasma levels	—
Medullary	—	—	High catecholamines in single plasma or urine samples	Response to sympathetic nervous system suppressant

ACTH, corticotropin.

ASSESSMENT OF ADRENAL FUNCTION

The various forms of adrenal hypo- and hyperfunction are relatively rare, but because of the multiple and diffuse effects of adrenal hormones, many more patients than the few who actually have these diseases may be suspected of having them. Thus, although few will have adrenocortical hyperfunction, some of the large number of women with central obesity and primary hypertension will be suspected of having cortisol excess (Cushing's syndrome) and will merit an assessment to exclude it. Therefore, screening tests to assess adrenal function are needed rather frequently. If these screening tests are positive, more definitive tests may be needed to confirm the presence of the disorder and to determine its precise form (Table 14-9). In addition to biochemical tests, insights into anatomical localization and type of adrenal pathology may be obtained by various X-ray and isotopic scanning procedures such as CT and MRI.

As a general approach to screening for either hypo- or hyperfunction, simple measurements of plasma or urine concentrations of adrenal hormones under basal conditions are usually inadequate, mainly because of the wide range of values seen in normal individuals. In screening for hypofunction, the presence of low levels of the adrenal hormone along with high levels of the physiological stimulating hormone (e.g., ACTH for glucocorticoids and renin–angiotensin for mineralocorticoids) may be useful. Better results are obtained by measuring plasma levels after an appropriate stimulus, such as ACTH for glucocorticoids and diuretic-induced acute volume depletion for mineralocorticoids. For more definitive evidence, the responses of either plasma or urine levels of the hormones are measured after repeated administration of the appropriate stimulus.

To screen for hyperfunction, attempts at rapid suppression of the adrenal hormones are made. For glucocorticoid excess, the response of plasma cortisol to a single dose of the exogenous glucocorticoid dexamethasone (1 mg at bedtime) is usually adequate, although others prefer to use the 24-hour urine free cortisol instead. For mineralocorticoid excess, the response of plasma aldosterone to acute volume expansion by a short infusion of normal saline is measured. For more definitive testing, the responses of either plasma or urine levels of the hormones after more prolonged attempts at suppression are used.

There are few indications to test for deficiencies of adrenal androgens and even fewer to test for catecholamine deficiency. Excesses of androgens derived from adrenal precursors are seen with congenital adrenal enzymatic defects. Catecholamine-secreting tumors (pheochromocytomas) are detected by measuring plasma and/or urine levels of the catecholamines or their metabolic products.

In summary, the assessment of adrenal function is similar to that of other endocrine disorders. Hypofunction is best diagnosed by attempting to stimulate with the appropriate physiological trophic agent, and hyperfunction by suppressing with the appropriate physiological maneuver.

SUGGESTED READING

Barnes PJ: Anti-inflammatory actions of glucocorticoids; molecular mechanisms. Clin Sci 94:557–572, 1998.

Boumpas DT, Chrousos GP, Wilder RL, Cupps TR, and Balow JE: Glucocorticoid therapy for immune-mediated diseases: basic and clinical correlates. Ann Intern Med 119:1198–1208, 1993.

Cooper M and Stewart PM: The syndrome of apparent mineralocorticoid excess. Q J Med 91:453–455, 1998.

Findling JW and Raff H: Diagnosis and differential diagnosis of Cushing's syndrome. Endocrinol Metab Clin North Am 30:729–747, 2001.

Funder JW: Glucocorticoid and mineralocorticoid receptors: biology and clinical relevance. Annu Rev Med 48:231–240, 1998.

Grinspoon SK and Biller BMK: Laboratory assessment of adrenal insufficiency. J Clin Endocrinol Metab 79:923–931, 1994.

Guyton AC: The adrenocortical hormones. In: Textbook of Medical Physiology, 8th ed., AC Guyton, ed., Saunders, Philadelphia, pp. 667–678, 842–854, 1991.

Keegan CE and Hammer GD: Recent insights into organogenesis of the adrenal cortex. Trends Endocrinol Metab 13:200–208, 2002.

Merke D and Kabbani M: Congenital adrenal hyperplasia: epidemiology, management, and practical drug treatment. Paediatr Drugs 3:599–611, 2001.

Moneva MH and Gomez-Sanchez CE: Pathophysiology of adrenal hypertension. Semin Nephrol 22:44–53, 2002.

Nieman LK: Diagnostic tests in Cushing's syndrome. Ann NY Acad Sci 970:112–118, 2002.

Rainey WE, Carr BR, Sasano H, Suzuki T, and Mason JI: Dissecting human adrenal androgen production. Trends Endocrinol Metab 13:234–239, 2002.

Sandeep TC and Walker BR: Pathophysiology of modulation of local glucocorticoid levels by 11beta-hydroxysteroid dehydrogenases. Trends Endocrinol Metab 12:446–453, 2001.

White PC: Disorders of aldosterone biosynthesis and action. N Engl J Med 331:250–258, 1994.

White PC: Steroid 11β-hydroxylase deficiency and related disorders. Endocrinol Metab Clin North Am 30:61–79, 2001.

White PC and Speiser PW: Congenital adrenal hyperplasia due to 21-hydroxylase deficiency. Endocr Rev 21:245–291, 2000.

15

Calcium Homeostasis

HOWARD J. HELLER

Ionized calcium plays a pivotal role in many physiological and biochemical processes, including the contraction of muscles, the clotting of blood, and impulse conduction in the heart and nervous system. Moreover, it acts as a secondary messenger within the cell to initiate other cascades important for cell signaling and both exocrine and endocrine secretion. The major storage sites for calcium in the body are the teeth and skeleton. These hard tissues, which contain 99% of the body's calcium (approximately 1 kg), provide the structure necessary for mastication, locomotion, and protection of internal organs. In the blood, calcium is found in three forms—ionized (50%), protein-bound (40%), and soluble complexes (10%). Unlike the other two forms of calcium, the protein-bound fraction, which is primarily bound to albumin, is not filtered by the kidney. In normal individuals, the range of serum total calcium is 8.5 to 10.3 mg/dl. In a given individual, however, the diurnal variation of serum calcium is limited to 0.3 mg/dl. This chapter reviews calcium homeostasis in the extracellular fluid, the integrated response to calcium stressors, and disorders of calcium metabolism.

CALCIUM HOMEOSTASIS: ORGAN LEVEL

The bone, kidneys, and intestines are the most important calcium-transporting tissues and play an important role in calcium homeostasis (Fig. 15-1). These three corners of the calcium homeostasis triangle are individually discussed below.

Bone

The bone is a dynamic tissue that is constantly changing. From birth until the completion of puberty, bone lengthens and changes shape by a process called *modeling*. In the adult skeleton, *remodeling* is the process used to repair damaged areas, to strengthen sites of stress or injury, and to remove unnecessary bone from sparsely used skeletal sites. The entire skeleton is demolished and refabricated by this process within 10 years. There are two main types of bone that remodel at different rates. *Cortical* bone, which makes up 80% of the bone mass, is highly calcified, dense tissue found mainly in the appendicular skeleton such as the arms and legs.

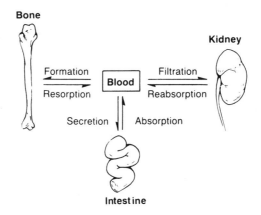

Fig. 15-1 Calcium homeostasis is regulated by the transfer of calcium between the blood and three major target organs.

Trabecular bone is found in marrow-containing areas such as the spine and metaphyses. Despite its limited share of the bone mass, trabecular bone comprises 80% of the surface area of the bone. This greater surface area explains the greater bone turnover or remodeling in trabecular bone (20%) relative to its cortical counterpart (4%).

The cellular organelle responsible for bone remodeling, the *basic multicellular unit* (BMU), was conceptualized by Harold Frost in the 1960s and augmented by later discoveries (Fig. 15-2). Chemical factors are believed to recruit *osteoclasts* to resorb or remove the old bone. Each osteoclast attaches to the bone via integrins. The cell polarizes so that a sealed space is formed between the osteoclast and the bone. Proton pumps, located just below the cell membrane in a structure called the *ruffled membrane,* acidify the space to dissolve the hydroxyapatite crystals in bone, and proteolytic enzymes (including cathepsin K and matrix metalloproteinase 9) cleave the structural proteins of the bone. After an average of 2 weeks and probably after it has resorbed the surface to a specific depth, the osteoclast releases from the bone and undergoes apoptosis. The formation phase is initiated by recruited osteoblasts derived from mesenchymal precursors. They follow the path of the burrowing osteoclasts to deposit osteoid, bone matrix proteins composed primarily of type I collagen, and to mineralize this matrix with calcium and phosphate that matures into hydroxyapatite crystals (chemical structure: $Ca_{10}(PO_4)_6(OH)_2$). The initial product is haphazardly arrayed (*woven bone*), but it is then reorganized into concentric layers (*lamellar bone*). Each osteoblast is active for about 3 months. As the bone is deposited and surrounds the cells, some osteoblasts undergo apoptosis, but others mature into *osteocytes*. Osteocytes, which make up 90% of the cell mass of the bone, are connected to one another and to flattened surface lining cells via cytoplasmic processes encased by bony *canaliculi*.

In general, the process of resorption and formation of the bone is tightly coupled to maintain bone mass. In the highly calcified cortical bone, the BMU forms tunnels, with the osteoclasts at the head of the tunnel, whereas, in trabecular bone,

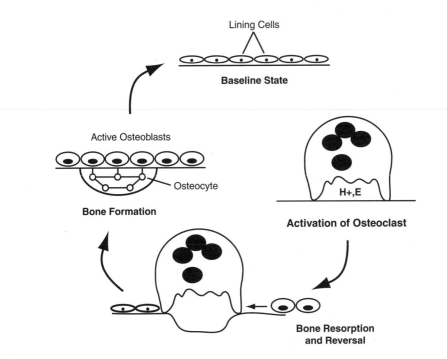

Fig. 15-2 Bone remodeling cycle. The process begins with recruitment and attachment of osteoclasts to the bone surface. The osteoclasts secrete acid (H$^+$ in the figure), which dissolves hydroxyapatite crystals, and proteolytic enzymes (signified by E in the figure), which dissolve the protein scaffolding along the bone, creating a resorption trench. Osteoblasts follow in the trench and reform the bone by depositing osteoid and mineralizing it. Within the new bone, some osteoblasts differentiate into osteocytes that, connected together by cytoplasmic processes, maintain the bone. When the remodeling cycle is complete, active osteoblasts mature into flattened lining cells.

the BMU forms trenches on individual tracebulae. The life span of the an individual BMU is about 6–9 months. At any given time point, there are approximately 1 million BMU active throughout the skeleton involving 10% to 20% of the skeleton.

It is currently believed that the osteocyte may act as a *mechanosensor* to drive bone turnover with net bone gain or loss in response to mechanical strain. The concept is that with a sensation of high strain, net bone formation ensues to reduce the strain to a given set point. As a clinical example, the bones of the dominant arm are exposed to greater strain, so it is not surprising that their density is 5% higher on average than that of the nondominant arm. In tennis players, the difference may reach 20%. Similarly, walking and running maintain or increase bone mass in weight-bearing locations. In contrast, a sensation of inadequate bone strain stimulates net bone resorption to increase the perceived strain until it reaches the established set point. Weightlessness of space flight and bed rest from spinal cord injury, which induce rapid bone loss from weight-bearing bones, provide meaningful illustrations.

It is important to review the derivation of osteoclasts and osteoblasts because abnormalities in this pathway result in clinical disease and may affect calcium homeostasis. A full description of the complicated cascades and the myriad factors is beyond the scope of this chapter, but the key factors will be highlighted. Osteoclasts derive from the monocyte/macrophage lineage (Fig. 15-3). It is recognized that factors including c-*fos* influence differentiation of macrophage precursors into osteoclasts, which are large multinucleated cells, because in the absence of these factors there is an abundance of macrophages but no osteoclasts. Interestingly, osteoclast formation *in vitro* requires the presence of bone marrow with osteoblasts or marrow stromal cells (likely precursors of osteoblasts). Secreted or found on the cell surface of osteoblasts and their marrow precursors, RANKL (receptor for activation of nuclear factor kappa B ligand) activates differentiation and proliferation of osteoclasts by binding RANK (receptor for activation of nuclear factor kappa B) on the preosteoclast surface. This process may be blocked by secreted OPG (osteoprotegerin), another osteoblast product, which acts as a decoy receptor for RANKL. Other factors, such as c-*Src*, are required to allow the differentiated osteoclast to reabsorb bone. Interestingly, absence of c-*Src* results in osteoclasts lacking the ruffled membrane. The absence or overexpression of the factors above results in pathological bone loss (osteoporosis, a condition in which low bone mass and disturbance of the skeletal architecture predispose to fracture) or bone gain (osteopetrosis, a condition in which the inability to remodel bone results in dense but brittle bone that encroaches the bone marrow space).

Osteoblasts derive from mesenchymal precursors that also give rise to fibroblasts, myocytes, and adipocytes (Fig. 15-4). Two of the important factors believed to stimulate the differentiation of the precursors to osteoblasts include BMP (bone morphogeneic protein) and CBFA-1 (core-binding factor 1). When BMP is injected

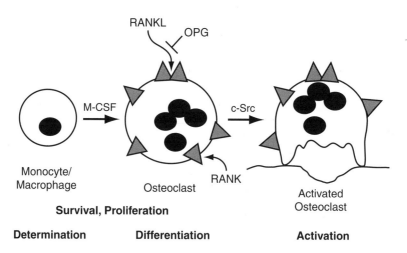

Fig. 15-3 Pathway for osteoclast differentiation. Precursors from the monocyte/macrophage line differentiate into osteoclasts after exposure to M-CSF (macrophage colony-stimulating factor) and RANKL (receptor for activation of nuclear factor kappa B ligand). The binding of RANKL to its osteoclast receptor, RANK (receptor for activation of nuclear factor kappa B), may be blocked by OPG (osteoprotegerin). Factors including c-*Src* are required to polarize the cell and resorb bone.

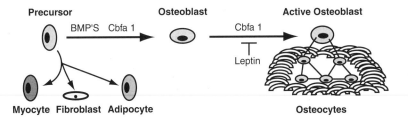

Fig. 15-4 Pathway for differentiation of osteoblasts and osteocytes. Mesenchymal precursors may differentiate into several cell types. Core-binding factor 1 (Cbfa 1) and several bone morphogenetic proteins (BMPs) may commit stromal precursors into the osteoblast cell line. In addition, Cbfa 1 activates osteoblasts to make bone, and leptin may block that process. Osteoblasts enclosed within the bone may differentiate into osteocytes connected by cytoplasmic processes or undergo apoptosis.

into muscle, bone may form. There are many BMPs with overlapping pleiotropic actions, and it is unclear how they act in normal bone physiology. In contrast, CBFA-1 is known to act specifically on osteoblasts and their precursors. In the complete absence of CBFA-1, osteoblasts do not form. In addition, osteoclasts are absent, providing further evidence that their formation requires differentiating factors from osteoblasts or osteoblast precursors.

Although the bone does not contribute to calcium homeostasis in normal individuals who are in a steady state (500 mg calcium enters bone for formation and 500 mg exits the bone after bone resorption), several conditions may shift the balance toward net bone resorption or bone formation. The net bone resorption found in osteoporosis or after prolonged bed rest shifts calcium out of the bone. The excess shift of calcium into the extracellular fluid would result in hypercalcemia if it were not counterbalanced by other organ systems. In contrast, the net bone formation of osteopetrosis shifts calcium into bone, which would result in hypocalcemia if uncompensated.

Kidneys

The kidneys play a very important role in calcium homeostasis. They filter an enormous amount of calcium daily. Of the 10 g calcium that is filtered, 98%–99% is reabsorbed. Thus, average urinary calcium excretion is 100 to 200 mg/day. The majority of calcium (60%–70%) is reabsorbed in the proximal tubule. In the thick ascending loop of Henle, another 20% is reabsorbed. In the distal tubule, 5%–10% is reabsorbed, and the remainder is reabsorbed in the collecting ducts. It is believed that the key active transcellular reabsorption of calcium occurs at the distal tubule; at other sites, the rule is passive intercellular movement of calcium driven by maintenance of a lumen-positive transepithelial potential difference.

Many factors affect the ability of the kidney to reabsorb calcium. If renal filtration decreases due to volume depletion or declining renal function, less calcium is lost into the urine. Alternatively, if renal filtration increases due to volume overload, more calcium is excreted into the urine. Parathyroid hormone, which is described in more detail later, improves renal calcium reabsorption. Acidosis or a dietary acid load impairs renal calcium reabsorption; alkalosis and a dietary alkali load produce the opposite effect. Excess dietary intake of salt enhances calcium excretion by increasing extracellular fluid volume and by impairing renal calcium reabsorption. Increased serum calcium and magnesium increase renal calcium excretion. Finally, drugs affect urinary calcium excretion. Loop diuretics, such as furosemide, increase renal calcium losses. Thiazide diuretics, which act on the distal tubule, and lithium reduce urinary calcium.

On a molecular level, much has been learned about active renal calcium reabsorption at the distal tubule, which is believed to be the main site of regulation. A brief discussion is presented here, but a detailed description is beyond the scope of this chapter. The rate-limiting step is the traversal of the luminal membrane via epithelial calcium channels (ECaC1 < ECaC2). Calcium enters across a favorable electrochemical gradient. Intracellularly, calbindins (calbindin-D_{28K} and calbindin-D_{9K}) bind the free calcium. This both protects the cell against toxic levels of ionized calcium and maintains its electrochemical gradient. Moreover, calbindins facilitate the diffusion of the calcium across the cell to the basolateral membrane. Calbindins are present in calcium-transporting tissues such as the intestine and kidney, and their concentration correlates with the magnitude of calcium transport. At the basolateral membrane, plasma membrane calcium ATPase (PMCA), which binds calcium more tightly than the calbindins, pumps calcium out of the cell. In addition, but to a lesser degree, calcium may be pumped out of the cell in exchange for sodium by the Na^+/Ca^{2+} exchanger.

Intestines

Calcium absorption varies by location in the gastrointestinal tract. The stomach does not absorb calcium, but it facilitates the absorption of calcium by solubilizing the mineral in acid. The rate of calcium absorption is greatest at the duodenum and falls along the small intestine. Even so, more calcium is absorbed at the jejunum because its transit time is longer than that of the duodenum. The colon is capable of absorbing calcium, but enclosure of calcium within stool prevents significant absorption.

Calcium absorption may be active across the cell or passive between cells. Active absorption is very efficient, but the magnitude of calcium transported plateaus since it is transporter dependent. The efficiency of passive calcium absorption is much less than that of active absorption, but it plays a greater role in high dietary calcium absorption since the fraction of calcium absorbed is maintained. Thus, active calcium transport is most important at lower dietary calcium intakes, and passive calcium transport is the major route of calcium absorption at higher calcium intakes (Fig. 15-5).

Calcium absorption varies both acutely and chronically according to the dose or intake of calcium and other dietary factors. The effect of acute and chronic intake will be discussed below in the section on physiological regulation. Several other dietary factors may affect calcium absorption. Soluble fiber and phosphate may inhibit calcium absorption by binding it within the intestinal lumen. Certain sugars may enhance calcium absorption acutely.

On a molecular level, the mechanism for active intestinal calcium absorption is believed to be very similar to that at the distal tubule except for the absence of

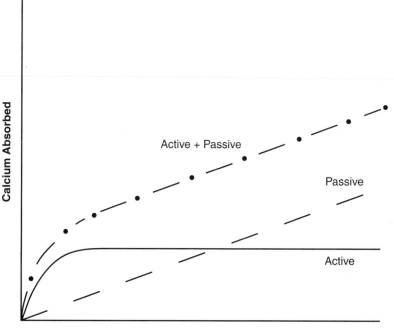

Fig. 15-5 Relative contributions of active and passive absorption in the intestine. At low doses, most of the calcium is absorbed by the active process (solid line). As the dose of calcium increases, active but not passive transport (dashed line) of calcium plateaus. At large doses of calcium, the main component of total calcium absorbed (dash-dot line) derives from passive absorption.

calbindin-D_{28K}. As the rate-limiting step, calcium crosses the luminal membrane via epithelial calcium channels (ECaC1 < ECaC2) along a favorable electrochemical gradient. Cytoplasmic calbindin-D_{9K} binds the free calcium and facilitates its diffusion across the cell. At that site, PMCA pumps calcium out of the cell. A small amount of calcium also may exit the cell via the Na^+/Ca^{2+} exchanger.

REGULATION OF CALCIUM HOMEOSTASIS

Serum calcium is regulated by hormonal control, the calcium sensor, and both physiological and physicochemical mechanisms.

Hormonal Regulation

Three hormones directly regulate calcium metabolism—parathyroid hormone (PTH), 1,25-dihydroxyvitamin D (1,25-$(OH)_2$ D), and calcitonin. In humans, however, calcitonin does not seem to play a major role. Other hormones, local factors or cytokines, which are not involved in the regulation of serum calcium concentration, also affect calcium metabolism.

Parathyroid Hormone

Parathyroid hormone is produced by the parathyroid glands, which are generally located posterior to the thyroid glands. Usually, there are four glands, each approximately the size of a pea, but there may be as few as two glands or up to eight glands in 5% of the population. Parathyroid hormone is derived from a prohormone. First, pre-pro-PTH is made within the cell. The 112-amino acid chain is then cleaved to pro-PTH. The final 84-amino acid polypeptide product is derived from cleavage of a signal peptide. Parathyroid hormone is not stored in the cell but is excreted soon after synthesis. Once in the blood, PTH is rapidly cleaved to other fragments with varying activities. The serum half-life of intact PTH is therefore <5 minutes. Thus, regulation of serum PTH is targeted on its synthesis rather than its release or degradation. Secreted PTH binds its G protein–associated receptor, the PTH/PTHrP receptor or type I PTH receptor, at the cell surface of target tissue cells. The receptor may transduce the signal along different pathways. In one pathway, signal transduction occurs through G_s, with resulting activation of adenylate cyclase, production of cytoplasmic cyclic adenosine monophosphate (cAMP), and activation of protein kinase A. Another pathway through G_q may activate phospholipase C and protein kinase C and may release intracellular ionized calcium stores.

Production of PTH is regulated by several factors, and its main action in adults is to raise serum calcium. The most important regulator of PTH is the ionized calcium concentration. As ionized calcium rises in the blood, serum PTH is directly and increasingly suppressed. Moreover, a feedback loop further protects against hypercalcemia. Parathyroid hormone stimulates production of 1,25-$(OH)_2$ D, which then, in a feedback loop, directly inhibits PTH synthesis. In contrast, hypocalcemia potently stimulates PTH synthesis. A rising concentration of phosphate in the blood raises serum PTH directly and also indirectly by binding calcium.

Parathyroid hormone acts on several organ systems to raise serum calcium and lower serum phosphate (Table 15-1). The hormone mobilizes calcium from the bone by enhancing bone resorption more than bone formation. It decreases urinary calcium losses by augmenting renal calcium reabsorption. Indirectly, PTH increases intestinal calcium absorption by augmenting production of 1,25-$(OH)_2$ D. Serum phosphate tends to fall with increasing serum PTH primarily as a result of increasing renal phosphate wasting.

1,25-Dihydroxyvitamin D

The active form of vitamin D, 1,25-$(OH)_2$ D, is produced by a complicated pathway involving the skin, liver, and kidneys (Fig. 15-6). First, 7-dehydrocholesterol in the skin is converted to previtamin D_3 by ultraviolet light, and this product is converted to vitamin D_3 by isomerization. This process is directly impaired in the elderly. At northern latitudes in the winter, the lack of sufficient ultraviolet light prevents adequate synthesis of vitamin D. In patients with highly pigmented skin, a greater duration of exposure to ultraviolet light is required for adequate vitamin D production because melanin also absorbs these wavelengths. Vitamin D_3 is transported in the blood by vitamin D-binding protein (VDBP) to the liver, where it is

Table 15-1 Effect and Regulation of Calciotropic Hormones

Hormone	Bone resorption	Bone formation	Renal Ca reabsorption	Intestinal Ca absorption	Stimulating factors	Inhibiting factors
PTH	↑↑	↑	↑	—	$\downarrow$Ca, $\uparrow$P, $\downarrow$ 1,25-(OH)$_2$ D	$\uparrow$Ca, 1,25-(OH)$_2$ D
1,25-(OH)$_2$ D	↑	↑, —, ↓	↑[a]	↑	$\downarrow$P, $\uparrow$PTH	$\uparrow$P, $\downarrow$PTH
Calcitonin	↓	—	↑[b]	↑, ↓	$\uparrow$Ca	$\downarrow$Ca

[a]If vitamin D deficient.

[b]At pharmacological doses.

Ca, calcium; 1,25-(OH)$_2$ D, 1,25-dihydroxyvitamin D; P, phosphate; PTH, parathyroid hormone.

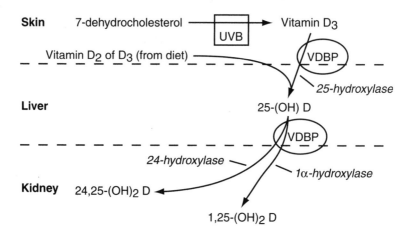

Fig. 15-6 Pathway for synthesis of 1,25-dihydroxyvitamin D (1,25-(OH)$_2$ D). In the skin, 7-dehydrocholesterol is converted by ultraviolet B (UVB) irradiation and isomerization into vitamin D$_3$. Vitamin D$_3$ is then transported to the liver by vitamin D-binding protein (VDBP) and is hydroxylated by 25-hydroxylase. Vitamin D$_2$ or D$_3$ may also be absorbed from the diet and transported to the liver in the portal circulation. Then 25-(OH)D is transported by VDBP to the kidney, where it may be converted to the active compound by 1α-hydroxylase or started on the catabolic pathway by 24-hydroxylase.

25-hydroxylated. Vitamin D$_2$ (plant sources) and vitamin D$_3$ (animal sources) may also reach the liver after dietary ingestion via the portal circulation. 25-Hydroxyvitamin D (25-(OH)D) is then transported to the kidney by VDBP. Most of the 25-(OH)D is shunted to the first step of the degradation pathway by 24-hydroxylase (CYP24) into 24,25-dihydroxyvitamin D at the level of the kidney and all over the body. A small amount of 25-(OH) D is converted to the active hormone, 1,25-(OH)$_2$ D, by the 1-alpha-hydroxylase (or CYP1α) in a tightly regulated process almost exclusively at the kidney. Secreted 1,25-(OH)$_2$ D is believed to cross the cell membrane of target tissue cells and to bind the ligand-binding domain of the vitamin D receptor (VDR). With its heterodimeric partner, a retinoid-X receptor, and accessory coactivators, the VDR complex up-regulates or down-regulates transcription of various genes after binding vitamin D response elements within the promoter region of those genes by the DNA-binding domain of VDR.

Several factors affect vitamin D synthesis. Hypophosphatemia and high serum PTH stimulate production of the active hormone, and other opposite conditions suppress it. In addition, the active hormone not only feeds back to inhibit its own production (suppresses PTH and the 1-alpha-hydroxylase), but also enhances its own degradation by up-regulating transcription of 24-hydroxylase.

Similar to PTH, 1,25-(OH)$_2$ D raises serum calcium, but it also raises serum phosphate (Table 15-1). Its primary action is to increase intestinal calcium absorption, but it also increases bone resorption. Renal calcium reabsorption is increased by 1,25-(OH)$_2$ in vitamin D–deficient animals. However, additional increases in the hormone do not boost renal calcium reabsorption further. Although 1,25-(OH)$_2$ D directly increases intestinal phosphate absorption and renal phosphate reabsorption to a modest degree, its main effect on serum phosphate is probably better explained by its direct suppression of PTH secretion.

Calcitonin

The role of calcitonin in humans is unclear, but in fish the hormone plays an important role in calcium metabolism (Table 15-1). The 32-amino acid polypeptide is derived from the C cells of the thyroid glands. Secretion of calcitonin is stimulated by hypercalcemia and gastrin. Since gastrin release is also increased by calcium, calcitonin has been postulated to prevent postprandial hypercalcemia. Binding of calcitonin to its receptor on the surface of osteoclasts generates the hormone's main action to decrease bone resorption. In humans, calcitonin seems to play a minor role in calcium metabolism. Calcitonin insufficiency (postthyroidectomy) or excess (medullary thyroid carcinoma) has been shown to have no effect on bone mineral density. However, pharmacological doses of calcitonin effectively decrease bone turnover in humans, and parenteral or intranasal formulations are approved to treat osteoporosis, hypercalcemia, and Paget's disease of the bone, a disease characterized by high bone turnover, bone pain, and bone deformities. At pharmacological doses in humans, calcitonin may also increase renal calcium excretion.

Other Hormones and Local Factors

Several other hormones and local factors may affect calcium metabolism. We will discuss these individually.

Estradiol. Estradiol acts in several ways to improve calcium retention, but it is not believed to regulate serum calcium directly. It prevents bone resorption, increases renal calcium reabsorption, and augments intestinal calcium absorption. After menopause, rapid bone loss occurs transiently for 3–7 years, and then the rate of bone loss returns to baseline. For this reason, investigators have postulated that estrogen acts on a mechanosensor in the bone. In this model, estrogen deficiency desensitizes the mechanosensor strain set point so that higher levels of strain are required for sensation. As a result, bone is lost until the resulting greater strain reaches a new set point. Late after menopause, the commonly observed secondary hyperparathyroidism may also be due to the lack of estrogen. This likely represents physiological compensation for impaired intestinal calcium absorption and renal calcium conservation. However, the long-term cost is bone loss.

Testosterone and Dihydrotestosterone. The role of testosterone and dihydrotestosterone is not as clear. Although androgen deficiency results in rapid bone loss similar to that produced by estrogen deficiency, and although this bone loss is reversed by treatment with testosterone, new evidence has suggested that the majority of this effect is due to simultaneous loss of estradiol, which is formed from secreted testosterone. Men with a mutation in the aromatase enzyme, which is necessary to convert testosterone to estradiol, have very low bone mass despite normal testosterone concentrations. Similarly, men with inactivating mutations in the estrogen receptor alpha gene have low bone mass. On the other hand, it is difficult to directly test the effect of testosterone administration because it may be converted at the level of the bone to estradiol by aromatase. However, a role for testosterone has been identified in the bone to increase the width of certain bones over time by adding to the outer surface of the bone, which provides a mechanical advantage in the bones of men.

Glucocorticoids. Glucocorticoids are known to have several effects on calcium homeostasis, but serum calcium is not affected due to compensatory changes. In the short term, high doses increase renal calcium loss by reducing renal calcium reabsorption. Intestinal calcium absorption is decreased by steroids via a vitamin D–independent action. The combined effects on the kidney and the intestine may cause compensatory secondary hyperparathyroidism in some patients. However, the main effect of glucocorticoids is on the bone. These hormones increase bone resorption, decrease bone formation, and cause apoptosis of osteoblasts and osteocytes. Of these mechanisms, the last two appear to be most important. When a patient is treated with glucocorticoids, rapid bone loss occurs within the first 6 months, and then bone loss continues at a slower rate.

Growth Hormone and Thyroid Hormone. The actions of growth hormone and thyroid hormone are not as well characterized as those discussed above. Growth hormone increases both bone resorption and bone formation, but greater stimulation of bone formation generally leads to gain in bone mass. Patients with growth hormone deficiency have low bone mass, and their bone mineral density rises with growth hormone treatment. In contrast, acromegalic patients who have excessive secretion patterns of growth hormone tend to have low bone mass, probably because of concomitant changes caused by the pituitary tumor such as hypogonadism. Insulin-like growth factor-I (IGF-I) is believed to be an important osteoblastic growth factor. Thyroid hormone increases bone reabsorption and bone loss. The resulting higher ionized calcium suppresses PTH, 1,25-$(OH)_2$ D, and intestinal calcium absorption. Modest hypercalcemia may occur in 10%–20% of patients with Graves' disease (see Chapter 13).

Local Factors. Several local factors may affect the bone and calcium homeostasis. Interleukin (IL)-1, IL-6, tumor necrosis factor (TNF), OPG, RANK-L and other factors are involved in osteoclastogenesis. After menopause, up-regulated cytokines such as IL-1, IL-6, and TNFα promote differentiation within the osteoclast cell line. In addition to a larger pool of preosteoclasts, bone reabsorption is further driven by up-regulation of RANK and diminished secretion of OPG. By secreting cytokines, malignant cells within the bone may also promote osteoclastic bone resorption and hypercalcemia.

Parathyroid hormone–related peptide (PTHrP) may also affect calcium metabolism. It is a paracrine factor that is widely expressed in tissues, and is believed to play many important physiological roles including arborization of the lacteal system in the breast and maintenance of smooth muscle tone in blood vessels and multiple organs. In the bone, it plays a critical role in embryogenesis to prevent premature ossification of the forming bone. In malignant states, PTHrP may be so overexpressed that it is measurable in the blood and acts similarly to PTH as an endocrine hormone. The first 13 amino acids of PTHrP are almost identical to those of PTH (Fig. 15-7), but there is no homology in the remainder of the 141-amino acid structure. Interestingly, PTHrP exerts its hormonal action via the PTH/PTHrP

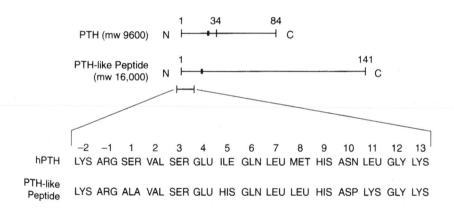

Fig. 15-7 Comparison of the structure of native human parathyroid hormone (PTH) with that of PTH-related protein (1 to 141). The striking homology in the first 13 amino acids allows both peptides to bind the type I PTH receptor, despite limited further homology. (From Stewart AF and Broadus AE: In: *Advances in Endocrinology and Metabolism*, Vol. 1, EL Mazzaferri, RS Bar, and RA Kreisberg, eds., Mosby, St. Louis, p. 7, 1990.)

receptor and similarly increases bone resorption. Thus, hypercalcemia may result from malignancies that overexpress PTHrP.

Regulation by the Calcium-Sensing Receptor

The seminal discovery that calcium may be directly sensed by a receptor was made only in the past decade. For many years, it had been noted that dispersed parathyroid cells exhibited a set point so that peak PTH secretion fell by 50% at a given ionized calcium level. Ed Brown and colleagues finally cloned the calcium-sensing receptor (CaSR) in 1993. Subsequently, it was shown that inactivating mutations caused hypercalcemic disorders (familial hypocalciuric hypercalcemia, neonatal severe hyperparathyroidism) and activating mutations caused hypocalcemia (autosomal dominant hypoparathyroidism).

The CaSR is located in the parathyroid glands, C cells of the thyroid, kidney, intestine, and focal areas of the brain. It may also be present in bone. At the level of the parathyroid gland, a rise in serum calcium activates the CaSR and results in suppression of PTH secretion. On the other hand, hypocalcemia results in higher serum PTH since less inhibition is provided by the CaSR. As a further balance against hypercalcemia, the CaSR in the C cells of the thyroid are set up exactly in reverse. The CaSR activation results in calcitonin secretion, which lowers serum calcium, and lack of CaSR activation reduces calcitonin release. Although the CaSRs are diffusely localized within nephrons, their highest expression and likely their main action appear to be at the ascending limb of Henle. As serum calcium rises beyond the set point, reabsorption of calcium is suppressed by renal CaSR and urinary calcium excretion is thereby amplified. One may speculate about the existence of a similar process in the intestine that accounts, in part, for the immediate adaptation of intestinal calcium absorption with varying loads of calcium, as described in the next section. Perhaps, the CaSR may also play a role in observed physiological control mechanisms in the bone that seem to involve a sensation of calcium. For example, the osteoclast is directly inhibited by high calcium concentrations produced by bone resorption. Thus, a CaSR may act as a short feedback to avoid hypercalcemia. Some investigators have found evidence of the CaSR in the bone or bone marrow, but others have not. The role of the CaSR in the brain is not intuitively obvious, but it is interesting to remember that that there are multiple central nervous system symptoms of hypercalcemia, to be described in the section below on hypercalcemia.

The above discussion of CaSR focuses on calcium, but the reader should understand that the CaSR would perhaps be better named a *polycation-sensing receptor*. It is known that the sensor binds gadolinium and neomycin more avidly than calcium. Magnesium also binds the receptor, but not as well as calcium. Several clinical observations may be explained as potential physiological consequences of this observation. First, hypermagnesemia often accompanies hypercalcemia in patients who have inactivating mutations of the CaSR, and hypomagnesemia and hypocalcemia arise in patients with activating mutations. Second, in patients without CaSR mutations, either high serum calcium or magnesium induces renal wasting of both calcium and magnesium. Finally, magnesium excess decreases secretion of PTH.

PHYSIOLOGICAL REGULATION

At the organ level of the three important calcium transporting tissues, adaptation allows correction of serum calcium to baseline.

At the kidney, filtered calcium is almost completely reabsorbed when blood calcium is low. As blood calcium rises, increasingly activated calcium sensors decrease renal calcium reabsorption. At a certain threshold, excreted calcium rises geometrically with small increments in blood calcium. Serum PTH affects the curve. Lack of the hormone shifts the curve to the left so that hypercalciuria occurs at lower concentrations of serum calcium. In contrast, with high serum PTH, higher serum calcium is required for each level of urinary calcium excretion.

The small intestine demonstrates two levels of control, immediate and long-term. It is well known that the fraction of calcium absorbed will differ according to the quantity given. At very small amounts, such as 20 mg, 80%–100% is absorbed. With larger amounts, such as 100 and 500 mg, less is absorbed—40%–60% and 20%–40%, respectively. One explanation is that the active calcium absorption plateaus at relatively low intakes of calcium and that higher intakes rely increasingly more on inefficient passive absorption (Fig. 15-5). Another possibility is that calcium sensors play a role. The CaSR has been found in the small intestine, and there may be others as yet unidentified. With long-term dietary changes in the intake of calcium, adaptation is believed to be regulated by changes in calciotropic hormones. For example, poor calcium intake will lead to lower blood calcium and, in turn, to higher serum PTH and 1,25-$(OH)_2$ D, which then boosts intestinal calcium absorption. The opposite occurs when dietary calcium intake is excessive.

Since 99% of the body's calcium is stored in the bone, the skeleton plays a major role in maintaining calcium homeostasis. At steady state, the amount of calcium entering the bone (bone formation) equals the amount exiting (bone resorption). When blood calcium is low, higher serum PTH and 1,25-(OH)$_2$ D result in net bone loss (bone resorption exceeds bone formation). When blood calcium is high, lower serum PTH and 1,25-(OH)$_2$ D produces less bone resorption, and net bone gain occurs until the bone is replenished. There also is cellular evidence that osteoclasts are inhibited by high local calcium concentrations, suggesting that calcium sensors may provide a short feedback loop within the bone.

Physicochemical Effect

At very high levels of blood calcium or phosphate, *metastatic calcification* (deposition of calcium phosphate) occurs in the soft tissues. The location of the involved tissues varies. With hypercalcemia, metastatic calcification occurs in lung, conjunctiva, lining of the stomach, and/or endothelium of arteries. The distribution is different in the setting of hyperphosphatemia. It may occur in cerebral basal ganglia, lens, or dermis. Either hypercalcemia or hyperphosphatemia may calcify the kidneys or periarticular tissues.

Integrated Response to Calcium Stressors

Hypercalcemic Challenge

The body is well protected against hypercalcemic challenges. When dietary calcium suddenly increases, a smaller fraction of each dose is absorbed immediately. If this adjustment is not sufficient, ionized calcium will rise and, via the CaSR, will suppress serum PTH and, in turn, 1,25-(OH)$_2$ D (Fig. 15-8). Moreover, calcitonin secretion will be stimulated by activation of calcium sensors within the C cells of the

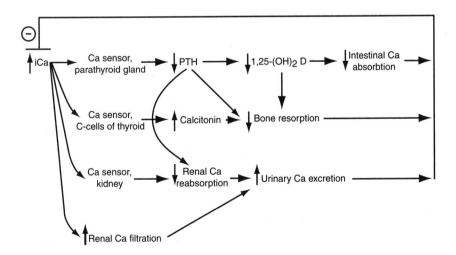

Fig. 15-8 Integrated response against hypercalcemia. Ca, calcium; 1,25-(OH)$_2$ D, 1,25-dihydroxyvitamin D; PTH, parathyroid hormone.

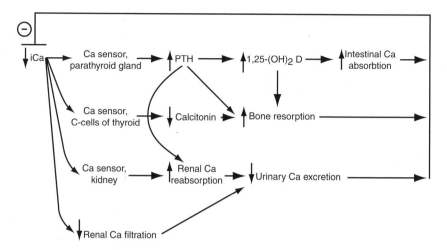

Fig. 15-9   Integrated response against hypocalcemia. Ca, calcium; 1,25-$(OH)_2$ D, 1,25-dihydroxyvitamin D; PTH, parathyroid hormone.

thyroid. These hormonal changes correct serum calcium by reducing intestinal calcium absorption, bone resorption, and renal calcium reabsorption. The CaSR further corrects hypercalcemia by augmenting urinary calcium excretion. Hypercalcemia may also occur due to excessive renal calcium reabsorption or bone resorption. Again, the response of the calciotropic hormones will restore calcium homeostasis. Thus, a hypercalcemic challenge from only one organ system (intestine, kidney, or bone) cannot generate sustained hypercalcemia. Since the kidney plays the largest role in calcium balance, some element of reduced renal calcium excretion is usually present in hypercalcemic patients.

Hypocalcemic Challenge

Hypocalcemic challenges from a single organ system are also easily rectified. The most common challenge is inadequate intake of calcium. A greater fraction of the dietary calcium will be absorbed, but if this adjustment is inadequate, hypocalcemia will be sensed by the CaSR, stimulating PTH secretion (Fig. 15-9). Serum 1,25-$(OH)_2$ D will rise, and serum calcitonin will be suppressed. Serum calcium is then corrected by enhanced intestinal calcium absorption, bone resorption, and renal calcium reabsorption. The diminished activation of the renal CaSR will enhance renal calcium reabsorption further. A similar pathway protects against hypocalcemia mediated by decreased skeleton calcium mobilization or increased renal calcium losses. Hypocalcemia results if organs in the calcium homeostasis triangle are unable to compensate fully for the challenge.

DISORDERS OF CALCIUM METABOLISM

Hypercalcemia

A variety of clinical associations, symptoms, and signs may accompany hypercalcemia (Table 15-2), but there is no specific finding. The severity of symptoms is

Table 15-2 Symptoms of Hypercalcemia by Organ System

Organ or system	Symptom
Nervous system	Fatigue, lethargy, coma, depression, psychosis, reduced concentration
Musculoskeletal system	Weakness, pain in bone or joints, fracture
Gastrointestinal system	Polydipsia, anorexia, nausea, emesis, weight loss, constipation, abdominal pain
Kidney	Polyuria, nocturia, hematuria,[a] dysuria[a]

[a]Kidney stones require long-standing disease.

related to the rapidity with which hypercalcemia developed. For example, a normal volunteer infused with calcium would become lethargic or even comatose once serum calcium exceeded 14 mg/dl. In contrast, subjects with hypercalcemia that has developed due to a slow-growing parathyroid carcinoma may present with minimal changes in mental status even when calcium exceeds 19 mg/dl.

Hypercalcemia is commonly classified in terms of the three key organ systems involved (Table 15-3). Although numerous causes of hypercalcemia are listed, this chapter will focus on the two most common ones: primary hyperparathyroidism and hypercalcemia of malignancy. Other uncommon causes of hypercalcemia, explaining the remaining 10% of cases, will be briefly discussed.

Mechanisms of Hypercalcemia

Primary Hyperparathyroidism. Excess secretion of PTH affects the three corners of the calcium homeostasis triangle. Parathyroid hormone directly increases bone resorption and renal calcium reabsorption and indirectly augments intestinal calcium absorption. Despite increased renal calcium reabsorption, most patients with primary hyperparathyroidism (PHPT) have elevated urinary calcium due to the increased filtered load of calcium.

Most commonly, PHPT results from a single adenoma, but in 10%–20% of cases, it may be due to adenoma or hyperplasia in multiple glands. Approximately 30%–50% of patients with hyperplasia have familial disease (multiple endocrine

Table 15-3 Mechanisms of Hypercalcemia

General source	Mechanism	Cause
Increased calcium input	↑ Bone resorption	Hyperparathyroidism, malignancy, granulomatous disorders, immobilization, hyperthyroidism, intoxication with vitamin A or D
	↑ Intestinal calcium absorption	Hyperparathyroidism, granulomatous disorders, intoxication with vitamin D, milk-alkali syndrome
Decreased calcium removal	↓ Renal calcium excretion	Renal failure, volume depletion, hyperparathyroidism, familial hypocalciuric hypercalcemia, milk-alkali syndrome, thiazides, lithium
	↓ Bone formation	Immobilization

neoplasia type 1 and type 2a, familial hyperparathyroidism jaw-tumor syndrome, and familial isolated hyperparathyroidism). Rare causes of PHPT include carcinoma of a parathyroid gland (<1%) or true ectopic secretion by another tumor (<10 cases reported).

Patients with hyperparathyroidism may present clinically with any of the listed symptoms of hypercalcemia (Table 15-2); however, about 80% have mild elevations in serum calcium and symptoms that are absent or too vague to be firmly attributed to their disease, such as fatigue or constipation. Prior to widespread screening of serum calcium, PHPT was a rare very symptomatic disease presenting with kidney stones, bone pain or fracture, abdominal pain (associated with pancreatitis and peptic ulcer disease), and psychiatric manifestations (depression, pyschosis, lethargy). Today the most common complication is nephrolithiasis, which occurs in 20% of patients. A pathognomonic but uncommon (<2%) finding on X-ray is subperiosteal bone resorption. More commonly, bone mineral density, a measure of the bone mass, is low, especially at the cortical bone of the arm. Very rarely and only with severe disease, patients may present with proximal muscle wasting, hyperreflexia, and tongue fasciculations. The possibility of parathyroid carcinoma should be considered in patients with severe hypercalcemia (>14 mg/dl), high elevations in serum PTH (10× normal), significant anemia, severe symptoms (especially involving two or more organs), and rapid progression (even these cases tend to progress over years rather than weeks, however).

Primary hyperparathyroidism may be confused with other hypercalcemic conditions. *Familial hypocalciuric hypercalcemia* (FHH), which is caused by inactivating mutations of the calcium sensor, is a benign disease characterized by high serum calcium, high-normal PTH, and low urinary calcium. It is important to differentiate FHH from PHPT because, unlike PHPT, which may be cured by removal of the offending gland, hypercalcemia will persist in patients with FHH unless the patients are rendered hypocalcemic by removal of all four parathyroid glands. Moreover, FHH is not associated with complications of PHPT such as kidney stones and osteoporosis. There are several clues that suggest FHH over PHPT. In FHH, hypercalcemia occurs at birth and is inherited in an autosomal dominant pattern. Serum PTH is usually high normal, but it may be up to twice the upper limit of normal. A key difference between the two hypercalcemic disorders is that urine calcium is low (<100 mg/day) in most patients with FHH, while it is high (>200 mg/day) in most patients with PHPT. Similar to the pattern found with calcium, patients with FHH tend to have high serum and low urine magnesium. In contrast, patients with PHPT tend to have hypomagnesemia. A final unusual diagnosis to consider is Jansen's disease, which is caused by activating mutations to the PTH/PTHrP receptor. Patients have congenital findings consistent with PHPT plus a metaphyseal chondrodysplasia since PTH plays a role in bone modeling. However, serum PTH is appropriately suppressed.

Hypercalcemia of Malignancy. The three main mechanisms of hypercalcemia of malignancy (PTHrP, local factors, and $1,25$-$(OH)_2$ D) are discussed below. The most common causes include lung or breast carcinoma (60%), renal cell carcinoma (10%–15%), head and neck squamous cell carcinoma (10%), and myeloma or lymphoma (10%). An alternative way to consider hypercalcemia of malignancy is the percentage of specific tumors that causes hypercalcemia—breast cancer 20%–40%, lung cancer 5%–15%, myeloma >30%, lymphoma 2%.

1. *Mediated by PTHrP.* Hypercalcemia induced by PTHrP, also known as *humoral hypercalcemia of malignancy* (HHM), is the most common cause of hypercalcemia of malignancy (80% of cases). Fuller Albright was the first to recognize HHM in 1941. The patient, who had a single bone metastasis from renal carcinoma, presented with hypercalcemia and hypophosphatemia. With his typical foresight, Albright hypothesized that the tumor released a factor similar to PTH, since it was unlikely that a single bone metastasis would cause enough local destruction to explain the hypercalcemia. Several lines of evidence have since proven him correct. Parathyroid hormone–related peptide is expressed only in neoplasms associated with HHM. Local implantation of such tumors in animal models results in hypercalcemia before metastases occur, and this is reversed by antibodies to PTHrP. Finally, the majority of patients with HHM have elevated PTHrP. It is believed that the other patients with HHM may have a biologically active fragment of PTHrP that is not immunologically detectable. Tumors that cause HHM include squamous carcinomas, carcinomas of the breast, kidney, and bladder, and some lymphomas.

   Although the actions of PTHrP are similar to those of PTH, there are also several differences between them. Since PTHrP binds to the same receptor as PTH, the similarities are expected. Similar to patients with PHPT, those with HHM have elevated serum calcium, low-normal to low serum phosphate, and elevated urinary calcium, phosphate, and cAMP. Parathyroid hormone raises serum 1,25-$(OH)_2$ D by stimulating renal 1-α-hydroxylase. Likewise, serum 1,25-$(OH)_2$ D rises in normal subjects infused with PTHrP. However, serum 1,25-$(OH)_2$ D in patients with HHM is generally low for unclear reasons. Patients with HHM also tend to have more hypercalciuria than those with PHPT. Patients with PHPT have increased bone resorption and formation, whereas those with HHM have increased bone resorption but decreased formation. Some have hypothesized that these difference in action between PTH and PTHrP may be explained by the existence of other unknown receptors with specific affinity for one factor or the other. Alternatively, tumors may secrete additional factors that affect calcium homeostasis.

2. *Local osteolytic hypercalcemia (LOH).* In about 20% of patients with hypercalcemia of malignancy, elaboration of paracrine factors by the tumor in the skeleton causes hypercalcemia. These factors, which include IL-1, IL-6, TNF, prostaglandin E_2 (PGE_2), and RANKL, drive osteoclastogenic bone resorption and bone loss. If these are coupled with impaired renal calcium excretion, hypercalcemia may result. Tumors believed to cause LOH include multiple myeloma, breast carcinoma, and lymphoma.

3. *Vitamin D–mediated hypercalcemia.* Rarely, lymphomas contain 1α-hydroxylase and may produce 1,25-$(OH)_2$ D in large enough quantities to cause hypercalcemia. This hormone drives intestinal calcium absorption and bone resorption. The body compensates by increasing renal calcium excretion. With renal impairment or severe overload, hypercalcemia may result.

Other Causes of Hypercalcemia. Several uncommon causes of hypercalcemia are listed in Table 15-3. Vitamin D–mediated hypercalcemia, either by excess intake or by excess production, is the most common of these causes. The hypercalcemia is mediated by increased intestinal calcium absorption and, to a lesser degree, increased bone resorption. Hypercalcemia occurs only after the kidney's excretory reserve is overwhelmed. Vitamin D, ingested from the diet or supplements or produced in skin, is converted to 25-(OH)D. However, the renal 1-α-hydroxylase is normally so tightly regulated that 1,25-(OH)$_2$ D should not increase in hypercalcemic patients despite excess substrate. Since 25-(OH)D is much less potent at the vitamin D receptor, hypercalcemia requires very high concentrations in 25-(OH)D–driven disease. This occurs only after a pharmacologically excess intake of 25-(OH)D or vitamin D, which is readily converted to 25-(OH)D in the liver. In contrast, 1,25-(OH)$_2$ D may be produced in granulomatous tissue in multiple disorders (most commonly sarcoidosis and tuberculosis) or prescribed by a physician. In these cases, serum 25-(OH)D is low or normal but 1,25-(OH)$_2$ D is elevated. Patients with hypercalcemia from granulomatous disease tend to have other symptoms related to their disease to suggest the diagnosis.

There are several other reported causes of hypercalcemia. Vitamin A intoxication and hyperthyroidism increase bone resorption; hypercalcemia occurs when renal calcium excretion is overwhelmed. Alkali, thiazides, and lithium decrease renal calcium excretion. When these are coupled with excess calcium intake or bone resorption, hypercalcemia ensues. Long-term therapy with lithium is also associated with primary hyperparathyroidism. The milk-alkali syndrome results from a huge intake of calcium and alkali (often from milk and antacids). Over time, the high delivery of calcium and alkali to the kidney additionally causes renal insufficiency. After several weeks of immobilization, from spinal cord injury for example, hypercalcemia may gradually develop. Immobilized subjects have increased bone resorption (early) and decreased bone formation. Again, hypercalcemia develops only when the renal excretion of calcium is overwhelmed. In addition, it has been noted that hypercalcemia of immobilization is more common in conditions with very high bone turnover, such as childhood (active bone modeling and remodeling) or metabolic bone diseases such as Paget's disease (osteitis deformans).

Clinical Assessment of Hypercalcemia

The history and physical exam may be very helpful in diagnosing the cause of hypercalcemia. Long-standing asymptomatic disease is more consistent with primary hyperparathyroidism, and recent onset of hypercalcemia with multiple symptoms implicates hypercalcemia of malignancy. For rarer causes of hypercalcemia, a history of calcium intake, medications (particularly calcium, antacids, vitamins A or D, diuretics, and lithium), bed rest, a family history of hypercalcemia, or symptoms/ physical findings consistent with hyperthyroidism or granulomatous disease may pinpoint specific diagnoses.

The clinician must confirm that the patient is hypercalcemic. Ionized calcium is the clinically relevant form of the mineral because it is directly involved in cellular processes and sensing mechanisms. Thus, one may confirm hypercalcemia by measuring ionized calcium. One may also measure total calcium and serum albumin, the primary protein binder of calcium. Thus, if albumin is low, ionized calcium will be proportionately higher, and if it is elevated, ionized calcium will be proportionately lower. To determine if total calcium is truly elevated, the *adjusted serum calcium* is derived by adding 0.8 mg/dl of calcium for every 1 g/liter decrement in serum albumin. If albumin is elevated, one should instead subtract 0.8 mg/dl of calcium from total calcium for every 1 g/liter increment in serum albumin. Acidosis shifts protein-bound calcium to the ionized phase, whereas alkalosis shifts calcium to the protein-bound fraction. Thus, the adjusted serum calcium may not be accurate in patients with moderate acidosis or alkalosis.

Once hypercalcemia is established, serum PTH (normal range on a commonly used assay, 10–65 pg/ml) should be measured (Fig. 15-10). If it is inappropriately elevated for hypercalcemia (>50 pg/ml), the diagnosis of primary hyperparathyroidism is clear. However, one should at least consider FHH, which represents about 0.5% of patients with presumed primary hyperparathyroidism. In addition to its clinical characteristics, FHH commonly presents with elevated serum calcium, inappropriately normal to modestly elevated PTH (up to two times the upper limit of normal), hypermagnesemia (50%), and low urinary calcium and magnesium. If PTH is 30–50 pg/ml, the patient likely has primary hyperparathyroidism, but the diagnosis is unclear and further testing or long-term follow-up will establish the diagnosis. If PTH is suppressed (<20 pg/ml), hyperparathyroidism is ruled out and other diagnoses should be considered.

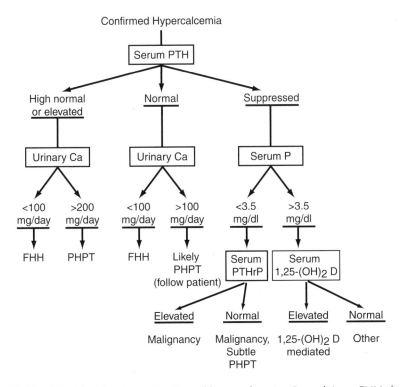

Fig. 15-10 Algorithm for the evaluation of hypercalcemia. Ca, calcium; FHH, familial hypocalciuric hypercalcemia; P, phosphate; 1,25-(OH)$_2$ D, 1,25-dihydroxyvitamin D; PHPT, primary hyperparathyroidism; PTHrP, parathyroid hormone–related peptide.

Serum phosphate is very useful to differentiate the cause of hypercalcemia in patients with suppressed serum PTH. If serum phosphate is low (<3.5 mg/dl), one should consider PTHrP-mediated hypercalcemia. Serum PTHPrP will be elevated in the majority of patients. However, the available assays for PTHrP are not as powerful as those for PTH. Therefore, some patients with presumed PTHrP-mediated hypercalcemia have normal serum PTHrP. Thus, while an elevated serum PTHrP secures the diagnosis of PTHrP-mediated hypercalcemia, a normal measurement does not rule it out. Nevertheless, these patients almost always have known cancer or symptoms suggestive of cancer. On the other hand, if serum phosphate is elevated, several other causes of hypercalcemia must be considered. The history and physical examination, as discussed above, are especially useful in this setting to facilitate diagnosis. If one of these diagnoses seems possible, several tests may be useful to confirm the diagnosis, including measurement of vitamin A, $1,25\text{-}(OH)_2$ D, 25-(OH)D, and thyroid-stimulating hormone. Since it is the third most common cause of hypercalcemia, serum $1,25\text{-}(OH)_2$ D should be measured in unclear cases. An elevated serum $1,25\text{-}(OH)_2$ D may indicate extrarenal production of the hormone or direct exogenous intake.

Treatment of hypercalcemia depends on its severity. For mild and asymptomatic elevations of serum calcium, only increased fluid intake is important. For symptomatic disease, the patient should be volume repleted by intravenous saline to enhance renal calcium excretion. Parenteral bisphosphonates and/or calcitonin are additional options for severely symptomatic disease. Rarely, hemodialysis may be needed.

Hypocalcemia

Hypocalcemia, which results when calcium exiting the system exceeds calcium input, may result in several clinical manifestations. The most common symptoms relate to neuromuscular excitability. The first symptoms, paresthesias, occur particularly in perioral and acral (hands and feet) areas. Numbness and tingling also occur with hyperventilation in normal individuals because ionized calcium falls when respiratory alkalosis shifts free calcium to the albumin-bound fraction. Muscular cramping usually starts at the hands and feet (carpopedal spasm) but may occur elsewhere, and the tetany may generalize across the body with severe hypocalcemia. Smooth muscle spasm may lead to abdominal pain, bronchospasm, and laryngospasm. The last two conditions result in wheezing and shortness of breath. Severe hypocalcemia may also result in confusion or even psychosis. Conduction abnormalities in neurons may result in seizures. Hypocalcemia also may affect heart function, resulting in palpitations due to arrhythmia or shortness of breath and other symptoms of congestive heart failure.

Physical findings of neuromuscular excitability may be induced at the bedside in patients with hypocalcemia. *Chvostek's sign* is a contraction of the side of the face that occurs after tapping on the facial nerve 1–2 cm anterior to the external auditory meatus. When the test is floridly positive, the facial muscles on the same side contract at the eye, nose, and lips. Chvostek's sign is not pathognomonic for hypocalcemia. In fact, 10% of normal subjects may show a mild response, such as twitching of the lips toward the side of the tapping. Unlike hypocalcemic patients, their response is usually fatiguable; repeated tapping progressively extinguishes the response. *Trousseau's sign*, a carpal spasm elicited by inflating a blood pressure cuff on the arm 20 mm above systolic blood pressure for 3 minutes, is more specific for hypocalcemia. Adduction of the thumb, extension of the phalanges, and flexion of the metacarpophalangeal joints and the wrist characterize the spasm.

Mechanisms of Hypocalcemia
The following section groups the causes of hypocalcemia by the main mechanisms— lack of PTH effect, lack of vitamin D effect, and binding or redistribution of calcium (Table 15-4).

Lack of Parathyroid Hormone Effect. The most common cause in this category is postsurgical hypoparathyroidism, in which parathyroid glands are removed usually due to aggressive resection of thyroid cancer with acceptable tumor-free margins. Autoimmune destruction is the second most common cause of lack of PTH effect. Although these patients may have isolated hypoparathyroidism, they often have multiple accompanying abnormalities such as moniliasis, hypoadrenalism, diabetes mellitus, Hashimoto's thyroiditis, hypogonadism, autoimmune hepatitis, and vitiligo. A mutation in the autoimmune regulator gene has been shown to cause polyglandular autoimmune syndrome type I. The parathyroid glands may be congenitally absent in the 22q11.2 deletion syndrome (DiGeorge, velocardiofacial, and conotruncal anomaly face syndromes). The causative microdeletions of chromosome 22q also result in varying degrees of facial dysmorphism, hypothyroidism, cardiovascular defects, and immunosuppression. Infiltration of the parathyroid glands with iron

Table 15-4 Mechanisms of Hypocalcemia

General source	Mechanism	Specific examples
Lack of parathyroid hormone (PTH) action	Decreased PTH production	Lack of gland formation, surgical removal, autoimmune destruction, infiltration, activating mutation of the calcium-sensing receptor, hypomagnesemia
	Resistance to PTH	Pseudohypoparathyroidism, hypomagnesemia
Lack of vitamin D action	↓ Vitamin D	Poor sunlight or intake
	↓ 25-(OH)D	Anticonvulsants, diarrhea, nephrotic syndrome, mutation in 25-hydroxylase
	↓ 1,25-(OH)$_2$ D	Renal failure, mutation in 1-α-hydroxylase, certain phosphate-wasting disorders
	Resistance	Mutation in the vitamin D receptor
Binding/redistribution	Hyperphosphatemia, citrate	Renal failure, rhabdomyolysis, tumor lysis syndrome, blood transfusions
	Alkalosis	Hyperventilation, bicarbonate administration
	Bone hunger	Post-parathyroidectomy, post-cure of hyperthyroidism, diffuse osteoblastic metastases

(hemachromatosis), copper (Wilson's disease), amyloid, or tumor may decrease their function. A recently discovered familial cause of hypoparathyroidism involves activating mutations of the CaSR. In these patients, serum PTH is suppressed even when serum calcium is relatively low. Hypomagnesemia may cause resistance to and, with increasing severity, decreased secretion of PTH. Finally, patients may have resistance to PTH. Due to the unexpected elevation of serum PTH in these patients with serum mineral abnormalities of hypoparathyroidism (hypocalcemia, hyperphosphatemia), this condition has been termed *pseudohypoparathyroidism*. Parathyroid hormone acts through a G protein–coupled receptor. Therefore, it is not surprising that one cause of pseudohypoparathyroidism is an inactivating mutation of the α_s subunit of that G protein.

Hypoparathyroidism may be recognized by laboratory abnormalities and additional clinical findings. In addition to its function of raising serum calcium, PTH lowers serum phosphorus by enhancing renal phosphorus excretion. Therefore, patients with lack of PTH effect have both hypocalcemia and hyperphosphatemia. The hyperphosphatemia may result in additional clinical manifestations due to soft tissue calcium deposition. Patients with hypoparathyroidism may have cataracts, calcification of the basal ganglia in the brain, and even moderate to severe cerebral calcification and mental retardation. Basal ganglia calcification may result in Parkinson's disease. As described by Fuller Albright, patients with certain types of pseudohypoparathyroidism have other clinical manifestations including short stature, obesity, and shortened metacarpals and metatarsals. The ring finger is the most commonly involved digit. When only the fourth metacarpal is shortened, the patient's fist may demonstrate the *knuckle, knuckle, dimple, knuckle* sign. Patients with pseudopseudohypoparathyroidism have these physical findings without abnormalities of serum calcium, phosphate, or PTH. Interestingly, the distribution of pseudohypoparathyroidism and pseudopseudohypoparathyroidism in families implicates imprinting. Pseudohypoparathyroidism results when the mutation is inherited from the mother, and pseudopseudohypoparathyroidism occurs when it is inherited from the father.

Lack of Vitamin D Effect. There are several causes of decreased vitamin D effect.

1. *Inadequate nutrition/sunlight.* Vitamin D_3 is present in only a few foods, including vitamin D–fortified milk (100 IU/cup), cod liver oil, and fatty fish such as salmon. Thus, it is difficult to achieve sufficient intake (600–800 IU/day per various experts; 400 IU per the current recommended daily allowance) from dietary sources alone. Vitamin D may also be produced in the skin with adequate ultraviolet light exposure. However, several conditions make it much more difficult to achieve sufficient vitamin D production by the skin. In Boston and at more northern latitudes, ultraviolet light exposure is insufficient to allow vitamin D production in the winter. Moreover, the production of vitamin D by skin requires greater ultraviolet light exposure with increasing skin pigmentation. Finally, the ability of the skin of aged subjects to produce vitamin D is impaired.
2. *Impaired production.* Inadequate 25-hydroxylation of vitamin D may rarely occur due to a lack of the enzyme or severe liver disease. Impaired pro-

duction of 1,25-$(OH)_2$ D rarely occurs due to lack of renal 1α-hydroxylase or certain phosphate-wasting disorders. More commonly, it occurs with renal failure. In patients with hypocalcemia from hypoparathyroidism, 1,25-$(OH)_2$ D production is suppressed due to low serum PTH and high serum phosphate.

3. *Catabolism or loss.* This is a more common cause of vitamin D insufficiency that is not widely recognized. Drugs, such as phenobarbital and phenytoin, increase catabolism of 25-(OH)D. Vitamin D substrates may be lost in the stool or urine. Fat malabsorption impairs the absorption of vitamin D, a fat-soluble vitamin. Vitamin D is normally secreted into the bile and reabsorbed in the ileum. Diarrhea may interrupt this enterohepatic loop by increasing bowel motility. In proteinuric states, vitamin D insufficiency results because VDBP with its bound vitamin D and 25-(OH)D is expelled into the urine.

4. *Resistance.* The key effects of vitamin D are mediated via its nuclear receptor, the VDR. Not surprisingly, mutations in VDR result in a resistant state characterized by low serum calcium and phosphate but elevated serum PTH and 1,25-$(OH)_2$ D.

Binding/Redistribution of Calcium. A common cause of hypocalcemia is binding. Phosphate binds calcium well, and if the level of the calcium-phosphate product is high enough, the salt will precipitate in soft tissues. Elevated serum phosphate may occur due to reduced urinary excretion in renal failure or by a shift out of other compartments, such as massive lysis of tumor cells or necrosis of muscle with tissue injury (rhabdomyolysis). Citrate, a preservative in blood to prevent clotting by binding calcium, may cause symptomatic hypocalcemia by lowering ionized calcium even though total calcium remains in the normal range. Similarly, alkalosis may reduce ionized calcium, but not total calcium, by increasing binding to albumin. In patients with pancreatitis, one postulated cause of hypocalcemia is calcium saponification of the fatty acids within the partially digested fatty organ. Finally, calcium may shift into bone. After surgical cure of primary hyperparathyroidism, for example, repair of the demineralized bone may be so active that hypocalcemia persists for weeks despite aggressive treatment with calcium and vitamin D.

Clinical Assessment of the Patient with Hypocalcemia

Clinical Assessment of Hypocalcemia. Although the diagnosis of hypocalcemia is usually made by measuring serum total calcium, one must rule out pseudohypocalcemia caused by hypoalbuminemia. Moreover, patients with alkalosis and normal serum total calcium may have true symptoms of hypocalcemia due to the shift of ionized calcium to the protein-bound fraction. Therefore, it is sometimes necessary to measure ionized calcium directly.

Once true hypocalcemia is confirmed, the history and physical exam may provide helpful clues to its underlying cause. A specific congenital defect may be suspected by onset of hypocalcemic symptoms early in life and by a positive family history. Vitamin D deficiency should be suspected based on poor intake/sunlight exposure, diarrhea, old age, hyperpigmented skin, or residence in northern latitudes.

A history of surgery at the neck, cancer, or recent trauma should be sought. A history and physical findings suggestive of other endocrinopathies or complications from hemachromatosis, Wilson's disease, or amyloidosis should be hunted.

Laboratory results must then confirm the suspected cause of hypocalcemia (Fig. 15-11). If specific diagnoses are uncovered by the history and physical exam, they may be directly tested. Otherwise, the most clinically useful test, in patients with normal renal function and no obvious contributing redistribution, is serum phosphate. Elevated serum phosphate (>3.5 mg/dl) indicates a diminished PTH effect, and serum PTH should be measured. If PTH is low, deficient production or severe hypomagnesemia is likely. If, on the other hand, PTH is highly elevated, resistance should be suspected. In contrast, low serum phosphate (<3.5 mg/dl) implicates diminished action of vitamin D. In compensation, PTH should be elevated. Vitamin D insufficiency is confirmed by low serum 25-(OH)D. If serum 25-(OH)D is normal, then serum 1,25-(OH)$_2$ D should be measured. If 1,25-(OH)$_2$ D is low, deficiency of 1α-hydroxylase is established, but if 1,25-(OH)$_2$ D is high, resistance to vitamin D is diagnosed.

The level of serum calcium and phosphate determines the best treatment, but all patients should be carefully followed long-term for optimal management. Patients with low serum phosphate should be treated with calcium and vitamin D. Serum calcium <7.0 mg/dl in a newly diagnosed patient and moderately symptomatic hypocalcemia should also be treated with intravenous calcium. Intake of dairy products, excellent sources of calcium and phosphate, should be encouraged in these patients. Moreover, calcium supplements should be ingested apart from meals to avoid binding phosphate. In contrast, dairy products should be avoided and calcium supplements given with all meals to control serum phosphate in patients with hy-

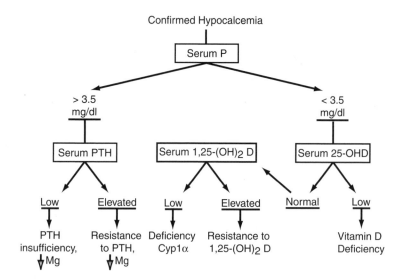

Fig. 15-11   Algorithm for the evaluation of hypocalcemia. Mg, magnesium; 1,25-(OH)$_2$ D, 1,25-dihydroxyvitamin D; 25-OHD, 25-hydroxyvitamin D; PTH, parathyroid hormone.

perphosphatemia. Intravenous calcium should be given with extreme caution, if at all, in patients with hyperphosphatemia due to the risk of soft tissue deposition of calcium phosphate, a condition that in its extreme form may require endotracheal intubation. It is also important to remember that PTH augments renal calcium reabsorption. Therefore, treated patients with hypoparathyroidism are at risk for hypercalciuria and kidney stones.

SUGGESTED READING

Bastepe M and Juppner H: Pseudohypoparathyroidism. New insights into an old disease. Endocrinol Metab Clin North Am 29:569–589, 2000.

Bell NH: Vitamin D-endocrine system. J Clin Invest 76:1–6, 1985.

Bouillon R, Van Cromphaut S, and Carmeliet G: Intestinal calcium absorption: molecular vitamin D mediated mechanisms. J Cell Biochem 88:332–339, 2003.

Breslau NA, McGuire J, Zerwekh JE, Frenkel E, and Pak CYC: Hypercalcemia associated with increased serum 1,25-dihydroxyvitamin D in three patients with lymphoma. Ann Intern Med 100:1–7, 1984.

Breslau NA and Zerwekh JE: Pharmacology of vitamin D preparations. In: *Vitamin D*, D Feldman, F Glorieux, and W Pike, eds., Academic Press, San Diego, CA, pp. 607–618, 1997.

Bronner F: Mechanisms of intestinal calcium absorption. J Cell Biochem 88:387–393, 2003.

Brown EM, Pollak M, and Hebert SC: Physiology and cell biology update: sensing of extracellular Ca^{2+} by parathyroid and kidney cells: cloning and characterization of an extracellular Ca^{2+}-sensing receptor. Am J Kidney Dis 25:506–513, 1995.

Ducy P, Schinke T, and Karsenty G: The osteoblast: a sophisticated fibroblast under central surveillance. Science 289:1501–1504, 2000.

Frost HM: Tetracycline-based histological analysis of bone remodeling. Calcif Tissue Res 3:211–237, 1969.

Garcia-Ocaña A, Vasavada RC, Takane K, De Miguel F, and Stewart AF: Parathyroid hormone–related protein. In: *Disorders of Bone and Mineral Metabolism*, FJ Coe and MJ Favus, eds., Lippincott Williams & Wilkins, Philadelphia, pp. 129–156, 2002.

Heaney RP, Weaver CM, and Fitzsimmons ML: Influence of calcium load on absorption fraction. J Bone Miner Res 5:1135–1138, 1990.

Heller HJ and Pak CYC: Primary hyperparathyroidism. In: *Disorders of Bone and Mineral Metabolism*, FJ Coe and MJ Favus, eds., Lippincott Williams & Wilkins, Philadelphia, pp. 516–534, 2002.

Manolagas SC: Birth and death of bone cells: basic regulatory mechanisms and implications for the pathogenesis and treatment of osteoporosis. Endocr Rev 21:115–137, 2000.

Marx SJ: Hyperparathyroid and hypoparathyroid disorders. N Engl J Med 343:1863–1875, 2000.

Naveh-Many T and Silver J: Regulation of parathyroid hormone gene expression by hypocalcemia, hypercalcemia and vitamin D in the rat. J Clin Invest 86:1313–1319, 1990.

Nordin BE and Peacock M: Role of kidney in regulation of plasma-calcium. Lancet 2: 1280–1283, 1969.

Parfitt AM: Osteonal and hemi-osteonal remodeling: the spatial and temporal framework for signal traffic in adult human bone. J Cell Biochem 55:273–286, 1994.

Perez E and Sullivan KE: Chromosome 22q11.2 deletion syndrome (DiGeorge and velocardiofacial syndromes). Curr Opin Pediatr 14:678–683, 2002.

Pollak M, Brown EM, Chou Y-HC, Herbert SC, Marx SJ, Steinman B, Levi T, Seidman CE, and Seidman JG: Mutations in the human Ca^{2+}-sensing receptor gene cause familial hypocalciuric hypercalcemia and neonatal severe hyperparathyroidism. Cell 75:1297–1303, 1993.

Pollak MR, Brown EM, Estep HL, McLaine PN, Kilfor U, Park J, Hebert SC, Seidman CE, and Seidman JG: Autosomal dominant hypocalcemia caused by a Ca^{2+}-sensing receptor gene mutation. Nat Genet 8:303–307, 1994

Riggs BL, Khosla S, and Melton LJ III: Sex steroids and the construction and conservation of the adult skeleton. Endocr Rev 23:279–302, 2002.

Silverberg SJ, Gartenberg F, Jacobs TP, Shane E, Siris E, Staron RB, and Bilezikian JP: Longitudinal measurements of bone density and biochemical indices in untreated primary hyperparathyroidism. J Clin Endocrinol Metab 80:723–728, 1995.

Stewart AF, Adler M, Byers CM, Segre GV, and Broadus AE: Calcium homeostasis in immobilization: an example of resorptive hypercalcuria. N Engl J Med 306:1136–1140, 1982.

Sutton ALM and MacDonald PN: Vitamin D: more than a "bone-a-fide" hormone." Mol Endocrinol 17:777–791, 2003.

Teitelbaum SL: Bone resorption by osteoclasts. Science 289:1504–1508, 2000.

Thomas MK and Demay MB: Vitamin D deficiency and disorders of vitamin D metabolism. Endocrinol Metab Clin North Am 29:611–627, 2000.

16

Glucose, Lipid, and Protein Metabolism

ROBERT L. DOBBINS
MICHAEL A. COWLEY
DANIEL W. FOSTER

The maintenance of life requires a constant supply of substrates that are used to generate energy and preserve the structure of cells and tissues. The process in principle is quite simple, yet the individual metabolic pathways and the regulation of fluxes through the pathways can be complex. Energy is derived when fuel substrates are oxidized to carbon dioxide and water in the presence of oxygen, generating adenosine triphosphate (ATP). A portion of the ingested foodstuff is also utilized, either directly or after transformation into other substrates, to repair and replace cell membranes, structural proteins, and organelles. The remainder is stored as potential energy in the form of glycogen or fat. Under normal circumstances, each individual remains in a near-steady state where weight and appearance are stable over prolonged periods. Despite the outward evidence of stability, fuel metabolism changes dramatically several times a day during alternating periods of feeding and fasting. An anabolic phase begins with food ingestion and lasts for several hours. Energy storage occurs during this period when caloric intake exceeds caloric demands. The catabolic phase usually begins 4 to 6 hours after a meal and lasts until the person eats once again. During this phase, utilization shifts from exogenous to endogenous fuels, a change heralded by the mobilization of substrate stored in liver, muscle, and adipose tissue.

Both anabolic and catabolic phases exhibit characteristic hormonal profiles and biochemical processes (Fig. 16-1). In the anabolic phase that follows ingestion of a mixed meal, substrate flux is directed from the intestine through the liver to storage and utilization sites. Glucose, triglyceride, and amino acid concentrations increase in plasma, whereas those of fatty acids, ketones, (acetoacetic and β-hydroxybutyric acids), and glycerol decrease. Both glycogen and protein synthesis begin in liver and muscle, while fatty acid synthesis and triglyceride esterification are stimulated in hepatocytes and adipose tissue. In the catabolic phase, the biochemical activities are reversed and the flux of fuel is from storage depots to liver and other utilization sites. Glucose and triglyceride levels in plasma decrease, whereas those of certain amino acids, long-chain fatty acids, and ketones increase. Glycogen breaks

State	Hormones	Fuel Source	Process
Anabolism	↓ Insulin	Diet	Glycogen Synthesis
	↑ Glucagon		Triglyceride Synthesis
	↑ GI Peptides		Protein Synthesis
	↑ Leptin		
Catabolism	↓ Insulin	Glycogen	Glycogenolysis
	↑ Glucagon	Fat Depots	Gluconeogenesis
	↑ Catecholamines	Muscle Protein	Lipolysis
			Ketogenesis
			Proteolysis

Fig. 16-1   Fuel metabolism in anabolic and catabolic phases. GI, gastrointestinal.

down, glycolysis is impaired, gluconeogenesis is activated (first in liver and then in kidney), lipogenesis and triglyceride synthesis cease, and lipolysis in the adipocyte increases manyfold. Fatty acid oxidation is enhanced in most tissues, and ketone body formation is initiated in the liver. Finally, proteolysis is activated in muscle to supply amino acids as substrate for gluconeogenesis.

When food is readily available and nutritionally balanced, the only risk during the anabolic phase in the normal individual is that it may be entered too frequently or maintained so long that obesity results. Ingesting particular foods causes symptoms in individuals having inborn errors of metabolism such as fructose intolerance or intestinal lactase deficiency, but these anabolic-phase diseases are rare. In contrast, famine is potentially dangerous, for without adaptations, death or permanent brain injury may occur because of a fall in plasma glucose concentrations to levels insufficient for sustaining central nervous system (CNS) function. Indeed, prevention of hypoglycemia is the primary factor driving acute metabolic changes that accompany the catabolic phase.

Two changes maintain plasma glucose within the normal range in the absence of food (Fig. 16-2). First, the liver produces glucose by initially breaking down hepatic glycogen stores, but additional substrate is subsequently formed via gluconeogenesis, a process in which amino acids, lactate, pyruvate, and glycerol are converted to glucose. The second major change is the conversion of tissues other than the CNS to a lipid economy. Most tissues utilize long-chain nonesterified fatty acids (NEFA) directly, but the CNS cannot and must rely on an alternative substrate derived from fatty acids. Approximately 25% of NEFA are taken up by the liver for conversion to ketone bodies that are efficiently oxidized by the CNS as a substitute for glucose or fatty acids. In the presence of ketone bodies at concentrations usually found after several days of fasting, the brain functions normally despite levels of glucose low enough to result in loss of consciousness or convulsions in the absence of glucose. This protective mechanism is not available during the first few hours of a fast because ketogenesis is not activated immediately by the absence of food. However, the shift to utilization of lipid substrates is critical for surviving a prolonged fast because the liver, even at maximal glucose production, cannot provide adequate carbohydrate to sustain all tissues in the body simultaneously. Al-

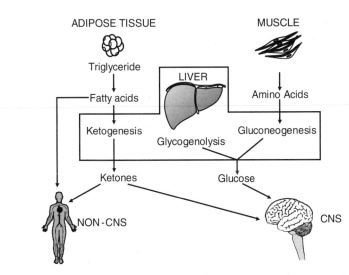

Fig. 16-2 The catabolic sequence. The liver becomes a net glucose producer first via glycogen breakdown and subsequently by gluconeogenesis. Glucose is preserved for use by the central nervous system (CNS) because other tissues (non-CNS) preferentially utilize long-chain fatty acids and their derivative products, the ketone bodies. Ketones can also be used by the brain. Glycerol (released by lipolysis), pyruvate-lactate (from muscle glycogen), and amino acids (released by proteolysis) are additional substrates for gluconeogenesis (not shown in the figure). See text for details.

though adaptation to famine is often overlooked under our current social conditions, these mechanisms allow human beings to survive for long periods in the total absence of food, provided that water is available. For example, most nonobese adults have 100,000–150,000 kcal stored as fat that, at a utilization rate of 2000 kcal/day, would ensure survival for 50–75 days.

COMPLEX HORMONAL COORDINATION OF SUBSTRATE METABOLISM

Historically, the endocrine pancreas has been considered the penultimate regulatory organ of fuel metabolism. It releases two key hormones, insulin and glucagon, that serve as the primary acute mediators of anabolism and catabolism, respectively. While there is no complementary hormone for insulin, the catabolic functions of glucagon are shared with epinephrine, norepinephrine, cortisol, and growth hormone. Glucagon and its partners are often designated *counterregulatory hormones*, indicating that they oppose insulin action and protect the body against hypoglycemia. Because counterregulatory responses are critical for maintaining an adequate supply of glucose, it is not surprising that the release of these hormones is regulated in part by the CNS. In fact, most norepinephrine reaches target sites via local release from sympathetic nerve endings rather than through the bloodstream. Akin to norepinephrine, local tissue production of cortisol may have greater importance in some tissues than plasma cortisol levels. Data suggest that the autocrine conversion of cortisone to cortisol by 11β-hydroxysteroid dehydrogenase-1 in adipose tissue, specifically omental fat, may play an important role in metabolic abnormalities associated with central adiposity.

More recent findings indicate that the pancreas is only one of many endocrine organs that interact with the CNS to regulate the complex activities associated with maintaining substrate balance. The brain integrates signals released by classical endocrine organs, adipose tissue, and the gastrointestinal tract to coordinate feeding behavior, physical activity, energy expenditure, and substrate selection. Newly recognized endocrine factors may very well hold the key to understanding how food intake and energy expenditure are balanced. A rapid rise in the plasma concentrations of insulin and the stomach hormone ghrelin, which stimulates a feeling of hunger, are among the first endocrine changes that occur around the time of a meal. First-phase or cephalic-phase insulin secretion occurs just prior to food ingestion, priming the body to rapidly absorb the sugars that are released by the actions of salivary amylase. Second-phase insulin secretion is stimulated primarily by plasma glucose, which rises as food is digested and absorbed. Ghrelin levels are suppressed by meals but not by gastric loading, diminishing the signals of hunger to the brain. Meal-related signals like cholecystokinin (CCK) and glucagon-like peptide 1 (GLP-1) that are able to inhibit feeding acutely are also released transiently in response to food ingestion. Both GLP-1 and CCK have been implicated in conditioned taste aversion, and CCK seems to synergize with neural signals of gastric distention, suggesting that CCK and GLP-1 serve as short-term satiety signals. In addition, GLP-1 plays important roles in promoting insulin secretion and is the subject of several experimental strategies to combat diabetes. Within 15 minutes of food ingestion the levels of peptide tyrosine tyrosine 3-36 (PYY 3-36) begin to rise, and remain stay elevated for up to 6 hours. Fatty meals stimulate PYY 3-36 secretion more than carbohydrate-rich meals. The secretion of pancreatic polypeptide (PP) is also enhanced throughout all stages of digestion. Both PYY 3-36 and PP potently inhibit food intake, may be part of the signal that reduces feeding during the absorptive period following a meal, and by actions in the hypothalamus activate the sympathetic nervous system to *burn* some of the ingested energy. Interestingly GLP-1 and PYY 3-36 are secreted from the same cell type found in the mucosal epithelium of the small and large intestines, but the regulation of their secretion appears to be divergent. Perhaps the most important meal-related peptide is leptin, secreted by adipocytes. Leptin concentrations quickly increase following a meal, functioning as an acute satiety signal. Leptin levels are also increased in proportion to adiposity, providing a chronic signal that limits weight gain. Human obesity seems to be associated with resistance to leptin action.

Many meal-related satiety factors appear to act directly on the CNS through both the arcuate nucleus of the hypothalamus and the area postrema. Within the arcuate nucleus, signals such as PYY 3-36 or leptin can increase the activity of anorexigenic pro-opiomelanocortin (POMC) neurons by two mechanisms: depolarization through a nonspecific cation channel and reduced inhibition by orexigenic neuropeptide-Y/γ-aminobutyric acid neurons. In addition, many of these factors play important roles locally in the gut, coordinating the complex sequence of physiological changes necessary to turn ingested food into stored nutrients.

REGULATION OF INSULIN AND GLUCAGON SECRETION

The release of insulin and glucagon is coordinated so that substrate flow in the alternating anabolic-catabolic phases maintains plasma glucose levels within a narrow range. Concentrations of the two hormones ordinarily vary reciprocally so that glucagon concentrations in plasma fall as insulin levels rise and vice versa. Although many other nutrients and hormones can modulate islet cell responses, the plasma glucose concentration is the principal regulatory signal to both glucagon-producing α-cells and the insulin-producing β-cells. Insulin release becomes negligible at low plasma glucose concentrations below 80 mg/dl (4.5 mmol/liter). Above this level, insulin secretion increases nearly in proportion to the plasma glucose level. On the other hand, low plasma glucose concentrations <50 mg/dl (2.8 mmol/liter) enhance glucagon secretion, which declines as the plasma glucose level rises until maximal suppression is achieved at a value of 150 mg/dl (8.3 mmol/liter). Insulin and glucagon, per se, also have important roles in modifying glucose sensing in pancreatic islets. Tissue-specific inactivation of the insulin receptor in mouse β-cells results in a selective loss of glucose-stimulated insulin secretion and progressive impairment of glucose tolerance. While insulin stimulates it own synthesis and release from the β-cell, it simultaneously acts to impair glucagon release from the α-cell. However, this inhibitory effect of insulin on the α-cell can be overridden by hypoglycemia so that glucagon levels rise to protect against hypoglycemia when plasma glucose is lowered with an exogenous insulin injection. Glucagon augments insulin secretion in the presence of permissive glucose concentrations. The mechanism likely involves binding to the glucagon receptor on the β-cell, with subsequent enhancement of insulin release, possibly mediated by cyclic adenosine monophosphate (cyclic AMP).

Current understanding of the intracellular mechanisms regulating glucose-stimulated insulin release remains incomplete. Well established is the fact that glucose enters the β cell via the high-K_m glucose transporter, GLUT-2, and is rapidly phosphorylated by glucokinase. Subsequent glucose metabolism generates ATP, which closes the ATP-sensitive K^+ (K_{ATP}) channel (also designated Kir6.2) and depolarizes the β-cell membrane. Membrane depolarization activates L-type voltage-dependent calcium channels that increase intracellular calcium and stimulate translocation of preformed insulin secretory granules to the cell surface. The importance of the potassium-dependent mechanism of insulin secretion is supported by the therapeutic efficacy of sulfonylurea agents that interact with the K_{ATP} channel to inhibit K^+ efflux from the cell. What has only recently come to light is that potassium-independent mechanisms can also be employed by the β-cell. It is now clear that glucose can still stimulate insulin secretion when regulation of the K_{ATP} channel is prevented by exposure of cells to high concentrations of K^+ and the pharmacological agent diazoxide. The separate potassium-independent mechanism of stimulus–secretion coupling provides an alternate site for modulation of insulin secretion.

While glucose appears to be the preeminent regulatory signal coordinating islet hormone traffic, other fuels and hormones may gain importance under certain conditions. For example, in the fasted state, circulating ketones or fatty acids play a key role in pancreatic β-cell function. Fatty acids synergize with glucose to maintain a low but critically important output of insulin, and they are also essential for the robust secretion of insulin following termination of the fast. Amino acids that would be ingested as components of a high-protein meal stimulate both glucagon and insulin release. This is the only common physiological circumstance in which plasma insulin and glucagon concentrations rise simultaneously. In contrast, insulin increases and glucagon decreases following a pure carbohydrate meal. In addition to the effect of ingested nutrients, the passage of food through the gastrointestinal tract induces hormonal and autonomic nervous system signals that modulate insulin secretion. These incretins include cholecystokinin, secretin, gastrin, gastric inhibitory peptide, glucagon-like polypeptide 1, and acetylcholine. Endogenous incretins, controlled from the gastrointestinal tract, are thought to function in anticipatory fashion, readying the β-cell to release insulin promptly as the products of digestion enter the bloodstream. They also account for the fact that the insulin response to oral glucose is greater than that seen when the same amount of glucose is given intravenously. In contrast to the incretins, somatostatin produced by the pancreatic δ-cell serves as a powerful inhibitor of both insulin and glucagon secretion. It could conceivably act in a paracrine fashion within the islet, but in fact this likely does not occur. Hormone release would cease if α- and β-cells were exposed to the somatostatin levels present in pancreatic venous effluent, so it is believed that somatostatin acts as a true endocrine factor that is released into the systemic circulation. One interpretation is that its central role is to slow intestinal absorption of fat. In animals, blockade of somatostatin action by the infusion of anti-somatostatin antibodies accelerates the appearance of chylomicrons after a meal, suggesting enhanced absorption of triglycerides. As for cortisol, growth hormone, and thyroid hormone, it is believed that they modulate metabolism primarily through extrapancreatic effects.

In stress and exercise, insulin–glucagon interrelationships are altered by adrenergic mechanisms. Epinephrine released from the adrenal medulla and norepinephrine reaching the islets from sympathetic nerve endings block insulin release and stimulate glucagon secretion so that hepatic glucose production rises as much as fivefold over the rate seen after an overnight fast. Epinephrine and norepinephrine act via α_2-adrenergic receptors in the β cell, inhibiting insulin release, whereas in the α-cell their action is mediated by β-adrenergic receptors that cause a rise in cyclic AMP with stimulation of glucagon secretion. Without the sympathetically mediated changes in metabolism, hepatic glucose output would be insufficient to protect against hypoglycemia during strenuous exercise.

MECHANISM OF ACTION OF INSULIN AND GLUCAGON

Despite intensive study over many years, the complex mechanisms of insulin action are still not fully understood. As with other peptide hormones, the initial step involves binding to a specific receptor localized in the plasma membrane. The insulin receptor gene is located on chromosome 19 in humans and encodes for separate α- and β-subunits (molecular weight of 135,000 and 95,000, respectively) that form a β–α–α–β heterotetramer. The hormone-binding site is on the α-subunit, while the β-subunit possesses tyrosine kinase activity. Once insulin is bound, it stimulates autophosphorylation of the receptor and tyrosine phosphorylation of other proteins including insulin receptor substrate proteins (IRS-1 through 4), *Shc*, Gab-1, *Cbl*, and APS. Once phosphorylated, these factors act as signaling molecules for a host of subsequent events. For example, a pair of pathways is required for insulin-stimulated translocation of glucose transporter-4 (GLUT-4) to the cell surface in muscle and adipose tissue. Phosphorylation of IRS proteins causes activation of phosphatidylinositol-3-kinase (PI-3-kinase), which in turn initiates a cascade of phosphorylation events that ultimately turns on protein kinase B (Akt) and/or atypical protein kinase C isoforms. A second pool of insulin receptors phosphorylates the adapter protein APS and the proto-oncogene c-*Cbl*. *Cbl* interacts with *Cbl*-associated protein (CAP) and initiates the PI-3-kinase-independent arm of the signal cascade required for GLUT-4 translocation. Other actions of insulin are triggered after phosphorylation of *Shc* and Gab-1 and the subsequent activation of the proto-oncogene *ras* by exchanging guanosine triphosphate (GTP) for guanosine diphosphate (GDP). *ras*, in turn, activates a related protein, RAF-1, which then activates other kinases, mitogen-activated protein kinase kinase (MAPK-K) and mitogen-activated protein kinase (MAP-K), that promote gene transcription, mitogenesis, and protein synthesis. Thus, insulin action is exerted through a complex series of protein kinase pathways that can be terminated by protein tyrosine phosphatases.

The mechanism of action of glucagon is better understood than that of insulin. It rapidly raises intracellular levels of cyclic AMP. The hormone binds to the glucagon receptor and stimulates adenylate cyclase through a coupling mechanism utilizing a stimulatory guanine nucleotide-binding protein, G_s. An inhibitory guanine nucleotide-binding protein, G_i, also interacts with the system so that the balance between stimulatory and inhibitory subunits determines net activity of the cyclase (see Chapter 3). Cyclic AMP levels in liver rise very rapidly after exposure to glucagon and bind to inactive protein kinase A, thereby freeing the catalytic subunit that initiates phosphorylation of multiple proteins. Some of the effects of glucagon may also be mediated by cyclic AMP–independent events involving changes in intrahepatic calcium stores, but in either case, the net result is phosphorylation of key enzymes, an event that may either activate or inhibit them. For example, hepatic glycogen synthase is inactivated, whereas glycogen phosphorylase is activated, accounting for the fact that glucagon inhibits glycogen synthesis and stimulates glycogen breakdown.

ANABOLIC PATHWAYS

The normal diet contains carbohydrates, lipids, and proteins plus other vitamins and minerals. The absorption of substrates from food requires intraluminal and brush-border enzymes in the intestine to break down the more complex components into constituent sugars, fatty acids, and amino acids that can be concurrently absorbed at varying rates.

Carbohydrate

Starch, sucrose, and lactose are the important carbohydrates in the normal diet. In Western societies about 60% of the daily carbohydrate intake is in the form of starch; 30% is sucrose, a disaccharide composed of glucose and fructose; and 10% is lactose, a disaccharide pairing glucose and galactose. About 20% of the starch is made up of amylose, which consists of straight chains of glucose molecules in $\alpha 1 \rightarrow 4$ linkage. The remainder is amylopectin, which has branching chains that occur about every 25 molecules, the branch point representing an $\alpha 1 \rightarrow 6$ linkage. Digestion of starch begins in the oral cavity with salivary amylase and is continued by the pancreatic version of that enzyme in the intestine. The initial products from the amylose chains are maltotriose and maltose, whereas branched oligosaccharides averaging eight glucose units (called *α-limit dextrins*) are produced from amylopectin. The products of starch digestion, together with dietary lactose and sucrose, are hydrolyzed to single sugars by oligosaccharidases localized in the brush border of the intestinal mucosa. Glucose and galactose are transported across the intestinal membrane by an energy-requiring process after being bound to carrier molecules. The energy required for transport of the two monosaccharides is provided by the sodium transport system. Sodium moves from the lumen into the epithelium down the concentration gradient created as sodium ions are actively pumped from the basilar portion of the cells. The monosaccharides are dragged into the cell along with the reabsorbed sodium ions. Fructose is absorbed by a slightly different process called *facilitated diffusion*. A specific carrier protein is required, but its function is energy and sodium independent. Once inside the intestinal epithelial cell, fructose is phosphorylated and then converted to glucose.

As noted above, the ingestion of a meal is accompanied by anticipatory priming of the pancreas that makes insulin available to control the metabolism of glucose absorbed directly and of glucose produced by interconversion from fructose and galactose. A portion of dietary glucose is oxidized in the postprandial period for energy production, and the remainder is converted to glycogen and fat. In muscle cells, the glucose molecule is phosphorylated and incorporated directly into glycogen via the sequence glucose $\rightarrow$ glucose-6-phosphate (G-6-P) $\rightarrow$ G-1-P $\rightarrow$ uridine diphosphate (UDP)-glucose $\rightarrow$ glycogen. The same reaction sequence occurs in the liver, but a discrete path is equally responsible for repleting hepatic glycogen when a meal is ingested after an overnight fast (Fig. 16-3). For the *indirect pathway*, glucose is first metabolized to lactate and then reconverted via gluconeogenesis into G-6-P to form glycogen. The identity of the tissues responsible for metabolizing glucose to lactate remains unclear. It is likely that nonhepatic tissues (e.g., intestine, adipose tissue, CNS, red blood cells, skin) are partly responsible, but some of the lactate could arise in the liver itself, because the hepatic parenchyma is architecturally divided into zones of predominant glycolysis and predominant gluconeogenesis.

High concentrations of insulin in hepatocytes during a carbohydrate meal inhibit glucose-6-phosphatase, which shuts off the release of glucose from the liver and favors conversion of G-6-P to glycogen. Newly formed glycogen would be quickly broken down if glycogen phosphorylase activity were not suppressed as well. Glucose-induced phosphorylation of this enzyme yields its inactive form, phos-

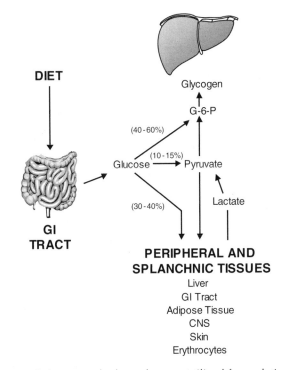

Fig. 16-3 Sources of glucose and other substrates utilized for repleting hepatic glycogen in the postprandial state. Glucose absorbed from the diet enters hepatic glycogen by two pathways. About 50% of glycogen is formed directly from ingested glucose without degradation. The remainder enters indirectly after conversion to lactate in peripheral and splanchnic tissues. A total of 15%–20% of glucose is converted to lactate in subcutaneous adipose tissue, skin, the central nervous system (CNS), and red blood cells. Lactate then returns to the liver and is converted to glucose-6-phosphate (G-6-P) via gluconeogenesis. A similar proportion of lactate arises from intestinal metabolism of either circulating or newly absorbed glucose. Essentially all muscle glycogen is formed by the direct pathway. GI, gastrointestinal.

phorylase *b* and depletes the active form, phosphorylase *a*. Increased insulin concentrations also turn on the insulin-stimulated protein kinase that phosphorylates a specific site of the protein phosphatase 1G complex. This specific phosphatase dephosphorylates glycogen synthase and converts it from an inactive to an active form. The combined effect of inhibition of G-6-P and activation of glycogen synthase accounts for the rapid glycogen repletion that characterizes the postprandial state.

Substantial evidence now supports the view that at physiological concentrations of plasma glucose, such as those seen after a normal meal, a significant fraction of hepatic glycogen arises from an indirect pathway. For many years it was believed that gluconeogenesis was shut down almost immediately after meal ingestion. This turns out not to be true; gluconeogenesis continues unimpaired for several hours after a meal. Indeed, it is likely that some basal rate of gluconeogenesis operates at all times. In humans, gluconeogenic flux has been found to increase earlier in the postprandial state than was once believed. Control of gluconeogenesis is ordinarily thought to be vested in the regulatory glycolytic intermediate fructose-2,6-bisphosphate (F-2,6-P$_2$); high levels of F-2,6-P$_2$ normally inhibit gluconeogenesis (see the discussion of gluconeogenesis below). In isolated hepatocytes, F-2,6-P$_2$ concentration rise rapidly after exposure to glucose, but in intact animals its concentration in the liver does not increase until glycogen stores are repleted. This late rise readily explains continued gluconeogenesis. In contrast, when fructose or sucrose is ingested, F-2,6-P$_2$ rises promptly to levels that should be inhibitory to gluconeogenesis, yet the process continues. This has been termed the *glucose paradox.*

Dietary carbohydrate not utilized for energy production is converted to glycogen first and then to fat. Triglyceride synthesis from carbohydrate takes place primarily in the liver, with lesser *in situ* synthesis occurring in adipose tissue. Thus, most glucose-derived fat is made in the liver and transported via lipoproteins to the adipocyte rather than being formed *de novo* in adipose tissue. The primary substrate is lactate derived from glucose. Pyruvate, which is formed from lactate in the cytosol, then enters the mitochondria and is decarboxylated to acetyl-coenzyme A (CoA) by the pyruvate dehydrogenase complex. Acetyl-CoA condenses with oxaloacetate to form citrate under the influence of citrate synthase. Citrate may proceed through the reactions of the tricarboxylic acid cycle, but a portion exits the mitochondria and is reconverted to acetyl-CoA and oxaloacetate in the cytosol by citrate cleavage enzyme. Acetyl-CoA is converted to malonyl-CoA under the influence of acetyl-CoA carboxylase, and the sequential addition of malonyl-CoA to an anchoring acetyl-CoA, carried out by fatty acid synthase, leads to the formation of palmitic acid. The latter (after conversion to its CoA ester) can then undergo changes such as elongation and desaturation. Importantly, malonyl-CoA, the basic building block of fatty acid chains, serves a regulatory purpose by switching off the enzyme carnitine palmitoyltransferase I (CPT I) and limiting the entry of the newly formed fatty acids into the mitochondria for oxidation. The sequence, in summary, is glucose $\rightarrow$ lactate/pyruvate $\rightarrow$ citrate $\rightarrow$ acetyl-CoA $\rightarrow$ malonyl-CoA $\rightarrow$ palmitate $\rightarrow$ other fatty acids. Once formed, the long-chain fatty acids are esterified to glycerol-3-phosphate, and the newly synthesized triglyceride is incorporated into a very-low-density lipoprotein (VLDL) molecule. Fatty acids are transferred from VLDL into adipocytes after hydrolysis of VLDL-borne triglycerides by endothelial-bound lipoprotein lipase (LPL). Adipose tissue also has the capacity to synthesize long-chain fatty acids *de novo* by the mechanism just described.

The transcriptional regulation of the developing adipocyte has become an area of intense research interest because of the clinical success of thiazolidinediones, a new class of insulin-sensitizing agents that have proven useful in treating type 2 diabetes. These agents are ligands that activate the peroxisome proliferator-activated receptor-gamma (PPARγ), a nuclear transcription factor promoting differentiation of adipocytes. Two separate members of the receptor family, PPARα and PPARδ, are believed to be activated by long-chain fatty acids so that they may serve as cellular *lipid sensors*. Activation of PPARδ favors adipogenesis and lipogenesis in adipose tissue. On the other hand, PPARα increases gene transcription of a number of enzymes responsible for fatty acid oxidation. Much information remains to be discovered regarding the importance of the PPAR family and other adipocyte differentiation factors such as the CCAAT/enhancer binding proteins and sterol regulatory element-binding proteins. These factors are not simply confined to adipose tissue. They are also components of signaling cascades in other insulin-sensitive tissues that are crucial for glucose and lipid metabolism, such as liver, skeletal muscle, and the β-cell.

Fat

Fat absorption is mediated by pancreatic lipase in the duodenum. The enzyme becomes active only after it forms a complex with triglyceride and colipase, a small protein molecule that is formed from its precursor, procolipase, by the action of trypsin. Complexing of lipase with colipase prevents the former's inactivation by intraluminal bile salts whose concentration increases after a meal. Pancreatic lipase splits off long-chain fatty acids from triglyceride, leaving a monoglyceride with the fatty acid in position 2. In the presence of bile salts, fatty acids and the 2-monoglyceride form a soluble complex called a *micelle*. Micelle formation, required because fatty acids and monoglycerides are poorly soluble in water, provides an efficient mechanism for delivering fatty acids through diffusion barriers of the intestinal mucosa to the absorptive surface of the intestinal epithelial cell. Inside the cell, triglycerides are re-formed and packaged into large, round lipoprotein particles called *chylomicrons*, which are rapidly secreted into the lymph to carry exogenous dietary lipids into the circulation. Medium- and short-chain fatty acids are not reesterified to triglycerides, nor are they transported out of the intestinal cell in chylomicrons; rather, they pass directly into the portal vein for transport to the liver as free fatty acids.

Chylomicrons are the largest lipoprotein particles found in the blood; about 90% of their bulk is made up of triglyceride. Clinically they can be separated from VLDLs, the endogenous fat transport molecules formed in the liver, by allowing plasma to stand overnight in the cold. Chylomicrons then separate out as a cream layer at the top of the tube with clear plasma underneath, whereas VLDL remains distributed throughout the plasma volume, giving the appearance of dilute skim milk. Chylomicrons contain a variety of apolipoproteins (apo) including AI, AII, and AIV. They also have a characteristic apo-B that is designated apo-B48. Apolipoprotein-B48 is a truncated form of apo-B100, another protein that is synthesized in liver and packaged within VLDL. Once in the plasma, the chylomicron's apolipoprotein composition changes rapidly; most of the A proteins are replaced by apo-CI, -CII, -CIII, and -E (Fig. 16-4). Apolipoprotein CII is a critical cofactor activating lipoprotein lipase (LPL), thereby ensuring rapid clearance of dietary fat from the plasma. Individuals with a congenital absence of either LPL or apo-CII display a severe hypertriglyceridemia phenotype when eating fat because of difficulty in clearing chylomicrons. Lipoprotein lipase is found on the luminal surface of capillary endothelial cells and acts in a fashion similar to that of pancreatic lipase described above, removing the long-chain fatty acids from positions 1 and 3 and leaving a 2-monoglyceride, which is then hydrolyzed intracellularly. The released fatty acids are transported into cells or bind to albumin in the plasma. Albumin binds over 99% of the fatty acids carried in plasma, so that the free, unbound fatty acid concentration lies in the range of 5–20 nM. The regulation of LPL activity in adipose tissue and skeletal muscle varies according to the nutritional status. In the postprandial period char-

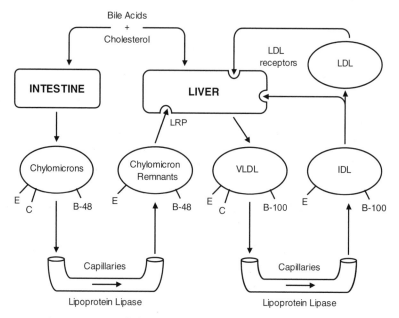

Fig. 16-4 The transport of dietary and endogenous fat. Capital letters stand for apolipoproteins. B-48 and B-100 refer to apolipoprotein B arising in intestine and liver, respectively. Dietary fat is transported to peripheral tissues as chylomicrons that pass to the liver after being stripped of triglyceride through the action of lipoprotein lipase. Uptake in the liver is mediated by a specific low-density lipoprotein (LDL) receptor-related protein (LRP) that interacts with apolipoproteins E. Very-low-density lipoprotein (VLDL) carrying endogenously synthesized fat follows a similar sequence, except that the remnant particle is designated *intermediate-density lipoprotein* (IDL). This can be taken up directly by the liver but is also the precursor for LDL. Both IDL and LDL are taken up by the LDL receptor. (Adapted with permission from Goldstein JL, Kita T, and Brown MS: N Engl J Med 309:289, 1983.)

acterized by elevated insulin and glucose concentrations, fatty acid storage in adipose tissue is favored by increased adipose tissue LPL activity relative to that of skeletal muscle. Increased catecholamines that typify the catabolic stress response accelerate LPL activity in muscle but not in adipose tissue.

In adipose tissue, most of the long-chain fatty acids are reesterified to glycerol derived from glucose (the original glycerol released from the chylomicron passes via plasma to the liver), but in muscle, heart, and other tissues, a significant portion of the fatty acid is oxidized for energy production. Most of the triglyceride in chylomicrons is removed in a single pass through tissues. Only 10%–15% of the original mass remains in the remnant particle that still contains cholesterol and cholesteryl esters that have not been released. The primary apolipoproteins left in the remnant are apo-B48 and apo-E. The remnant particle then passes to the hepatic sinusoids, where it is cleared from the plasma by a specialized receptor called *LDL receptor-related protein* (LRP) that interacts with apo-E after the particles have been bound to heparan sulfate proteoglycans on the microvillous surface of the hepatocytes. The affinity of this receptor for apo-E surpasses the affinity for the other apolipoproteins, and the LRP does not bind LDL.

A similar series of events occurs in the endogenous or hepatic pathway in which free fatty acids derived from diet, lipolysis in adipose tissue stores, or *de novo* synthesis in the liver are reesterified and packaged as VLDL. Lipoprotein lipase, again activated by VLDL-bound apo-CII, removes the majority of triglyceride from VLDL in a single pass through the tissues. The interactions between the many lipoprotein particles of the endogenous pathway are complex. The remnant particle of VLDL, called *intermediate-density lipoprotein* (IDL), exchanges apolipoproteins, cholesterol, and cholesterol esters with high-density lipoprotein (HDL) and is finally converted to low-density lipoprotein (LDL), the major cholesterol-carrying transport protein in the blood. Both IDL and LDL are then cleared from the plasma by the hepatocyte LDL receptor. Identical receptors are present on other tissues of the body, and binding of LDL to these receptors allows entry of cholesterol into cells for membrane synthesis and hormone formation. Partial or complete absence of the LDL receptor leads to familial hypercholesterolemia, a disease characterized by very high serum cholesterol levels and premature atherosclerosis. Low-density lipoprotein itself is innocent in atherogenesis because the delivery of LDL cholesterol to macrophages in plaques down-regulates LDL receptor expression and protects the cells from accumulating LDL cholesterol to form foam cells. Low-density lipoprotein becomes highly atherogenic only after oxidation to minimally modified LDL; the latter binds to a receptor distinct from the LDL receptor. The oxidized LDL receptor is known as the *acetyl LDL* or *scavenger* receptor, and it is not down-regulated by cholesterol excess.

High-density lipoprotein protects against atherosclerosis by removing cholesterol from blood vessels and by preventing the formation of oxidized LDL. High-density lipoprotein functions as an antioxidant opposing the oxidation of LDL. It binds to a potent endogenous antioxidant called *paraoxonase* and serves as a carrier for this molecule that protects against the generation of reactive oxygen species. In addition, HDL plays a key role in reverse cholesterol transport out of tissues (Fig. 16-5). The process begins with lipid-poor apo-AI synthesized by the liver or regenerated from mature HDL particles. Apolipoprotein-AI acquires free cholesterol and phospholipids through an interaction with the ATP-binding cassette transporter A1 (ABCA1) found on the surface of hepatocytes or other lipid-laden cells. The resulting disc-shaped nascent HDL particle can acquire more cholesterol via combined ABCA1 and diffusion pathways. The enzyme lecithen:cholesterol acyl transferase converts free cholesterol to cholesterol esters, forming the mature spherical HDL particle. Cholesterol is directly removed from circulating HDL by the liver and steroidogenic tissues or indirectly transported to the liver after being transferred to LDL by the cholesterol ester transfer protein.

Cholesterol Metabolism

Although cholesterol is not a fuel, a brief discussion of its metabolism is included here because it is intimately involved in triglyceride metabolism and because elevation of plasma cholesterol is a major risk factor in the development of atherosclerosis. Cholesterol in the body arises from two sources: diet and endogenous synthesis.

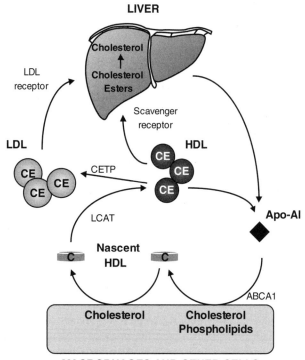

Fig. 16-5 Model depicting reverse cholesterol transport. The process begins with lipid-poor apolipoprotein-AI (Apo-AI) synthesized by the liver or regenerated from mature high-density lipoprotein (HDL) particles. Apo AI acquires free cholesterol and phospholipids through an interaction with the adenosine triphosphate (ATP)-binding cassette transporter A1 (*ABCA1*) found on the surface of lipid-laden macrophages, hepatocytes, or other cells. The resulting disc-shaped nascent HDL particle can acquire more cholesterol via combined *ABCA1* and diffusion pathways. The enzyme lecithen:cholesterol acyl transferase (LCAT) converts free cholesterol to cholesterol esters (CE), forming the mature, spherical HDL particle. Cholesterol is directly removed from circulating HDL by the liver and steroidogenic tissues or indirectly transported to the liver after being transferred to LDL by the cholesterol ester transfer protein (CETP). LDL, low-density lipoprotein.

The latter takes place via a linked series of enzymatic reactions starting from acetyl-CoA. An overview of the sequence is acetyl-CoA → acetoacetyl-CoA → hydroxy-methylglutaryl-CoA (HMG-CoA) → mevalonic acid → isopentenylpyrophosphate → squalene → lanosterol → desmosterol → cholesterol. The rate-limiting step is the conversion of HMG-CoA to mevalonic acid, a reaction catalyzed by the enzyme HMG-CoA reductase. The general rule is that dietary and synthetic sources of cholesterol are reciprocally related: when dietary cholesterol intake is high, cholesterol synthesis is low and vice versa. Another important clinical note is that the intake of saturated fat in the diet is more closely linked to elevated plasma cholesterol levels than is dietary cholesterol. Inhibitors of HMG-CoA reductase are the primary means of treating clinically significant hypercholesterolemia.

The average daily intake of cholesterol in Western diets is 300–500 mg plus 200–400 mg of plant sterols. The cholesterol is mostly esterified because of a high intake of eggs, dairy products, and meat. Esterified cholesterol is hydrolyzed before absorption by a pancreatic cholesteryl esterase that acts in the presence of bile acids. It is presumed that cholesterol is absorbed in the form of mixed micelles made up of bile salts, fatty acids, and phospholipid. The process has limited efficiency; absorption ranges from one-third to two-thirds of the ingested load. By means that are not well understood, cholesterol is transferred from the absorptive micelles to lipoproteins, the two major carriers being chylomicrons and HDL. The former predominates, particularly if the meal contains fat. As discussed earlier, absorbed cholesterol reaches the liver via the production of chylomicron remnants. Cholesterol taken up by the liver can be used for membrane synthesis, formation of bile acids, or export to extrahepatic tissues.

New findings are beginning to shed light on the mechanisms that direct the fate of cholesterol in the liver. The key regulatory components are the steroid regulatory element-binding proteins (SREBPs) and the SREBP cleavage-activating protein (SCAP). When the intracellular cholesterol content rises, SCAP suppresses proteolytic cleavage of SREBPs, thus limiting synthesis of LDL receptors and limiting the activity of HMG-CoA reductase and other enzymes. In this manner, SCAP and the SREBPs serve as the putative cholesterol sensors of the hepatocytes regulating the import of cholesterol as well as the intracellular synthesis of new cholesterol. Two members of the nuclear hormone receptor superfamily regulate the incorporation of cholesterol into bile acids. Activation of liver X-receptor (LXR) isoforms mediates dietary cholesterol–induced expression of 7α-hydroxylase (Cyp7a1), the rate-limiting step of bile acid synthesis, whereas accumulated bile acids activate the farnesoid X-receptor (FXR) and impair Cyp7a1 expression. Finally, dietary cholesterol, like newly synthesized cholesterol, can be repackaged into VLDL molecules in hepatocytes, which are converted to LDL molecules, as described in the previous section. Low-density lipoprotein is the principal means by which cholesterol reaches extrahepatic tissues for membrane synthesis and, in the endocrine glands, for steroid hormone formation.

Elucidation of the LDL receptor pathway has provided insight into a general mechanism whereby a variety of larger molecules pass from the plasma into cells. The system is called *receptor-mediated endocytosis*. Specificity is determined by the LDL receptors localized in specialized areas of the plasma membrane called *clathrin-coated pits*. The receptor, bearing its LDL, is then pinched off to form a coated vesicle. The vesicle next merges with lysosomes, and lysosomal enzymes rapidly degrade LDL to constituent amino acids with release of cholesteryl esters. The latter are hydrolyzed to free cholesterol. Empty LDL receptors cycle back to the cell surface. The speed of the process is quite remarkable, each receptor making the trip from coated pit to lysosome and back to the plasma membrane in 10 minutes. Normally, about 60%–70% of cholesterol traffic enters the cell via the LDL receptor, but about one-third traverses a nonspecific uptake pathway. Disturbances in the LDL receptor cycle ordinarily cause difficulty because cholesterol concentrations in plasma rise, leading to atherosclerosis via conversion of LDL to oxidized LDL. Interestingly, even the complete absence of the LDL receptor system is not accompanied by clinical hormonal deficiency states, presumably because the combination of endogenous cholesterol synthesis and entry of cholesterol by receptor-independent pathways satisfies cellular needs.

Protein

The absorption of protein is more complicated than the absorption of fat and carbohydrate. Protein digestion starts in the stomach through the action of pepsin. Pepsinogen is secreted into the stomach by mucosal and chief cells, and is converted to active pepsin in the presence of acid. Pepsin digests protein for only 1 or 2 hours following meal-stimulated acid secretion; this acid is later neutralized in the proximal duodenum by pancreatic bicarbonate. Most protein digestion takes place in the duodenum, where inactive pancreatic proteases are activated by enterokinase on the duodenal mucosa. Duodenal protein digestion is the result of the sequential action of endopeptidases followed by that of exopeptidases to produce single amino acids and oligopeptides. The endopeptidases trypsin, chymotrypsin, and elastase act on proteins to produce peptides with basic, aromatic, or aliphatic COOH terminals, respectively. The exopeptidase, carboxypeptidase B, cleaves arginine and lysine from peptides with basic COOH terminals; carboxypeptidase A cleaves neutral amino acids from peptides with aromatic and aliphatic COOH terminals.

Ordinarily the combined activities of all the endo- and exopeptidases yield about 30% free amino acids and 70% oligopeptides, with a chain length ranging from two to six amino acids. Only amino acids, di and tri oligopeptides can be directly absorbed by the enterocytes. There are at least four sodium-dependant amino acid transporters, one for aromatic and aliphatic amino acids, one for basic amino acids, one for glycine, proline, and hydroxyproline, and one for dicarboxylic amino acids. The fate of the oligopeptides is complicated. Brush border enzymes break down some of them and others are transported into the cell, where cytoplasmic peptidases complete the digestive process. The high-specific-activity amino-oligopeptidase of the brush border has its action blocked by the presence of a proline in the penultimate position of the oligopeptide chain. This regulatory proline thus appears to determine whether intraluminal/brush border digestion is complete or whether intracellular digestion is required. Absorbed amino acids pass to the liver via the portal vein.

There is a noteworthy exception to the digestion of all proteins prior to absorption; for a short time after birth, neonates can absorb intact proteins. This transient ability is important because the newborn animal acquires passive immunity by absorbing immunoglobulins in colostral milk.

The rise in amino acid concentrations in arterial blood that follows a protein meal does not reflect the makeup of the ingested protein. Although branched-chain amino acids make up no more than one-fifth of the total residues in meat, about 60% of the increase in amino acids following the protein meal is made up of leucine, valine, and isoleucine. Presumably they escape uptake by the liver and are transported to muscle, where they serve as the major substrate for protein synthesis (Fig. 16-6). Increased plasma concentrations of amino acids stimulate muscle protein syn-

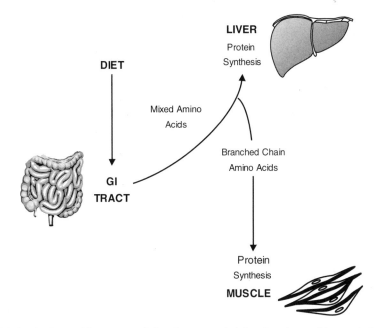

Fig. 16-6 Amino acid transport following a meal. Mixed amino acids reach the liver via the portal vein. Branched-chain amino acids preferentially pass through the hepatic circulation and account for 60% of the rise in amino acid concentrations in the general circulation. They appear to be utilized for protein synthesis under the influence of insulin. GI, gastrointestinal.

thesis. Half-maximal stimulation of protein synthesis occurs with plasma amino acid concentrations 60% higher than those normally seem in the postabsorptive phase of digestion. Little additional increase occurs when very high concentrations of amino acids are provided, and oxidation, ureagenesis, and gluconeogenesis dispose of the excess substrate. Insulin is permissive of protein synthesis, but elevated insulin concentrations do not cause further increases in protein synthesis. The mechanism is not completely understood, but at least one action of insulin is to stimulate the formation of *initiation complexes* that start the series of reactions leading to peptide formation. Net buildup of muscle following a meal is also a consequence of insulin-induced diminution in proteolysis; that is, insulin has the capacity to simultaneously stimulate protein synthesis and block protein breakdown.

CATABOLIC PATHWAYS

To review briefly, the catabolic phase of metabolism is a series of adaptations designed to ensure adequate fuels for body tissues in the absence of exogenous substrate. The preeminent concern is to maintain the plasma glucose at safe levels for the CNS until ketone concentrations rise into the protective range. If acetoacetic and β-hydroxybutyric acids are not present in sufficient concentrations, the brain is vitally dependent on glucose, and the absence of glucose is as devastating as the absence of oxygen. As noted earlier, the protective processes required are glycogen breakdown, gluconeogenesis, lipolysis, and ketogenesis.

Glycogenolysis and Gluconeogenesis

In the early postabsorptive state and the initial phases of fasting, maintenance of the plasma glucose depends mostly on glycogenolysis, but gluconeogenesis also makes an important contribution. Although glycogenolysis can be induced by cate-cholamines acting as β-agonists (and, in humans, to a small extent via α-receptors), it is generally accepted that the bulk of glycogen breakdown occurs through a glucagon-mediated rise in cyclic AMP. Activation of cyclic AMP–dependent protein kinase phosphorylates phosphorylase b, converting it to the active a form. Simultaneously, phosphorylation of glycogen synthase a converts it to the inactive b form. In consequence, glycogen formation ceases, avoiding a futile cycle of coexistent glycogen breakdown and formation. It is likely that glucose-6-phosphatase activity also increases in the catabolic phase, ensuring that G-6-P formed from glycogen will pass immediately into the plasma as free glucose. This would be a mirror image of the inhibition postulated to occur after feeding. The nature of regulation at the G-6-P reaction, if any exists, is not known. If the enzyme is not regulated, flux is probably substrate controlled; that is, a rise in G-6-P concentrations secondary to glycogen breakdown and impaired glycogen synthesis would drive the reaction.

The mechanisms by which carbon flow between G-6-P and pyruvate is controlled are now reasonably well understood. In the catabolic phase, glycolysis (G-6-P $\rightarrow$ pyruvate) is blocked and gluconeogenesis (pyruvate $\rightarrow$ G-6-P) is enhanced by the conversion of fructose-6-phosphate (F-6-P) to fructose-1,6-bisphosphate (F-1,6-P_2) (Fig. 16-7). Although most of the reactions of the glycolytic-gluconeogenic pathway are reversible, separate enzymes operate at this site. In the glycolytic pathway, F-6-P is converted to F-1,6-P2 via the enzyme 6-phosphofructo-1-kinase, whereas the reverse reaction, the major regulatory step in gluconeogenesis, is mediated by fructose-1,6-bisphosphatase. Glucagon control of the opposing reactions is effected by changing the concentrations of a regulatory intermediate, F-2,6-P_2, which is itself not a direct participant in glycolysis. Fructose-2,6-bisphosphate is formed from F-6-P by a bifunctional enzyme called *6-phosphofructo-2-kinase/fructose-2,6-bisphosphatase* (PFK2/FBPase2). This remarkable enzyme shifts from a kinase to a phosphatase when phosphorylated. When insulin levels are high and glucagon levels are low, the enzyme is dephosphorylated and functions as a kinase, which leads to the synthesis of F-2,6-P_2. When insulin levels fall and glucagon concentrations increase, the enzyme is phosphorylated, kinase activity is lost, and phosphatase activity appears. This decreases synthesis and increases hydrolysis of F-2,6-P_2, with the result that its concentration in the hepatocyte rapidly falls. When F-2,6-P_2 levels are high, phosphofructokinase activity is stimulated and glycolysis is active, whereas fructose bisphosphatase is inhibited, blocking gluconeogenesis. The catabolic sequence can be summarized as follows: increased glucagon $\rightarrow$ increased cyclic AMP $\rightarrow$ increased cyclic AMP–dependent kinase $\rightarrow$ increased phosphorylation of PFK2/FBPase2 $\rightarrow$ decreased F-2,6-P_2 $\rightarrow$ decreased glycolysis and increased gluconeogenesis. Activation of gluconeogenesis ensures

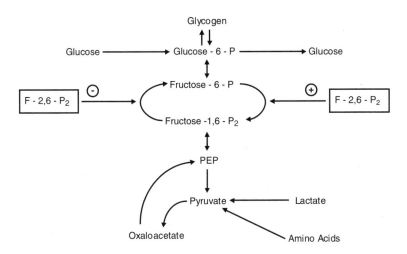

Fig. 16-7 The regulation of glycolysis and glyconeogenesis. Fructose-2,6-bisphosphate (F-2,6-P$_2$) stimulates glycolysis by activating phosphofructokinase, which converts fructose-6-phosphate (fructose-6-P) to fructose-1,6-bisphosphate (F-1,6-P$_2$) and inhibits gluconeogenesis by deactivating fructose-1,6-bisphosphatase, which converts F-1,6-P$_2$) bisphosphate to F-6-P. Glucose-6-P, glucose-6-phosphate; PEP, phosphoenolpyruvate.

sustained hepatic glucose production after preformed glycogen is depleted, while the block in glycolysis indirectly allows the liver to become a ketogenic organ, as described below.

In quantitative terms, hepatic glucose production averages about 12 μmol/kg body weight per minute after an overnight fast. The conventional view is that most of the glucose derives from glycogenolysis, but recent evidence has opened a new debate by pointing to gluconeogenesis as the primary mechanism contributor to glucose output at this stage. The gluconeogenic substrates include lactate, glycerol, and amino acids. Lactate derives from two sources. The first is lactate produced within the liver and gastrointestinal tract. The second is from glucose incompletely oxidized in peripheral tissues. Glucose passes from the liver to peripheral tissues, where it is metabolized to pyruvate-lactate. A portion of the pyruvate undergoes terminal oxidation to CO_2 and water with energy production, but the remainder of the pyruvate-lactate returns to the liver. Lactate concentrations in plasma are 10 times higher than those of pyruvate, so that it is the principal member of the couple. The glucose → lactate → glucose sequence is known as the *Cori cycle*.

Glycerol, which is a relatively minor contributor to gluconeogenesis, is released from triglycerides hydrolyzed in adipose tissue via the activity of hormone-sensitive lipase. The major substrate for gluconeogenesis is amino acids, which flow from muscle. Alanine and glutamine account for over 50% of the amino acids released, although alanine represents only about 7% of the total amino acid residues in muscle (Fig. 16-8). The explanation for the excess release of alanine from muscle is thought to be a transamination reaction wherein branched-chain amino acids (leucine, isoleucine, and valine) donate their amino groups to pyruvate derived from muscle glycogen. A teleological explanation might be that alanine is the best pre-

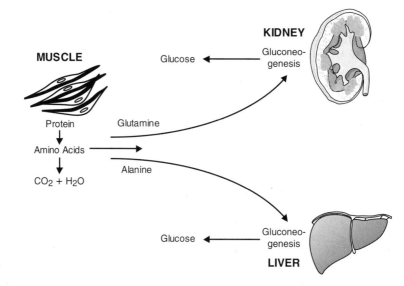

Fig. 16-8 Release of amino acids from muscle and their use in gluconeogenesis. Glutamine and alanine are the primary amino acids delivered to the liver and kidney for conversion to glucose. See text for details.

cursor for hepatic gluconeogenesis, entering the gluconeogenic sequence after reversed transamination to pyruvate. Glutamine is taken up primarily by extrahepatic splanchnic tissues and is also utilized for gluconeogenesis in the kidney after prolonged fasting. Studies in humans suggest that it may be a more significant substrate for hepatic gluconeogenesis than was previously thought.

The signals for proteolysis in muscle are not completely understood. It is likely that both insulin deficiency and the presence of counterregulatory hormones play a role. For example, small physiological increments in plasma cortisol concentrations clearly stimulate proteolysis. Catecholamines (and perhaps glucagon) probably have similar effects. Protein breakdown occurs by both lysosomal and nonlysosomal pathways. At least a portion of the latter is calcium dependent.

Unlike carbohydrates and fat, the body lacks a pure storage form of protein. Therefore, amino acids utilized in gluconeogenesis come from the breakdown of enzymes, transport molecules, and structural proteins in skeletal muscle. Their loss places cellular integrity at risk. Indeed, in most cases, death from starvation is due to protein wastage, often from cardiac arrhythmias. It thus becomes crucial that that the body adapt to a fast by increasing the reliance on oxidation of fatty acids and ketones. The metabolic shift reduces the demand for glucose and the consumption of gluconeogenic substrates. This is reflected in a lessening of the negative nitrogen balance that is so characteristic of starvation. How the muscle is notified to diminish proteolysis is not clear. One possibility is that rising free fatty acid concentrations stimulate insulin release from the β-cell and that it is insulin that is the antiproteolytic signal.

However, refeeding studies with fructose indicate that this sugar alone, in the absence of an increase in plasma insulin levels, also reverses all manifestations of starvation, including protein breakdown, suggesting that insulin is not an obligatory mediator for cessation of proteolysis. Conceivably the message is carried through amino acid concentrations in plasma. A diminished need for glucose, either because of refeeding or because of fat oxidation, might slow the uptake of alanine and other amino acids by the liver, leading to a transient rise in plasma and subsequently in muscle amino acid concentrations. This might somehow activate a negative feedback sequence that would blunt protein breakdown. Although it is clear that proteolysis slows with prolonged fasting, the mechanisms must be considered speculative at this time.

When the catabolic state induced by fasting is reversed by feeding, there is a complete reversal of the metabolic changes just described. The triggering event is almost certainly a rise in the [insulin]:[glucagon] ratio. As discussed above, gluconeogenesis continues for several hours after feeding, allowing hepatic glycogen repletion to take place in large measure via an indirect rather than a direct pathway. Continued gluconeogenesis is not difficult to explain after glucose feeding, as $F-2,6-P_2$ levels do not rise for several hours, as noted earlier. Conversely, with sucrose refeeding, $F-2,6-P_2$ levels rise early, yet gluconeogenesis is not impaired. There are two possible explanations. First, there might be a regulatory intermediate substance or transcriptional events that can override normal $F-2,6-P_2$ inhibition of gluconeogenesis. Second, the measured rise in $F-2,6-P_2$ might not be uniform in all hepatocytes; that is, some zones of the liver would contain cells that do not manifest an early rise in $F-2,6-P_2$ and thus continue gluconeogenesis.

Lipolysis and Ketogenesis

The switch to a lipid economy in the catabolic phase of metabolism requires changes in both adipose tissue and liver. The hydrolysis of triglycerides in the adipocyte delivers long-chain fatty acids, together with glycerol, into the circulation. Two-thirds to three-fourths of the mobilized fatty acids are utilized directly, and the remainder are taken up by the liver for conversion to ketone bodies. Under normal anabolic conditions the liver produces only tiny amounts of acetoacetic and β-hydroxybutyric acids. Dietary fatty acids entering the hepatocyte are simply esterified to triglycerides and transported into the circulation as VLDL. After a few hours of fasting, or under the influence of counterregulatory hormones induced by stress, fatty acid oxidative capacity is activated and significant ketone body production becomes possible, provided that long-chain fatty acids are available. Full-blown ketosis requires both an adequate delivery of free fatty acids (FFA) to the liver and activation of the enzyme system that converts these substrates to acetoacetic and β-hydroxybutyric acids. Failure of either substrate delivery or enzyme activation causes ketogenesis to fail. Once the liver is activated, rates of ketone body production are simply the consequence of the rate of delivery of long-chain fatty acids. Qualitatively, there is no difference in the metabolic adaptations in adipose tissue and liver that accompany the very mild ketosis of a brief fast and the raging ketoacidosis of uncontrolled type 1 diabetes mellitus. The differentiating determinant is that FFA concentrations are much higher in the latter state due to the complete absence of insulin.

The hydrolysis of triglycerides in adipocytes is due to activation of an intracellular lipase generally designated *hormone-sensitive lipase* to distinguish it from the extracellular lipoprotein lipase responsible for hydrolysis of triglyceride in plasma lipoproteins. Hormone-sensitive lipase is inhibited by insulin and adenosine and activated by counterregulatory hormones. In humans, catecholamines from the circulation and sympathetic nerve terminals appear to play the primary role in activation. Epinephrine and norepinephrine act through cyclic AMP–stimulated protein kinase in classic fashion. Removal of the insulin inhibitory effect, expected from a fall in plasma insulin accompanying the catabolic phase, is also important. The quantitative contribution of the removal of insulin inhibition in relation to the positive activating effects of catecholamines has not been completely worked out. Experimentally, hormone-sensitive lipase can also be inhibited by adenosine and ketone bodies. Some evidence suggests that the effects of adenosine may be physiologically important.

Fatty acid oxidation can be divided into two components: a transport component required to get long-chain fatty acids into the mitochondria and the intramitochondrial component (β-oxidation) that cleaves the long-chain fatty acid to acetyl-CoA. In most tissues, the fatty acid–derived acetyl-CoA undergoes terminal oxidation to CO_2 and water in the tricarboxylic acid cycle for the generation of energy. In the liver, however, the bulk of the acetyl-CoA in the catabolic phase is converted to ketones (Fig. 16-9). Transport appears to be rate limiting under most cir-

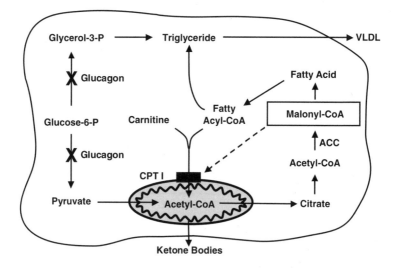

Fig. 16-9 The regulation of ketogenesis. In the transition from anabolic to catabolic phases glucagon blocks glycolysis, thereby interrupting flux over the sequence glucose-6-phosphate (glucose-6-P) → pyruvate → acetyl-coenzyme A (CoA) → citrate → acetyl-CoA → malonyl-CoA. In addition, glucagon, via activation of 5′-adenosine monophosphate (AMP)–activated protein kinase, and long-chain fatty acyl-CoA inhibits the activity of acetyl-CoA carboxylase (ACC). The fall in malonyl-CoA produced by the ACC step disinhibits carnitine palmitoyltransferase I (CPT I), the rate-limiting step in fatty acid oxidation, thereby activating the ketogenic pathway. Fatty acids delivered to the liver from adipose tissue are thus preferentially oxidized to the ketone bodies, acetoacetic and β-hydroxybutyric acids. The fall in malonyl-CoA simultaneously limits fatty acid synthesis. Glycerol-3-P, glycerol-3-phosphate; VLDL, very-low-density lipoprotein.

cumstances so that any fatty acids traversing the inner mitochondrial membrane are rapidly oxidized. When long-chain fatty acids are taken up by diffusion or specific fatty acid transporters on the cell surface, they are converted to CoA derivatives, with ATP as an energy source. The long-chain fatty acyl-CoA cannot penetrate the inner mitochondrial membrane, however; it requires a transesterification step in which CoA is exchanged for carnitine, a carrier molecule in lipid transport. The transesterification is carried out by an enzyme located on the outer mitochondrial membrane called CPT I. Fatty acylcarnitine is then transported across the inner mitochondrial membrane by a translocase enzyme and reconverted to the CoA derivative under the influence of CPT II. The newly reformed fatty acyl-CoA appears to be committed to oxidation in the β-oxidative sequence. The activity of CPT I is regulated in large measure by the cytosolic concentration of malonyl-CoA. Under catabolic conditions, malonyl-CoA concentrations rapidly fall, thereby activating fatty acid oxidation, whereas lipogenesis simultaneously ceases as a result of a deficiency of substrate. The fall in malonyl-CoA is mediated in part by glucagon. One component of the mechanism is inhibition of glycolysis caused by the fall in F-2,6-P$_2$. The interruption of flux from G-6-P to pyruvate reduces citrate production in the mitochondria, which in turn leads to failure of acetyl-CoA generation in the cytosol. Because malonyl-CoA is formed from the carboxylation of acetyl-CoA under the influence of the enzyme acetyl-CoA carboxylase, malonyl-CoA concentrations decrease, disinhibiting fatty acid oxidation. Glucagon also inhibits acetyl-CoA carboxylase (through cyclic AMP–mediated phosphorylation), as do long-chain fatty acyl-CoA concentrations, which also rise in liver during the catabolic adaptation (under some circumstances the carboxylase can also be inhibited by AMP-dependent protein kinase). With refeeding, malonyl-CoA concentrations are restored to anabolic levels, thereby deactivating CPT I. The simultaneous rise in insulin, which inhibits lipolysis, normalizes the substrate wing of the process. Malonyl-CoA is also a regulatory molecule for fatty acid oxidation in nonhepatic tissues. In the pancreatic β-cell, its role in enhancing glucose-stimulated insulin secretion is controversial.

DERANGEMENTS IN GLUCOSE, LIPID, AND PROTEIN METABOLISM

Obesity

Obesity has reached epidemic proportions in developed countries, and the U.S. surgeon general recently issued a "call to action" to prevent and decrease it. Obesity is a serious breakdown of fuel homeostasis and is associated with a wide spectrum of comorbidities including osteoarthritis, hypertension, cardiac disease, cancer, and type 2 diabetes. Although excessive weight gain can occur only if there is an imbalance between calories consumed and calories expended, this simple logic belies the fact that there is genetically determined variability among individuals in how they dispose of ingested calories and also considerable variation in the number of calories ingested. From studies with normal and genetically obese rodents, early physiologists concluded that a circulating lipostatic factor, which is released from adipose tissue, interacts with hypothalamic neurons to decrease food intake. It was further postulated that insufficient production of the factor, or reduced hypothalamic responsiveness to the factor, would lead to obesity.

This line of reasoning received major experimental support with the discovery of the hormone leptin (from the Greek word *leptos*, meaning "thin"). It was shown that leptin is a 16 kDa protein that is produced in fat cells and secreted into the blood. Moreover, it was found that the morbid obesity of the *ob/ob* mouse stems from the absence of leptin production because of a mutation in the leptin gene. Not surprisingly, treatment of these animals with leptin corrected their hyperphagia, increased their metabolic rate, and restored normal body weight.

The leptin receptor gene encodes a long version and several truncated versions of the receptor. The long form has a 303-amino acid cytoplasmic tail that confers signaling properties and is present in a variety of tissues but is particularly abundant in the hypothalamus. In keeping with earlier predictions, the *db/db* mouse (and the Zucker *fa/fa* rat) has a mutation in the leptin receptor gene that results in failure to produce the long form of the receptor. As expected, leptin treatment of these animals has no effect on their hyperphagia, hypometabolism, or obesity.

There are two theories of how leptin influences physiology. The first postulates that leptin plays a gatekeeper role, and that only when sufficient leptin levels are attained does normal physiological function occur. In particular, it appears that reproductive function is suppressed until a critical threshold of body fat is attained; some students may be familiar with amenorrhea seen in elite female athletes and extreme dieters. In parallel, other behavioral, metabolic, and endocrine adaptations to starvation are suppressed once the critical leptin threshold is reached. A slightly different viewpoint is that leptin exerts a tonic and dominant inhibitory input to hypothalamic circuitry that functions to maintain body weight around a set point. Some researchers have described this circuitry as an *adipostat*, a physiological system for maintaining constant body fat levels. Two groups of neurons in the hypothalamus form the core of the adipostat circuitry. Leptin, and other signals of nutrient sufficiency or satiety, inhibit the activity of neurons that release neuropeptide Y and reciprocally activate POMC neurons that secrete α-melanocyte-stimulating hormone (α-MSH). Neuropeptide Y acts within the brain to stimulate feeding and decrease energy expenditure, and α-MSH inhibits feeding and increases energy expenditure. Thus leptin acts as a negative feedback signal to limit energy intake and fat deposition. The adipostatic circuitry is also sensitive to other signals of nutrient status. The adipostatic circuitry appears to exert behavioral, endocrine, and metabolic effects. The best-characterized actions occur via α-MSH activation of the melanocortin 4 receptor (MC4 R) to increase the activity of the sympathetic nervous system and simultaneously decrease the activity of the parasympathetic nervous system. Enhanced sympathetic activity would be expected to accelerate adipose tissue lipolysis through catecholamine stimulation of adrenergic receptors and to reduce malonyl-CoA levels in both fat and muscle cells. If, as is thought to be the case, there were a concomitant rise in uncoupling protein 2 or 3 activity in these tissues, conditions would be set for increased fat oxidation, elevation of the metabolic rate, and dissipation of fat stores.

The initial hope that leptin might provide a magic bullet for the treatment of human obesity has not materialized. A few humans with serious homozygous mutations in the leptin gene have been found, and these individuals lose weight rapidly with leptin treatment. In contrast, the vast majority of obese individuals have higher than normal circulating leptin levels and appear to be resistant to leptin action. Only a few hyperleptinemic obese individuals have a defect in their leptin receptor, so it is likely that leptin resistance will be polygenic and heterogeneous in character; an appropriate analogy might be to type 2, or insulin-resistant, diabetes. An intense effort is underway to decipher the signaling pathways involved in leptin action, and cases of monogenic obesity have been identified with mutations of the POMC, prohormone convertase 1, or the MC4 R genes. It is hoped that information from such individuals may provide rational new approaches to the pharmaceutical treatment of obesity and its many complications.

Diabetes Mellitus

Diabetes mellitus is an extremely common metabolic disease affecting 7% of the U.S. population. Its prevalence is much higher in certain groups, such as the Hispanic and Native American subpopulations. There are two main types of diabetes, type 1 and type 2. The former is much less common but has an earlier onset and is more severe.

Current understanding of type 1 diabetes mellitus (also known as *insulin-dependent diabetes*) suggests that the individual inherits a genetic susceptibility to the disease that is permissive but not causal. That multiple genes are involved has been suspected for some time and is reinforced by a recent search of the entire human genome, which revealed no fewer than 20 independent chromosomal regions with positive linkage to the disease. Of these, a particularly strong association was found with a gene located on the short arm of the sixth chromosome in the major histocompatibility complex. More than 90% of patients, when typed by a serological test, exhibit human leukocyte antigen (HLA) DR3, DR4, or the combination DR3/DR4. It is currently thought that genes on the DQ β-chain may be more closely linked to diabetes susceptibility than those in the DR region. Some alleles appear to be susceptibility genes and others resistance genes, while still others are neutral. Human leukocyte antigen associations appear less informative in individuals developing diabetes after the age of 20.

The pathogenesis of autoimmune type 1 diabetes is not precisely known. Leakage of cryptic antigens following a viral infection is one possibility. Alternatively, the mechanism of molecular mimicry may be involved. In molecular mimicry, homology between viral or food antigens and β-cell antigens fools the body's immune system into attacking itself. For example, a Coxsackie virus infection elicits an immune response. The cytotoxic T lymphocytes, armed against the viral antigens, cannot distinguish between the virus and the homologous amino acid segment in the β-cell, and thus attack and destroy the latter.

Symptoms appear when 90% or more of the insulin-producing capacity of the islets of Langerhans is destroyed. Immune destruction is probably carried out by both humoral and cellular mechanisms, but the latter is considered dominant. Islet cell antibodies can be demonstrated in the plasma long before symptomatic diabetes appears. The most important predictive antibodies recognize glutamic acid decarboxylase (GAD) and insulin. It had been hoped that early exposure to insulin or an altered peptide ligand of insulin might elicit tolerance in high-risk individuals with antibodies, but this promising strategy has not been efficacious in the clinical setting. The consequences of the immune destruction of the β-cell are an absolute deficiency of insulin and overproduction of glucagon secondary to removal of the normal insulin restraint. The predictable metabolic consequences are overproduction of glucose and ketones by the liver plus underutilization of glucose in nonhepatic tissues. In type 1 diabetes, because insulin production is impossible, hyperglycemia steadily increases, adipose tissue lipolysis becomes excessive, and subsequent overproduction of ketone bodies by the liver leads to a life-threatening ketoacidosis.

The more common type 2 diabetes mellitus (also called *noninsulin-dependent diabetes*) is generally associated with obesity. Insulin resistance is a major problem, and insulin deficiency is relative rather than absolute. Obesity is an identifiable cause of insulin resistance, but impaired insulin action is found in offspring of two parents with type 2 diabetes even when they are not overweight or diabetic. The mechanism of the intrinsic insulin resistance has not been worked out, although there is growing evidence that fat accumulation in the muscle cell plays a role. Early in type 2 diabetes, insulin levels are high in absolute terms but are insufficient to overcome insulin resistance. Later, insulin levels fall as hyperglycemia worsens. The nature of the β-cell defect leading to diminished insulin reserve is not known, but here again, an abnormal buildup of cellular lipids is thought to be one culprit. Because of the insulin resistance, glucagon levels are high and the [glucagon]:[insulin] ratio is elevated in terms of biological activity, even though the actual ratio may be near normal when assessed by radioimmunoassay. That is because the insulin present does not work well, leaving glucagon's actions unopposed. Once again, the hormonal changes are those characteristic of the catabolic state, and major hyperglycemia supervenes.

Ketoacidosis does not develop in type 2 diabetic subjects under most circumstances. Ketone levels may rise after prolonged periods of poor medical control, but in general, they never exceed the concentrations seen during the fasting state in normal individuals. Hyperglycemia may become extreme, exceeding 1000 mg/dl (55.6 mmol/liter), resulting in severe body fluid losses through the kidney. If adequate hydration is not maintained, affected individuals can develop a syndrome called *hyperosmolar, nonketotic diabetic coma*. *Hyperosmolar* indicates that massive water deficits caused by glucose-induced osmotic diuresis lead to increases in the plasma osmotic pressure from a normal level of 280–300 mOsmol/liter to values over 400 mOsmol/liter. The term *nonketotic* does not mean that ketone bodies are not measurable in the urine or plasma, but simply that their production is not high enough to cause ketoacidosis. Patients with hyperosmolar, nonketotic coma usually manifest altered consciousness or coma, convulsions, impaired kidney function, and sometimes pancreatitis and infections with gram-negative organisms. Mortality rates are very high.

The profound metabolic derangements of uncontrolled diabetes underline the importance of the control systems that normally govern fuel metabolism in the body. Although the metabolic disturbances of diabetes can usually be controlled well enough by dietary restriction and insulin therapy to prevent symptoms, it is almost impossible to maintain the plasma glucose within the normal range. Consequently, after many years of diabetes, patients become vulnerable to late degenerative complications involving the eyes, nerves, kidneys, and blood vessels. Thus, diabetes is a leading cause of blindness, kidney failure, amputations, strokes, and heart attacks. It is these complications that make it such a devastating illness.

Congenital Generalized Lipodystrophy

Congenital generalized lipodystrophy (CGL) is a rare autosomal recessive disorder characterized by the near absence of adipose tissue coupled with severe insulin resistance and even type 2 diabetes. Severe hyperinsulinemia and hypertriglyceridemia develop in childhood and adolescence, whereas plasma HDL and leptin concentrations are very low. Children with CGL also demonstrate accelerated growth, voracious appetite, increased basal metabolic rate, and advanced bone age. Mutations of the gene (*AGPAT2*) encoding 1-acylglycerol-3-phosphate-*O*-transferase have been identified in a number of CGL patients from different pedigrees. This enzyme forms a key intermediate of triacylglycerol and glycerophospholipid synthesis, but it is still not clear why this enzyme deficiency results in a distinctive redistribution of body fat. Adipose tissue in metabolically active depots such as subcutaneous adipose tissue, intra-abdominal and intrathoracic fat, and bone marrow is absent, but adipose tissue can be found in the retroorbital area, the palms and soles of the feet, and other sites where fat serves a *mechanical* function. Profound fatty infiltration of the liver, skeletal muscle, and heart has been noted, and it has been suggested that these deposits lead to insulin resistance and cardiomyopathy. Strong clinical evidence supporting the hypothesis that type 2 diabetes, even in the more general form, might result from abnormal accumulation of lipid in nonadipose tissues has been obtained from studies of CGL patients. Subcutaneous leptin replacement for 8–10 months alleviates the voracious appetite in these subjects and reduces the hepatic lipid content by 80% and the intramyocellular lipid content by 42%. The fall in cellular lipid content is accompanied by a twofold increase in insulin-mediated glucose disposal. The link between improved insulin action and the resolution of tissue steatosis is striking, but much investigation is needed before tissue lipid accumulation can be deemed a cause of insulin resistance.

Hyperglycemia of Severe Injury

Nondiabetic subjects who sustain extreme injuries such as massive burns or major trauma may develop hyperglycemia even in the face of normal pancreatic function. The stress of such injuries leads to an outpouring of epinephrine and norepinephrine, which block insulin release from the β-cell, stimulate glucagon production, activate glycogenolysis, stimulate lipolysis, and induce proteolysis. In short, severe injury can quickly convert a normal state, even in a person who has just eaten, into the catabolic response. Stress overrides normal metabolism and does so by provoking sustained release of counterregulatory hormones.

Tangier Disease

Tangier disease is a rare autosomal recessive disorder characterized by low plasma concentrations of HDL and LDL cholesterol and the presence of enlarged orange tonsils containing lipid-laden macrophages of the reticuloendothelial system. Other clinical features include corneal opacities, hepatosplenomegaly, neuropathy, and premature atherosclerosis. A series of metabolic studies indicates that the strikingly low HDL cholesterol levels in these individuals results from accelerated clearance of these particles rather than impaired synthesis. Mutations in the gene encoding for the ATP-binding cassette protein-1 are responsible for this disorder. The protein is stoichiometrically coupled to the process of cholesterol, and possibly phospholipid, efflux from cells into HDL particles so that homozygous loss-of-function mutations severely limit reverse cholesterol transport (heterozygous mutations also have a less severe phenotype). The resulting smaller HDL lipoproteins are believed to have accelerated clearance compared to larger HDL subpopulations. Phagocytic cells of the immune system accumulate intracellular lipids as the lysozymes degrade the cell membrane components of destroyed cells. Because these cells cannot efficiently unload the lipids onto HDL in the absence of *ABCA1* activity, they become dysfunctional and accumulate in the tonsils and spleen. Accumulation of lipid-laden macrophages in atherosclerotic lesions is postulated to underlie the premature development of advanced atherosclerotic disease.

Familial Hypercholesterolemia

Familial hypercholesterolemia is an autosomal dominant illness of humans that produces marked elevation of the plasma LDL and total cholesterol levels. The latter, in turn, causes premature atherosclerosis with myocardial infarctions occurring at an early age. In the more severe homozygous form of the disease (two abnormal genes for the LDL receptor), plasma cholesterol levels are in the range of 600–1200 mg/dl (15.5–31.0 mmol/liter), whereas the normal range is <200 mg/dl (5.2 mmol/liter). In heterozygous patients (one mutant allele), levels are in the 300–550 mg/dl (7.8–14.2 mmol/liter) range. In homozygous familial hypercholesterolemia, heart attacks commonly occur between the ages of 5 and 30 and have been reported as early as 18 months. In men with the heterozygous form of the illness, there is a 5% chance of having a heart attack by the age of 30, 51% by the age of 50, and 85% by the age of 60. The classic physical manifestation found in over three-fourths of affected individuals is lipid deposition (tendon xanthomas) on the Achilles tendons or the extensor tendons of the hands. Xanthelasma, lipid deposition in the skin around the eyes, and premature arcus corneae are additional characteristic physical findings. These deposits provide strong evidence of hypercholesterolemia, but they may be subtle and easily overlooked. Careful palpation of the Achilles tendon may reveal beaded xanthomas in patients who do not show typical deposits in the skin or over bony protuberances.

The elevation in plasma cholesterol is due in all cases to a genetic defect that produces an abnormal LDL receptor. Several types of defects are now known. Class 1 mutants synthesize no receptors. Class 2 mutants do not transfer LDL receptors efficiently from the endoplasmic reticulum to the Golgi apparatus so that the receptors are degraded in the cell before they can reach the cell surface. Class 3 mutants have LDL receptors that reach the cell surface but are unable to bind LDL. Class 4 mutants produce receptors that do not cluster in coated pits, thereby interrupting the normal metabolism of cholesterol.

Limiting the intake of saturated fat and cholesterol is an important component of the multifaceted treatment approach required in this condition. Combined drug therapy is almost always necessary. It is possible to increase LDL receptors in heterozygous patients by giving bile salt–binding resins. If endogenous cholesterol synthesis is then blocked by administering nicotinic acid or drugs that inhibit HMG-CoA reductase (statin drugs), substantial declines in plasma cholesterol can be obtained. Niacin may have an additional therapeutic benefit. Unfortunately, the drugs are not effective in the homozygous form because no normal gene is available to stimulate.

Hypertriglyceridemia

Elevated plasma triglycerides may appear as a primary genetic disease or secondary to other illnesses. Elevated triglycerides have two major detrimental effects. Acutely, they predispose to acute pancreatitis. Chronically, they lower HDL levels, predisposing to atherosclerosis. Acquired functional deficiencies of LPL often appear secondary to conditions such as diabetes mellitus, hypothyroidism, alcoholism, lupus erythematosus (caused by antibodies against LPL or its cofactor, heparin), and uremia. The most common genetic defects accounting for pure hypertriglyceridemia that appears at an early age are deficiencies of LPL or apo-CII. Lipoprotein lipase is a 448-amino acid protein that functions as a dimer attached to heparin sulfate proteoglycans on the surface of capillary endothelial cells. Functional activation of LPL requires binding to heparin and apo-CII. Clinically, LPL deficiency can be diagnosed in hypertriglyceridemic patients by demonstrating the absence of plasma lipase activity after heparin administration. The diagnosis of apo-CII deficiency can be made when specialized tests indicate that it is absent from the plasma apolipoprotein electrophoresis profile. Restriction of dietary fat is the mainstay of treatment for severely affected patients, and it is important to rule out the secondary causes of hypertriglyceridemia.

SUGGESTED READING

Atkinson MA and Maclaren NK: The pathogenesis of insulin dependent diabetes mellitus. N Engl J Med 331:1428–1436, 1994.

Batterham RL, Cowley MA, Small CJ, Herzog H, Cohen MA, Dakin CL, Wren AM, Brynes AE, Low MJ, Ghatel MA, Cone RD, and Bloom SR: Gut hormone PYY 3-36 physiologically inhibits food intake. Nature 418:650–654, 2002.

Brown MS and Goldstein JL: A receptor-mediated pathway for cholesterol homeostasis. Science 232:34–47, 1986.

De Feo P, Perriello G, De Cosmo S, Ventura MM, Campbell PJ, Brunetti P, Gerich JE, and Bolli GB: Comparison of glucose counterregulation during short-term and prolonged hypoglycemia in normal humans. Diabetes 35:563–569, 1986.

Farooqi IS, Jebb SA, Langmack G, Lawrence E, Cheetham CH, Prentice AM, Hughes IA, McCamish MA, and O'Rahilly S: Effects of recombinant leptin therapy in a child with congenital leptin deficiency. N Engl J Med 341:879–884, 1999.

Friedman JM and Halaas JL: Leptin and the regulation of body weight in mammals. Nature 395:763–770, 1998.

Havel PJ: Peripheral signals conveying metabolic information to the brain: short-term and long-term regulation of food intake and energy homeostasis. Exp Biol Med 226:963–977, 2001.

Havel RJ and Rapaport E: Drug therapy: management of primary hyperlipidemia. N Engl J Med 332:1491–1498, 1995.

Horton JD, Goldstein JL, and Brown MS: SREBPs: activators of the complete program of cholesterol and fatty acid synthesis in the liver. J Clin Invest 109:1125–1131, 2002.

Kahn CR: Banting lecture: insulin action, diabetogenes, and the cause of type II diabetes. Diabetes 43:1066–1086, 1994.

Kather H, Bieger W, Michel G, Aktories K, and Jakobs KH: Human fat cell lipolysis is primarily regulated by inhibitory modulators acting through distinct mechanisms. J Clin Invest 76:1559–1565, 1985.

Kwiterovich PO: Clinical relevance of the biochemical, metabolic, and genetic factors that influence low-density lipoprotein heterogeneity. Am J Cardiol 90:30i–47i, 2002.

McGarry JD: What if Minkowski had been ageusic? An alternative angle on diabetes. Science 258:766–770, 1992.

McGarry JD and Brown NF: The mitochondrial carnitine palmitoyltransferase system: from concept to molecular analysis. Eur J Biochem 244:1–14, 1997.

McGarry JD and Dobbins RL: Fatty acids and insulin secretion. Diabetologia 42:128–138, 1999.

McGarry JD, Kuwajima M, Newgard CB, Foster DW, and Katz J: From dietary glucose to liver glycogen: the full circle round. Annu Rev Nutr 7:51–73, 1987.

Oram JF: Molecular basis of cholesterol homeostasis: lessons from Tangier disease and *ABCA1*. Trends Mol Med 8:168–173.

Philipson LH and Steiner DF: Perspectives. Pas de deux or more: the sulfonylurea receptor and K^+ channels. Science 268:372–373, 1995.

Pilkis SJ and Granner DK: Molecular physiology of the regulation of hepatic gluconeogenesis and glycolysis. Annu Rev Physiol 54:885–909, 1992.

Radziuk J and Pye S: Hepatic glucose uptake, gluconeogenesis and the regulation of glycogen synthesis. Diabetes Metab Res Rev 17:250–272, 2001.

Rennie MJ, Bohe J, and Wolfe RR: Latency, duration and dose response relationships of amino acid effects on human muscle protein synthesis. J Nutr 132:3225S–3227S, 2002.

Repa JJ and Mangelsdorf DJ: The role of orphan nuclear receptors in the regulation of cholesterol homeostasis. Annu Rev Cell Dev Biol 16:459–481.

Ruderman NB, Saha AK, Vavvas D, and Witters LA: Malonyl-CoA, fuel sensing, and insulin resistance. Am J Physiol 276:E1–E18, 1999.

Saltiel AR and Pessin JE: Insulin signaling in time and space. Trends Cell Biol 12:65–71, 2002.

Schuit FC and Pipeleers DG: Differences in adrenergic recognition by pancreatic A and B cells. Science 232:875–877, 1986.

Index